PRACTICAL GUIDE

Infectious diseases in cats

For this English edition:

Infectious diseases in cats. Practical guide.

Plaza Antonio Beltrán Martínez nº 1, planta 8 - letra I
(Centro empresarial El Trovador)
50002 Zaragoza - Spain

First printing: August 2017

This book has been published originally in Spanish under the title:
Enfermedades infecciosas felinas. Manual práctico
© 2015 Grupo Asís Biomedia, S.L.
ISBN Spanish edition: 978-84-16315-07-9

Translation:
Owen Howard

ISBN: 978-84-16818-83-9
D.L.: Z 1072-2017

Design, layout and printing:
Servet editorial - Grupo Asís Biomedia, S.L.
www.grupoasis.com
info@grupoasis.com

Servet is the publishing house of Grupo Asís

Warning:

Veterinary science is constantly evolving, as are pharmacology and the other sciences. Inevitably, it is therefore the responsibility of the veterinary surgeon to determine and verify the dosage, the method of administration, the duration of treatment and any possible contraindications to the treatments given to each individual patient, based on his or her professional experience. Neither the publisher nor the author can be held liable for any damage or harm caused to people, animals or properties resulting from the correct or incorrect application of the information contained in this book.

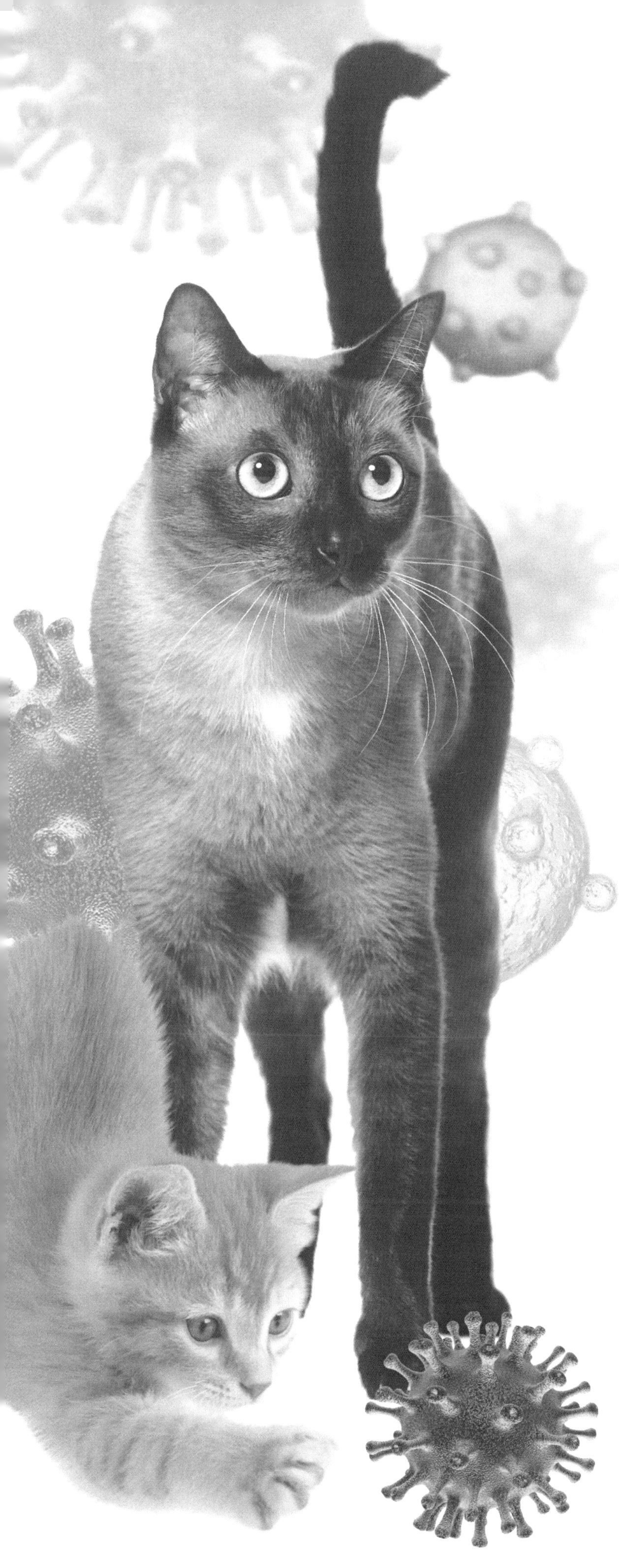

PRACTICAL GUIDE

Infectious diseases in cats

Valentina Aybar Rodríguez
Juanjo Vega Guerrero

SERVET

"When we thought we had all the answers, suddenly they changed all the questions."

Mario Benedetti

Acknowledgements

I want to thank my family, and in particular my grandparents for the values they passed on to me: Joselo, strength and honesty; Sylvia, happiness and an infinite capacity for unconditional love; Luis Emilio, energy and a love of life; Mili: intelligence.

To my parents, Luifer and Sylvia, for your love, principles, and values. We have grown together and lived through heartbreaking exile from Chile, something that has made us a unified family capable of overcoming all difficulties. I am grateful every day for having my sister Camila by my side. She may be the little sister, but I look up to her. I want to thank my friends for their support and companionship, as well as my little treasures, who have now grown up: Andrés, Juan, and Luis. You are my engines. My mother told me she learned to be a mother by becoming a grandmother. I learned to become a daughter by being a mother. The important thing is to keep learning every day. Thank you, I love you.

Valentina Aybar

I want to thank all the people who have been by my side during the writing of this book, especially my three children, Andrés, Juan, and Luis, as well as the rest of my family, in particular my father Joseph and my mother Marisa, both of whom have supported me unconditionally and to whom I owe everything. Thanks also to my true friends, who have never abandoned me.

Many thanks to my colleagues, with whom I have been able to orient my professional career in the direction I desired.

Finally, thanks to all those who have put their trust in me as a professional over the years. Thanks to them and their cats, I have progressed as a vet and have learned to love my profession.

Juanjo Vega

The authors

Valentina Aybar Rodríguez

Bachelor of Veterinary Science from the Complutense University of Madrid. AVEPA-certified in feline medicine. Certified as a specialist in feline medicine by the European School of Veterinary Postgraduate Studies: General Practitioner Certificate in Feline Medicine—GPCert (Feline Medicine).

She is a founding partner of the Ventas Feline Hospital, where she has worked since its inception in 1996, specialising in feline medicine with a particular focus on internal medicine, infectious diseases, medical diagnostic imaging, and anaesthesia.

She is a member of AMVAC (Madrid Association of Small Animal Veterinary Surgeons), AVEPA (Spanish Association of Small Animal Veterinary Surgeons), and GEMFE (Feline Medicine Specialist Group), as well as of international associations of feline medicine specialists: FAB (Feline Advisory Bureau) and ISFM (International Society of Feline Medicine).

She has spoken at many national conferences and has published articles on feline medicine in various media.

Juanjo Vega Guerrero

Bachelor of Veterinary Science, Complutense University of Madrid, 1994. AVEPA-certified in feline medicine. Certified as a specialist in small animal surgery by the European School of Veterinary Postgraduate Studies: General Practitioner Certificate in Small Animal SurgerySurgery—GPCert (SAS).

He is a founding partner of the Ventas Feline Hospital, where he has worked since its inception in 1996, offering services exclusively to feline patients, with a special emphasis on surgery, orthopaedics, neurology, and cardiology.

He is a member of AMVAC (Madrid Association of Small Animal Veterinary Surgeons), AVEPA (Spanish Association of Small Animal Veterinary Surgeons), and GEMFE (Feline Medicine Specialist Group), as well as of international associations of feline medicine specialists: FAB (Feline Advisory Bureau) and ISFM (International Society of Feline Medicine).

Currently he is secretary of the board of GEMFE and a member of the scientific committee of the association.

He has lectured on feline medicine at numerous conferences, both national and international, and has published articles in various Spanish feline medicine journals. In 2014 he formed part of the AVEPA team responsible for continuous training in feline medicine.

Foreword

It is a pleasure and honour to write the foreword to this book, *Practical guide: Infectious diseases in cats*. In Spain, as in other countries with long traditions of keeping cats as pets, feline medicine has become a discipline in its own right. Multiple factors have influenced the growth of this specialty. One of the most important was the emergence in the 1990s of a group of veterinary surgeons who began to feel that cats required distinct treatment to dogs, both in terms of patient management and technical aspects including diagnosis, treatment, and prevention of diseases.

This group of veterinary surgeons gave rise to the feline medicine group (GEMFE) of AVEPA, which has since become a designated specialty group. The authors of this book formed part of this group of veterinary surgeons who viewed feline medicine as a separate discipline, and even transformed their own workplace into a hospital exclusively for the care of cats, within the framework of the Cat-Friendly Practice programme.

Within feline medicine, infectious diseases, especially viral infections, are of particular importance given the associated morbidity and mortality. Every day, we deal with cats with distinct infections and viral diseases of major importance. These include acute infections with high mortality caused by viruses that are highly resistant in the environment (parvovirus), infections caused by viruses with low levels of resistance but which lie latent in many cats and can be reactivated silently (herpesvirus), and infections caused by viruses with a high capacity for mutation, which determines the type and severity of the resultant disease (calicivirosis or FIP). These diseases thus vary greatly in terms of the interpretation of diagnostic tests, treatment options, and prevention methods.

Applying a practical and scientifically rigorous approach, this clinical manual provides the reader with up-to-date knowledge necessary to understand the pathogenesis of these infectious diseases of cats, effectively establish a diagnosis, and select the best treatment and prevention strategies. Multiple case studies and graphical material including photos, diagrams, and tables, make for an easy-to-read text that can be rapidly consulted during daily clinical practice. Furthermore, the appendices detail the main diagnostic and treatment procedures used in the management of these infectious diseases.

In conclusion, this rigorously written practical manual, which reflects the wide-ranging clinical experience of two experts in feline medicine, constitutes an essential tool for the management of infectious diseases in cats.

Albert Lloret
Internal Medicine Service, Veterinary Teaching Hospital, Autonomous University of Barcelona
Member of the International Society of Feline Medicine (ISFM)
and the European Advisory Board on Cat Diseases (ABCD)

Preface

This book is a summary of our experience over the last 15 years in the clinical management of infectious diseases of cats, acquired working with cats from the street, from shelters, and from homes with many cats.

Our objective was to provide practical insight into the main infectious diseases of cats with which clinicians deal in daily practice, including diagnostic protocols, new treatments, and interventions that may improve the survival of affected animals including blood transfusions, parenteral feeding, placement of central venous catheters, and other techniques that may be of use in daily practice.

Within the appendices we have included general vaccination guidelines. These are based on the recommendations of the main international expert panels in the field and are the same guidelines we use in designing our vaccination protocols.

We hope you find the content useful.

Table of contents

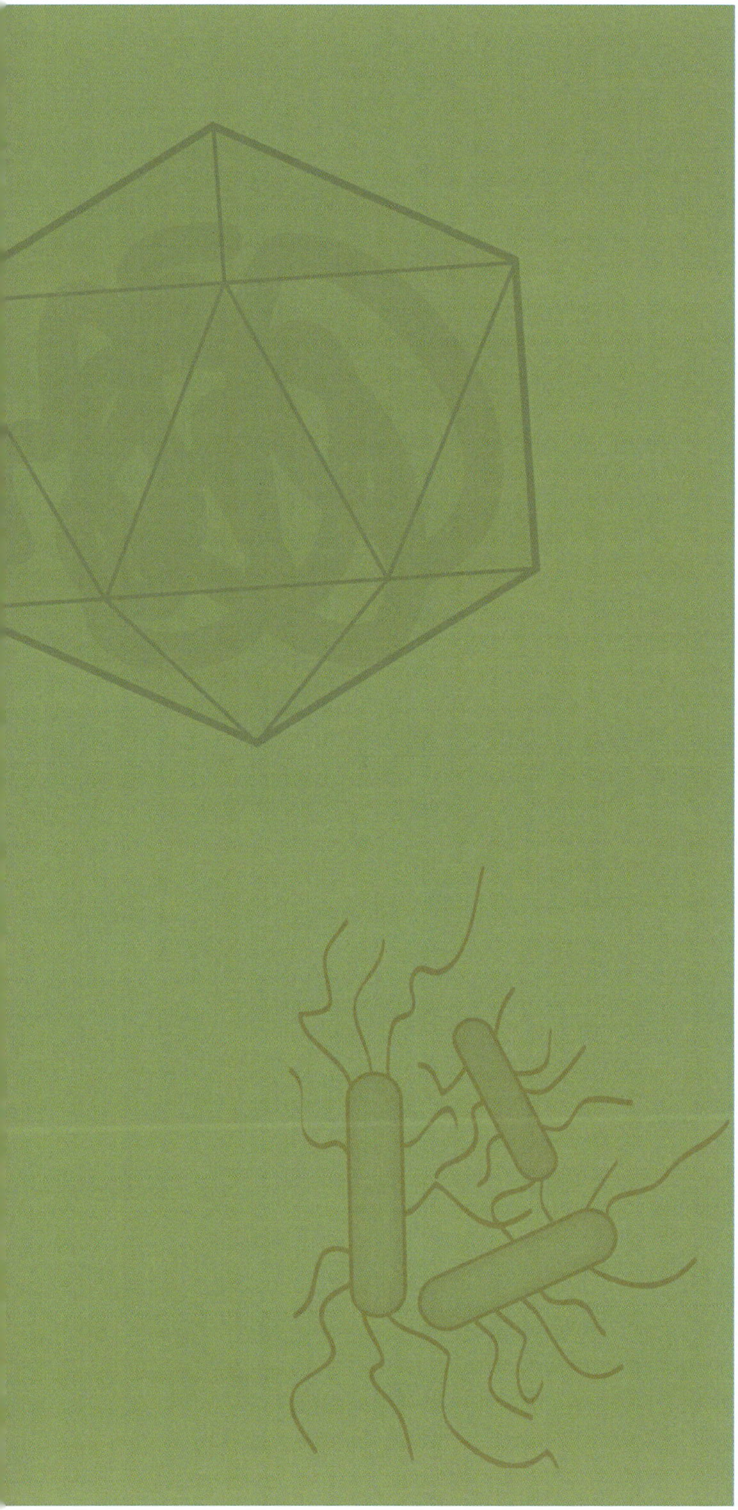

1 Feline panleukopaenia 1

Aetiology 2

Pathogenesis and clinical signs 3
Subclinical infection 3
Sudden death 3
Classic feline enteritis 3
Neurological signs 3

Laboratory diagnosis 4

Treatment 5
Supportive care 5
Specific antiviral therapy 5
Antiviral chemotherapy 5
Passive immunotherapy 5

Prevention 6
Vaccination 6
Sanitary period 6
Hyperimmune sera 6
Feline interferon ω 6

Prognosis 7

Frequent questions 8
Can a dog infect a cat? 8
Can a cat infect a dog? 8
If the result of the antigen test is negative, can I rule out FPV infection? 8
Can an animal that does not leave the house become infected? 8
Can a vaccinated cat become infected with FPV? 8
Why are neurological signs observed in kittens infected with FPV? 8
How is cerebellar hypoplasia diagnosed? Can it be contagious to other cats? 8

What vaccination schedule is recommended for an adult cat of unknown vaccination status? 8
What is the most appropriate treatment? Is it appropriate to use antibiotics? 8
What to do in case of an outbreak of FPV at the clinic 9

CASE STUDY 1: *PETETO* 10

Medical history 10
Physical examination 10
What are the most likely diagnoses? 10
What other tests should be performed? 11
Can feline panleukopaenia be ruled out? 11
What treatment can we propose? 11
Evolution 11

CASE STUDY 2: *RA* AND HIS TWO LITTERMATES 12

Medical history 12
Physical examination 12
What treatment options can be offered to *Ra*? 13
Evolution 13

2 Feline infectious peritonitis 15

Aetiology and pathogenesis 16

Diagnostic tests for FIP 17

Indirect tests 18
Complete blood count, albumin, globulin, and bilirubin 18
Effusion analysis 18
Ultrasonography 19
Albumin/globulin ratio 19
Ocular and neurological signs 19
Antibody titre in feline coronavirus 19
Rivalta's test 19
Acute phase proteins 19

Direct tests 20
Immunohistochemistry 20
Polymerase chain reaction (PCR) 22

Treatment 22

Immunity and prevention 22

References 24

CASE STUDY 1: *PAPILLÓN* 26

Medical history 26
Physical examination and diagnostic tests 26

3 Upper respiratory tract infections 31

Clinical signs 32

Pathogenic agents 33

Feline calicivirus (FCV) 33

Feline herpesvirus type 1 (FHV-1) 34

Chlamydophila felis 35

Diagnosis 35

Treatment 36

Supportive care 36

Antibiotics 37

Antiviral treatments 37

Prevention 38

References 38

CASE STUDY 1: *NIN* 39

Medical history 39

Physical examination 39

Differential diagnosis 40

Additional tests 42

Treatment 44

Follow-up 45

Discussion 45

Conclusion 47

References 47

4 Lower respiratory tract infections 49

Clinical signs 50

Diagnostic tests 50

Haematology 50

Biochemistry 51

Radiology 51

Bronchoalveolar lavage 52

Transtracheal aspiration 52

Fine-needle aspiration 54

Cytology 54

Microbiological tests 54

LRTI-causing bacteria 55

Mycoplasmas 55

Diagnosis 55

Treatment 55

Bordetella bronchiseptica 56

Treatment 56

Streptococcus spp. 56

Escherichia coli 57

Pasteurella spp. 57

Salmonella spp. 57

Mycobacterium spp. 57

Other bacteria 57

LRTI-causing parasites 58

Aelurostrongylus abstrusus 58

Diagnosis 58

Treatment 58

Eucoleus aerophilus 59

Toxoplasma gondii 59

Diagnosis 59

Treatment 59

LRTI-causing fungi 60

LRTI-causing viruses 60

Feline calicivirus 60

Feline herpesvirus 60

Pyothorax 61

Causes 61

Clinical signs 61

Diagnostic tests 62

Haematology and biochemistry 62

Radiology 62

Analysis of pleural fluid 63

Other diagnostic imaging tests 63

Diagnosis 64

Treatment 64

Systemic antimicrobial treatment 64

Thoracentesis 64

Pleural drainage tube or thoracostomy 64

Thoracotomy 64

Thoracoscopy 65

Prognosis 65

References 66

5 Feline immunodeficiency virus 69

Epidemiology 70

Pathogenesis 71

Clinical signs 72

Diagnosis 72

Virus isolation 72

Polymerase chain reaction (PCR) 72

Serology 72

Treatment 74

Supportive care 74

Antiviral treatment 74

Zidovudine or azidothymidine (AZT) 74

Plerixafor (AMD3100) 74

(R)-PMPDAP 74

Human interferon α 75

Feline interferon ω 75

Vaccination 75

References 76

CASE STUDY 1: *BREE* 77

Medical history 77

Physical examination and diagnostic tests 77

Recommended treatment 78

Follow-up 79

6 Feline leukaemia virus 81

Epidemiology 82

Pathogenesis 83

Immunocompetent cat 83

Immuncompromised cat 83

Clinical signs 84

Immunodepression 84

Anaemia 84

Cancer 85

Diagnosis 88

Virus isolation 88

ELISA (p27) 88

Immunochromatography 89

Immunofluorescent antibody test (IFA) 89

PCR for detection of provirus (DNA-PCR) 89

PCR for detection of viral RNA (RNA-PCR) 89

Serology 90

Interpretation of test results 90

Management of infection 90

Immunomodulators 91

Antiviral drugs 91

Feline interferon ω 91

Zidovudine (AZT) 91

Raltegravir 91

Prevention 91

References 93

CASE STUDY 1: *LUCAS* 94

Medical history 94

Physical examination and diagnostic tests 94

Recommended treatment 97

Follow-up 97

7 Intestinal protozoa of cats 101

Giardia 102

Clinical signs 102

Diagnosis 103

Treatment 103

Tritrichomonas foetus 104

Clinical signs 104

Diagnosis 105

Treatment 105

Prevention 105

Toxoplasma gondii 105

Clinical signs 106

Diagnosis 106

Treatment 107

Cystoisospora 108

Clinical signs 108

Diagnosis 108

Treatment 109

Cryptosporidium felis 109

Clinical signs 110

Diagnosis 110

Treatment 110

References 111

Recommended readings 111

Appendices 113

1 Fluid therapy 115

Physical examination 116

Treatment 116

Fluid 116

Solutions 117

Shock management 117

2 Vascular access routes 119

Central venous catheters 119

Selecting a catheter 120

General catheter care 120

How long can a catheter be left in place? 120

Intraosseous access 124

Material 124

Technique 124

3 Feeding in critical situations 127

Parental nutrition 127

Patient selection 128

Determination of parenteral nutrition needs 128

Caloric needs 128

Components of parenteral nutrition 129

Amino acids 129

Dextrose 129

Lipids 129

Minerals 129

Vitamins 129

Composition of mixtures used for parenteral nutrition 129

Administration 132

Complications 132

Interruption 133

4 Blood transfusion 135

Donor selection 135

Adverse reactions associated with blood group 136

Blood transfusion haemolysis 136

Neonatal isoerythrolysis 136

Collection of blood from donor 136

Transfusion volume 136

Administration 137

Adverse transfusion reactions 138

5 Punctures and drainage devices 139

Thoracentesis 139

Indications 139

Complications 139

Technique 139

Thoracic drainage 140

Objective 140

Indications 140

Complications 140

Preparing the patient 140

Technique 141

Postoperative care 143

Abdominocentesis 143

Indications 143

Complications 144

Technique 145

References 145

6 Feline oral disease 147

Clinical signs 147

Major oral diseases of cats 147

Periodontal disease 147
- Predisposing factors 148
- Treatment 148

Feline chronic gingivostomatitis 149
- Factors involved 151
- Diagnostic tests 153
- Management of chronic feline gingivitis 153
- Adjunctive treatment in specific cases 154
- Questionnaire for the evaluation of FCGS management 157

References 159

7 When to stop treatment 161

End of life 161

Responsibilities of the veterinary surgeon 162

Quality of life 162

Euthanasia 163

Rejection of euthanasia by owners 163

How can I know if my cat is suffering? 164

References 166

8 Vaccination 167

Types of vaccines 167

Inactivated vaccines 167

Modified live (attenuated) vaccines 168

Recombinant vaccines 168

Vaccination guidelines 168

House cats 168

Shelter cats 169

Trap-neuter-return (TNR) programme cats 169

Cats in catteries 169

References 171

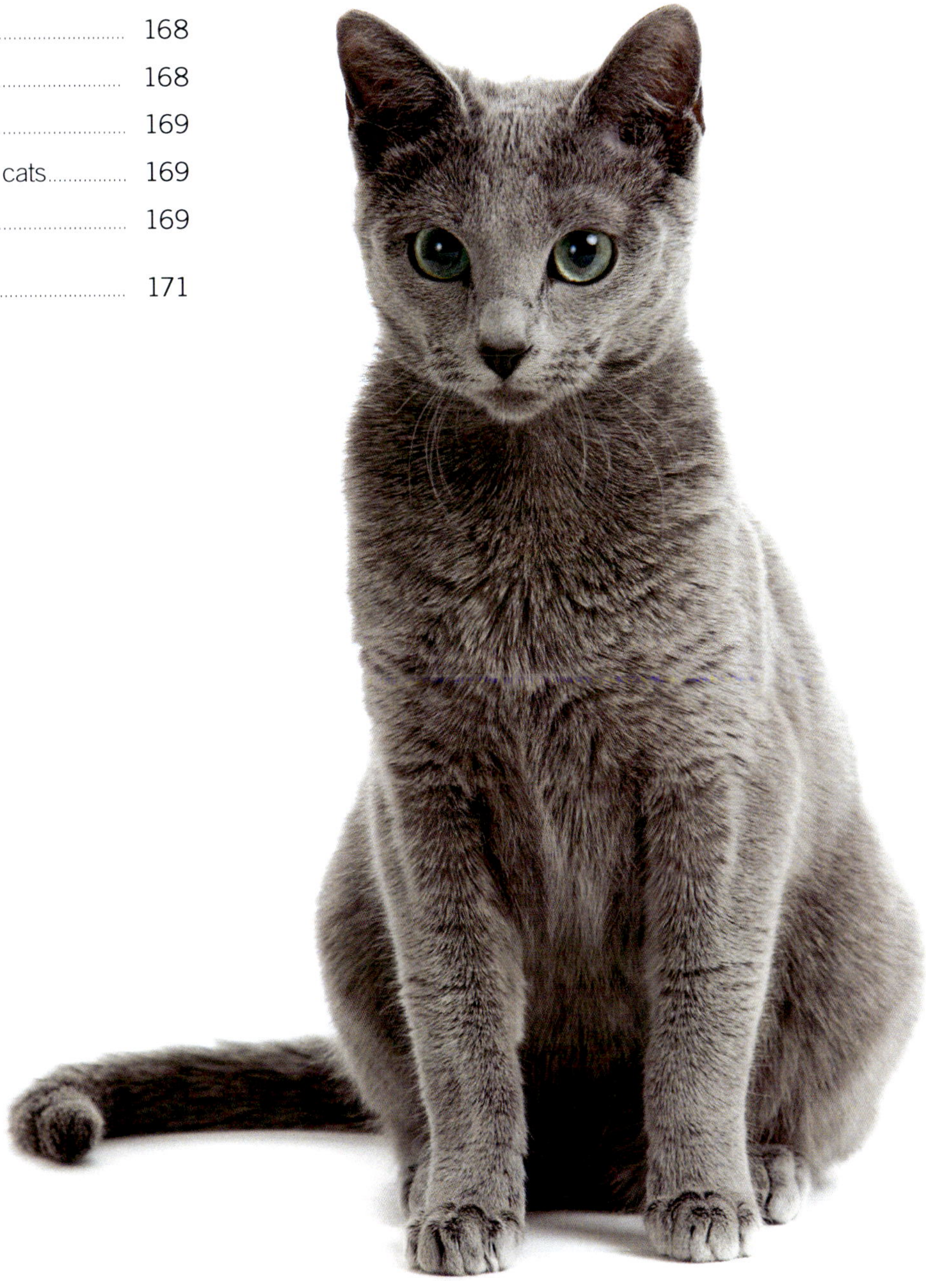

Feline panleukopaenia

Feline panleukopaenia

Feline panleukopaenia is a highly contagious viral disease that can cause serious conditions in isolated cats and, in particular, in communities. Data on the prevalence of the disease are scarce. However, this disease persists over time, and in certain areas the number of cases may have increased in recent years. The aim of this chapter is to cover several important aspects of this disease from a clinical practice perspective.

Feline panleukopaenia is caused by feline parvovirus (FPV), a single-stranded DNA virus. This virus is highly contagious for all members of the Felidae family. Control of this disease is complicated by environmental resistance, the shedding of high viral loads, and interspecies transmission.

The severity of clinical signs depends on the immune status of the animal and the presence of other concurrent diseases. Clinical presentations range from subclinical infection to the development of a hyperacute syndrome followed by sudden death. The classic clinical signs are fever, lethargy, and anorexia. Affected cats may present with vomiting and watery or bloody diarrhoea, and die from complications associated with secondary bacterial infections, such as sepsis, dehydration, and disseminated intravascular coagulation.

Some parvoviruses such as canine parvovirus type 1 (CPV-1) and FPV have undergone minimal evolution over time, while canine parvovirus type 2 (CPV-2) has demonstrated a marked capacity for adaptation and mutation, resulting in the development of three pathogenic strains: CPV-2a, CPV-2b, and CPV-2c.

A significant increase in the number of animals with FPV has been observed in the United States. Some authors attribute this increase to changes in vaccination protocols: the risk of vaccine-associated sarcomas has led to increased use of intranasal vaccines, which appear not to have the same efficacy as parenterally administered vaccines, especially in high-risk animals. On the other hand, new vaccination guidelines for both dogs and cats recommend completing primary vaccination at 14 to 16 weeks of age, based on studies that have shown greater persistence of maternal antibodies than previously assumed. It is therefore possible that these new protocols have not yet been implemented by most veterinary surgeons.

In Spain, there are no published data on the increase in the prevalence of this disease. However, our experience indicates an increase in the number of cats diagnosed with panleukopaenia in recent years (195 cases in 6 years).

Aetiology

FPV is a small (20 nm) single-stranded, non-enveloped DNA virus. It is transmitted via the faecal-oral route. Infected cats excrete virus intermittently for days or weeks.

Contagion occurs easily via clothing, shoes, and utensils; even flies have been shown to propagate infection.

Disinfection of contaminated sites is difficult, given the significant resistance of the virus to chemical disinfectants and physical agents. Disinfectants to which the virus is most sensitive include sodium hypochlorite, formaldehyde, and glutaraldehyde.

The virus begins to replicate in the oropharyngeal tissue. This single-stranded DNA virus requires dividing cells in S phase. Moreover, given the need for DNA polymerase enzyme to synthesise the complementary DNA strand, the virus requires tissues with high mitotic activity. Replication is followed by viraemia and dissemination of the virus through the bloodstream to the target organs: tonsils, mesenteric lymph nodes, lymphatic intestinal tissue, bone marrow, etc. Pathogenic consequences and clinical manifestations vary depending on the type of cells infected (Table 1).

Table 1. Pathogenic consequences and clinical manifestations of FPV depending on the tissue infected.

Infected tissue	Consequences	Clinical manifestations
Intestinal crypt epithelium	Collapse of villi	Enteritis
Lymph nodes and thymus	Lymphocyte apoptosis, thymic atrophy	Lymphopaenia
Bone marrow	Decrease in stem cell number	Pancytopaenia
Foetus	Foetal death	Abortion
Developing cerebellum	Cerebellar hypoplasia	Ataxia

Pathogenesis and clinical signs

The incubation period (from the moment the animal comes into contact with the virus until the appearance of clinical signs) ranges from 5 to 9 days. Four types of clinical manifestation are described.

Subclinical infection

Occurs in most infected cats. These animals show no clinical signs of disease.

Whether a cat develops clinical disease or not depends on numerous factors. The rate of mitosis of the intestinal crypt cells significantly influences the outcome of infection: low rates result in minimal intestinal lesions, whereas high rates, caused by stress or concomitant diseases, provide the virus with an ideal environment in which to replicate and to exert a more severe pathogenic effect. Even a change of diet can increase the rate of mitosis, facilitating viral replication. These factors may explain, for example, why adopted kittens develop severe enteritis and die, whereas kittens from the same litter that stay with the mother or in a shelter develop a milder clinical presentation, if any.

Sudden death

Sudden death is relatively common, especially in young kittens, unvaccinated cats, and animals in shelters or pet shops, etc.

Classic feline enteritis

Usually occurs suddenly. Owners often associate the clinical signs with poisoning. This clinical presentation is characterised by fever, anorexia, dehydration, vomiting, and in some cases bloody diarrhoea (Figs. 1 and 2). A complete blood count reveals signs of pancytopenia. Death may occur due to severe dehydration and loss of the intestinal barrier with bacterial overgrowth.

Neurological signs

The predilection of the virus for dividing cells makes the foetus especially vulnerable to the virus. Infection during in the first trimester of gestation can result in abortion with foetal resorption and death. Infections at later stages can cause cerebellar hypoplasia, hydrocephalus with signs of ataxia, intention tremor, and limb loss.

Laboratory diagnosis

Laboratory diagnosis includes isolation of the virus, viral antigen detection, detection of viral genetic material by PCR, and determination of serum antibodies:

- **Virus isolation:** performed using stool samples, although this is often difficult.
- **Antigen detection:** due to the antigenic similarity of the virus to CPV, the rapid immunochromatographic test used to detect CPV can also be used (Figs. 3 and 4). Studies conducted using certain tests have reported a positive predictive value of 100 % and a negative predictive value of 98 %. Positive results can be obtained up to two weeks after vaccination. Others have reported predictive values of 34 %. It is thus important to know what kind of test is being used to ensure that the diagnosis is reliable.
- **PCR:** can be performed using blood or stool samples. If the animal has diarrhoea it is preferable to perform the test using a blood sample.
- **Antibody detection:** ELISA and indirect immunofluorescence (IF) are the most commonly used methods. The disadvantage of this type of analysis when dealing with vaccinated animals is the difficulty in differentiating between vaccine antibodies and those produced in response to infection.

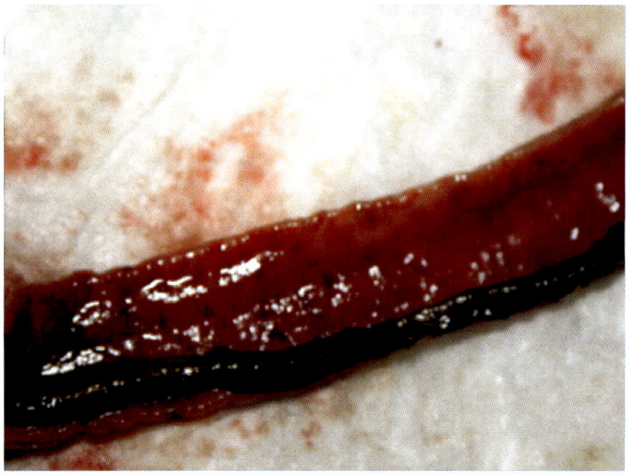

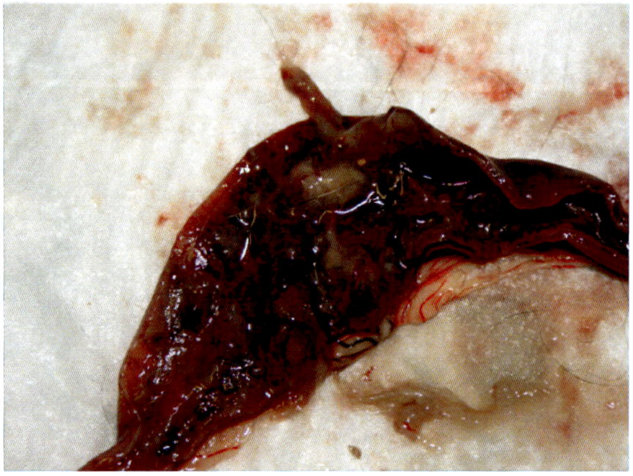

Figures 1 and 2. Severe necrosis of intestinal mucosa. Images obtained at necropsy of animals dead due to feline panleukopaenia.

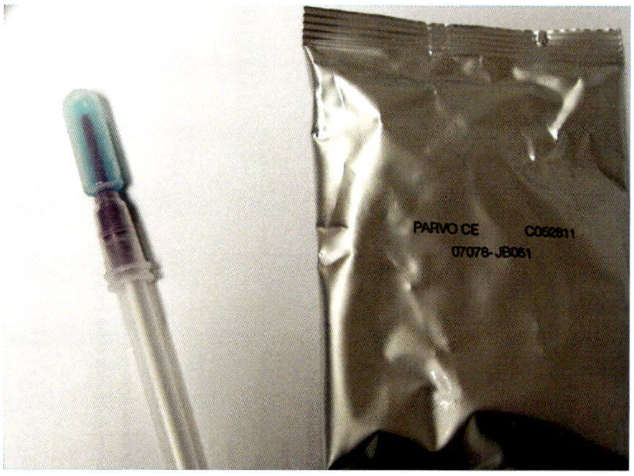

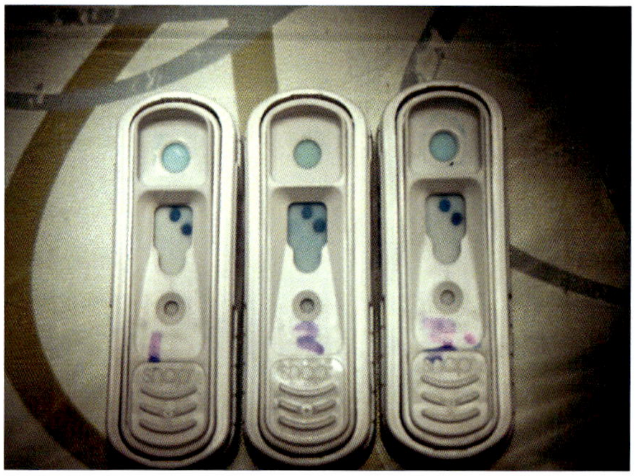

Figures 3 and 4. Diagnostic test for canine parvovirus antigen for the detection of feline panleukopaenia.

Treatment

If a cat is hospitalised in a veterinary clinic with a confirmed or suspected diagnosis of panleukopaenia, strict isolation should be considered given the characteristics of this virus, which could potentially contaminate the entire clinic (Figs. 5 and 6).

Supportive care

Treatment of clinical signs consists of:

1. **Fluid therapy:** intravenous fluid therapy and electrolyte control are important (see Appendix 1). Whenever possible, this is administered via a central venous catheter (see Appendix 2), since these animals will be hospitalised for an extended period of time and tend to present hypoalbuminaemia and peripheral oedema. In some cases the animal's condition may be critical, requiring intensive care (Fig. 7).
2. **Antibiotic therapy:** broad-spectrum antibiotics are used to prevent bacterial contamination caused by loss of the intestinal barrier. One option is to combine amoxicillin and clavulanate with a third-generation cephalosporin.
3. **Parenteral nutrition:** see Appendix 3.
4. **Antiemetics:** not only to control vomiting, but also to prevent any nausea and discomfort that the cat may experience.
5. **Transfusions:** whole blood or plasma (see Appendix 4).
6. **Analgesics:** it is very important to detect the presence of acute pain in cats and to know how to control it using opiates such as buprenorphine or fentanyl.

Specific antiviral therapy

Antiviral chemotherapy

Feline interferon ω: 2.5 MIU/kg IV every 24 hours for 3 consecutive days. While some studies have been conducted in dogs, no cat studies have produced a high level of scientific evidence.

Passive immunotherapy

Antibody transfer: this involves the subcutaneous administration of 1–3 ml/kg of serum or homologous plasma from animals that have recovered from

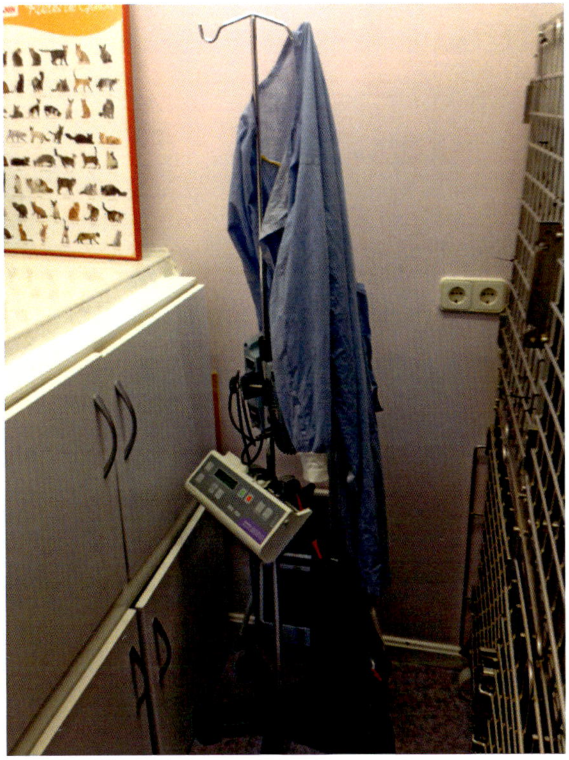

Figure 5. Equipment in the isolation area for infectious animals.

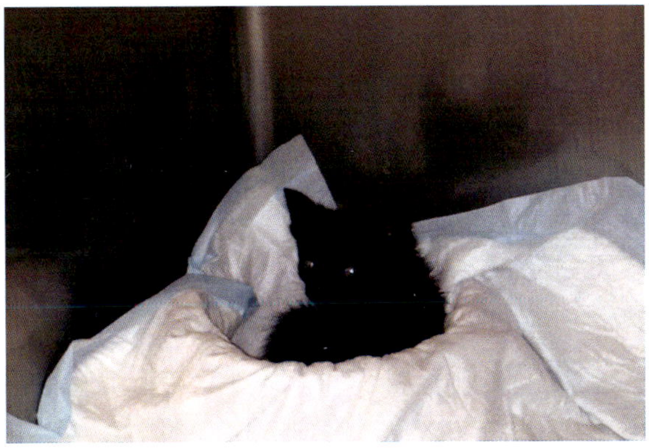

Figure 6. Hospitalised patient.

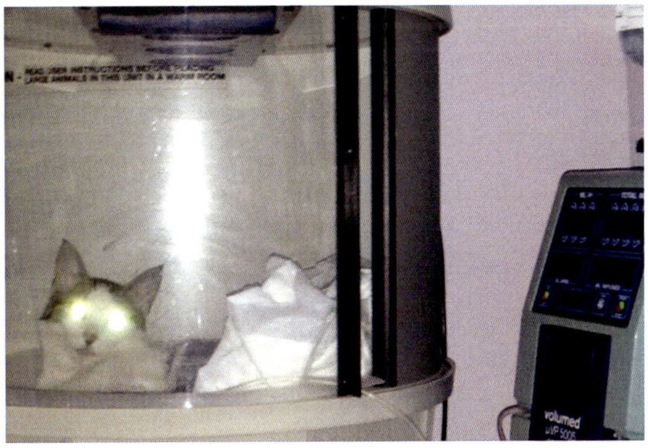

Figure 7. Intensive care area for animals in critical state.

infection or have high antibody titres following vaccination. Blood group should be determined beforehand. No studies of high scientific value have been published.

Prevention

Vaccination

Vaccination is the most effective means of preventing FPV infection. This is achieved using live attenuated vaccines starting at 8 to 9 weeks of life, administering doses every 3 weeks so that the final vaccine is administered after 16 weeks of age, followed by revaccination after 1 year. It is essential that all cats, even those that do not spend time outdoors, are adequately vaccinated.

Owing to the cat's epitheliochorial placenta, maternal antibodies are passed to the foetus at the end of gestation. It is thus very important that kittens adequately feed on colostrum during the first 8 hours of life in order to acquire these antibodies. Maternal antibody levels decrease from the 10th week of life. If animals are vaccinated too early in life, passive immunity may interfere with active immunity. This can result in the following scenarios:

- In animals that have nursed well, the recommendation is to vaccinate at 8 to 9 weeks of age and to always administer the last dose after 16 weeks.
- In animals that have not nursed during the first hours of life, it is advisable to vaccinate early (7–12 days of age) with an inactivated vaccine, which allows the formation of neutralising antibodies.
- Gestating cats should be vaccinated with inactivated vaccines.
- Certain considerations should be borne in mind when dealing with animals with retroviral diseases: health status permitting, administration of inactivated vaccines is recommended.

Live attenuated vaccines provide immunity within three days of vaccination.

The general vaccination protocol followed in our centre, based on the consensus of experts, is shown in Box 1.

Box 1. Vaccination schedule.

- **1st vaccine:** 8–9 weeks of age.
- **2nd vaccine:** 12 weeks of age.
- **3rd vaccine:** after 16 weeks of age.
- **Revaccination:** 1 year later.

Sanitary period

The implementation of an adequate sanitary period is essential to eradicate the virus, especially in feline communities. It is important to remember that the virus can persist in the environment for up to a year.

Disinfection can be achieved using sodium hypochlorite (diluted bleach) to reduce the viral load. The creation of contamination-free areas in places with high risk of infection, such as shelters, catteries, foster homes, and veterinary clinics, may be of interest.

Hyperimmune sera

These can be administered in advance of a situation of risk, although studies demonstrating the effectiveness of this approach are lacking.

Feline interferon ω

An Italian field study conducted in cats naturally infected with FPV found no significant differences in survival rate or clinical signs between a group of 23 cats pretreated with interferon and another group of 17 untreated animals.

Prognosis

In CPV infection, leukopaenia, lymphopaenia, monocytopaenia, and eosinopaenia are indicators of a poor prognosis. The prognosis is further complicated if concentrations of cortisol, thyroxine, and serum cholesterol decrease.

Systemic inflammatory response syndrome (SIRS) develops most often in dogs that will not survive, and have other concurrent viral, bacterial, or parasitic diseases that worsen the prognosis.

While corresponding data for FPV are limited, these types of studies in cats are important to help improve the treatment of infected animals, anticipate complications, and improve survival rates.

Results of a retrospective study

» At the Ventas Feline Hospital (Madrid), we conducted a retrospective study of 66 cats diagnosed with feline panleukopaenia between 2004 and 2010 in order to detect risk factors for FPV. The objective was to minimise contagion between animals and to identify prognostic factors associated with survival.

» Diagnosis was established by means of an antigen detection test, which detects both FPV and canine parvovirus CPV-2a and CPV-2b.

» At the moment of diagnosis, all cats underwent a complete blood count, a serial stool analysis, and tests for feline leukaemia virus and feline immunodeficiency virus. The medical history of all cats was recorded, as well as data pertaining to their living conditions (multiple homes, communities, outdoor or indoor living, etc.), and vaccination and parasite control status. Cats were classified as unvaccinated, vaccinated with full schedule (including the last vaccine administered from 16 weeks of age), or vaccinated without full schedule.

» The most common clinical signs of the disease and the presence of signs associated with other diseases were also recorded.

» The following are some of the key findings of our study:

- The survival rate was 52 %. The majority of animals were infected during the first year of life (81 %), mainly between 3 and 4 months of age. However, FPV was also diagnosed in adult cats (18 %) and in those without outdoor access (89 %). Of the cats infected with FPV, 32 % had received one or two shots, but none had received the complete vaccination schedule or had been vaccinated after 16 weeks of age.
- The following are the main clinical signs presented by cats at the moment of diagnosis: anorexia (84 %), lack of energy (59 %), vomiting (64 %), and diarrhoea (54 %).
- Cats with concomitant respiratory infections had a higher mortality rate (80 %).
- The most significant laboratory findings were leukopaenia (74 %) and hypoalbuminaemia (69 %).

Frequent questions

Can a dog infect a cat?

Cats can become infected by both FPV and by canine parvovirus (CPV-2a, CPV-2b, and CPV-2c). Both viruses can cause signs of panleukopaenia. Kits for faecal canine parvovirus antigen detection can detect wild and vaccine strains of both viruses.

Can a cat infect a dog?

This depends on the strain involved. A cat shedding antigen for CPV-2a or CPV-2b can infect a dog, whereas a cat shedding FPV cannot infect dogs.

If the result of the antigen test is negative, can I rule out FPV infection?

Even if the result of the faecal antigen test is negative, FPV infection cannot be ruled out. Viral shedding can occur over a short period of time, or intermittently, and the results can be negative if the test is performed 5 to 7 days after disease onset. Viraemia occurs before faecal shedding of the virus. Therefore, a negative result can be obtained if the test is performed too soon.

In the early stages of the disease, samples of blood or bone marrow can be analysed by PCR, which can produce a positive result for FPV earlier than the faecal antigen test.

Can an animal that does not leave the house become infected?

Yes. A cat that does not leave the house can be exposed indirectly via shoes or bags contaminated with faeces carrying canine or feline parvovirus, or any other object that serves as a vehicle of disease transmission.

Can a vaccinated cat become infected with FPV?

Yes, if the complete vaccination schedule has not been completed. Maternal antibodies are the most common cause of disease in vaccinated cats. Interference with maternal antibodies can occur if vaccination commences before maternal antibody levels diminish. Cats should be vaccinated at 9 weeks and 12 weeks, and the last dose should always be administered after 16 weeks. These "new" recommendations contained in vaccination guidelines are supported by experts in feline infectious diseases.

Why are neurological signs observed in kittens infected with FPV?

Neurological examination of these kittens reveals cerebellar disease. This is characterised by a normal mental state with symmetrical ataxia and hypermetric movements of the limbs and head. Intention tremor is also common in these animals. Because multiple kittens are usually affected in a given litter, this disease is sometimes mistaken for congenital heart disease. However, unlike other congenital neurodegenerative diseases, affected animals present with non-progressive cerebellar ataxia, caused by hypoplasia of the cerebellum resulting from intrauterine FPV infection. This becomes clinically evident when the kitten begins to walk.

How is cerebellar hypoplasia diagnosed? Can it be contagious to other cats?

Diagnosis can be established by magnetic resonance imaging (MRI) or by post mortem analysis, but no test can detect parvovirus given the absence of an active infection.

It is not contagious to other cats. These are cats that gradually adapt to neurological deficits and can lead a normal life.

What vaccination schedule is recommended for an adult cat of unknown vaccination status?

It is highly recommended to vaccinate the cat with a regimen of 2 vaccinations separated by 3 weeks.

What is the most appropriate treatment? Is it appropriate to use antibiotics?

Cats with feline panleukopaenia should be isolated and provided with intensive treatment. Intravenous fluids are the most important element of treatment. Metabolic acidosis and hypokalaemia should be corrected with fluid therapy. Ingestion of food and water should only be restricted if there is vomiting, and should be restored as soon as possible. Symptomatic medication should be administered if the cat presents with vomiting or nausea.

In cases involving **hypoproteinaemia, transfusion of whole blood or plasma may be required.** The albumin concentration should be maintained above 2 mg/dl. In cases involving oedema, transfusion of plasma or synthetic colloids is recommended. In severe cases parenteral nutrition may be required. Hypoalbuminaemia is a negative prognostic factor. Microenteral nutrition may help prevent hypoalbuminaemia. Affected animals may present with thiamin deficiency, in which case thiamin supplementation may be beneficial.

Destruction of the intestinal barrier can allow bacteria to pass into the bloodstream, resulting in sepsis in immunocompromised patients. Antibiotics specific for gram-negative and anaerobic bacteria should be administered intravenously.

What to do in case of an outbreak of FPV at the clinic

Since sick cats shed virus for up to three days before the onset of clinical signs, it is already too late to act at this point. Cleaning and disinfection measures should be part of the infectious disease control protocol of any veterinary clinic. Disinfectants are ineffective against biological material, which should be washed first with soap, followed by disinfectant. Unvaccinated animals should be handled with gloves and placed on clean surfaces (disposable pads). Doorknobs, computer keyboards, light switches, countertops, and any other surface not included in routine cleaning should be cleaned periodically. Personnel who handle sick animals should do so using gloves, gowns, and foot coverings and should use a colour code to mark contaminated material.

It is important to know the vaccination status of other animals that attend the clinic for scheduled appointments or surgeries.

KEY POINTS

» Kittens are highly susceptible to infection with FPV with the decrease in maternal antibody levels, before acquisition of vaccine antibodies.

» Animals should be vaccinated against FPV, using a vaccination protocol adapted to the circumstances of each animal, but always vaccinating after 16 weeks.

» Adult and indoor cats are also susceptible to FPV infection.

» The clinical presentation may vary; affected cats often present with anorexia and depression, without vomiting or diarrhoea.

» Rapid tests provide a reliable means of establishing diagnosis, but with a risk of false negatives. Results should be interpreted bearing in mind the clinical presentation and the animal's risk of exposure. PCR analysis of blood or bone marrow can be used to verify diagnosis.

» Affected animals should be hospitalised should receive continuous supportive treatment. The course of the disease is variable. Hospitalisation time ranges from 5 to 9 days.

» Concomitant pathological processes are associated with a worse prognosis, irrespective of the animal's age.

» Enteral nutrition is beneficial in cases of vomiting. If not possible, alternatives include parenteral or microenteral nutrition.

» Hypoalbuminaemia and leukopaenia may be negative prognostic factors.

» Nursing care is essential. Cats should be kept warm, dry, and clean.

» There is a high risk of hospital contamination.

CASE STUDIES

CASE STUDY 1: *Peteto*

Summary: non-neutered male cat of 5 months of age (Fig. 1).

Reason for consultation: weakness, anorexia.

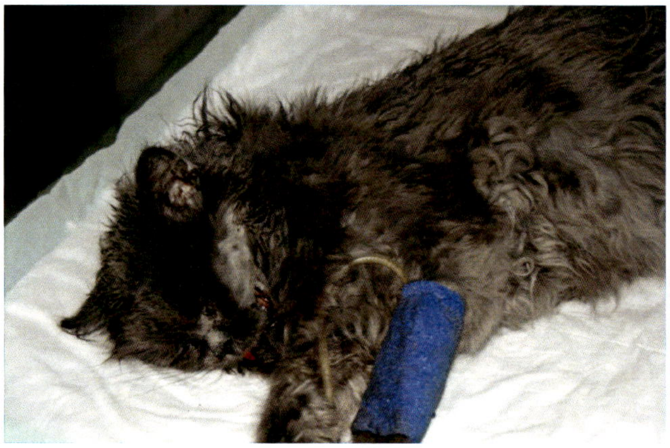

Figure 1. Patient after admission to the clinic.

Medical history

The cat is 5 months old, and had been adopted from a shelter 7 days beforehand. At 8 weeks of age, he had been vaccinated with an inactivated vaccine against panleukopaenia (FPV), herpesvirus (FHV), and calicivirus (FCV).

He has remained in hiding since arriving at its new home, and it is unclear whether he has eaten properly. The new owners had not brought the cat to the clinic earlier as they had assumed that the behaviour was normal for a cat in a new environment. However, *Peteto* had always been an active and friendly cat during his time at the shelter.

Physical examination

Clinical examination revealed the following: body condition 2/5, weight 1.7 kg, weakness, lethargy, dehydration (approximately 7 %), excessive salivation, abdominal pain on palpation, rectal temperature of 40.9 °C, bradycardia (60 beats per minute), and a capillary refill time >2 seconds. An emergency complete blood count is performed (Table 1).

What are the most likely diagnoses?

The following are the most common causes of gastrointestinal disease in young cats that are not adequately vaccinated and come from an environment of risk:

- Infectious.
- Parasitic.
- Dietary changes: food intolerance, ingestion of harmful substances, foreign bodies.

Feline panleukopaenia virus (FPV) is the most likely diagnosis in a young cat that has fever and severe leukopaenia, has been exposed to an environment of risk, and not been properly vaccinated.

Table 1. Results of complete blood count.

Complete blood count	Result	Reference
Erythrocytes	9.2×10^{12}/l	5–10 × 10^{12}/l
Platelets	123×10^{9}/l	175–400 × 10^{9}/l
Leukocytes	0.30×10^{9}/l	5.5–19.5 × 10^{9}/l
Neutrophils	0.11×10^{9}/l	2.5–12.5 × 10^{9}/l
Lymphocytes	0.10×10^{9}/l	0.4–6.8 × 10^{9}/l

What other tests should be performed?

ELISA for detection of canine parvovirus antigen in faeces, a test for *Giardia* spp., and serial analysis of stool samples for three days are recommended.

The following results are obtained:

- *Giardia* spp. test: negative.
- Faecal ELISA for canine parvovirus: negative/equivocal result (Fig. 2).
- As regards stool analysis, it is not considered prudent to wait three days for results in such an urgent case.

Can feline panleukopaenia be ruled out?

A negative or weakly positive result for antigen in faeces does not rule out infection with FPV. The virus is shed intermittently for a short period. Negative results can be obtained when the test is performed 5 to 7 days or more after disease onset. Because viraemia occurs before faecal shedding of the virus, negative results may be obtained in the early stages of the disease, before the onset of diarrhoea.

In the case of *Peteto*, a diagnosis of FPV is most likely, given the clinical signs and the presence of fever, the contaminated environment from which the cat came, its vaccination status (not vaccinated after 16 weeks), and the marked leukopaenia observed in the complete blood count.

What treatment can we propose?

Cats with panleukopaenia require complete isolation and hospitalisation with intensive care. Placement of a central venous catheter is advisable, if possible (Appendix 2).

Physical examination reveals peripheral perfusion problems, bradycardia, and hypotension, indicating a state of shock, probably hypovolaemic although possibly with a septic component. Cats in a state of shock present with bradycardia, as opposed to the compensatory tachycardia seen in other species.

Fluid replacement therapy is required to normalise blood volume (Appendix 1). Antimicrobial treatment is administered (metronidazole, 10 mg/kg IV every 12 hours, and ceftriaxone, 22 mg/kg IV every 12 hours).

Evolution

After 3 days of supportive treatment, enteral nutrition is instituted. *Peteto* improves significantly and is discharged.

Enteral nutrition should be started as soon as possible: nutrition of the cells of the intestinal epithelium is essential to fight against bacterial translocation and facilitates better recovery of intestinal lesions.

An examination conducted 10 days later reveals a normalised blood count and recuperation of normal bodyweight.

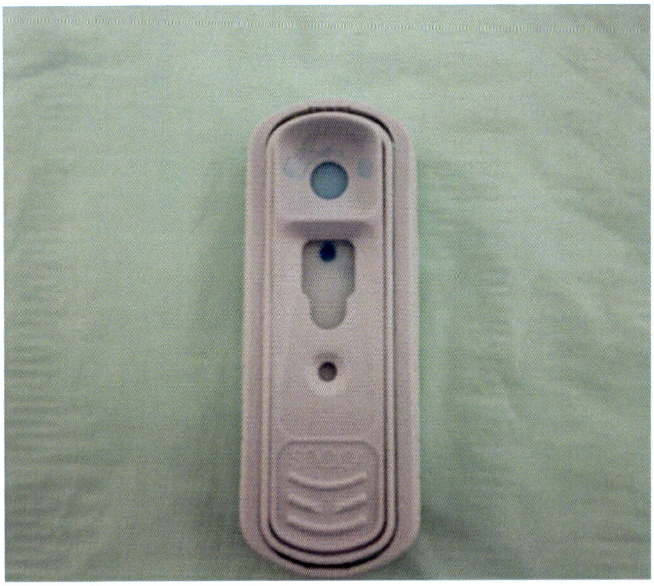

Figure 2. Inconclusive ELISA test for detection of canine parvovirus in faeces.

CASE STUDY 2: *Ra* and his two littermates

Review: domestic shorthair cats of 2 months of age (Fig. 3), neither vaccinated nor dewormed.

Reason for consultation: lack of energy.

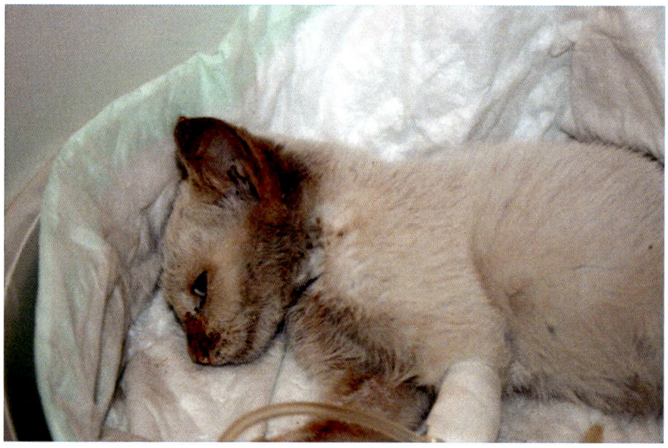

Figure 3. Patient after admission to the clinic.

Medical history

Ra is a two-month-old male domestic shorthair cat. He is brought to the clinic along with two other cats, all of whom were found in the street. All appear to be from the same litter. Since their arrival at their new home 10 days previously, all three have gained weight, playing and eating normally.

Three or four days before attending the clinic, *Ra* stopped playing and eating, and has since sat in the sandbox. His owners report no signs of loose stools, or any other information of note, apart from *Ra*'s general debilitated state.

Table 2. Results of complete blood count.

Complete blood count	Result	Reference
Erythrocytes	3.8×10^{12}/l	$5–10 \times 10^{12}$/l
Platelets	33×10^{9}/l	$175–400 \times 10^{9}$/l
Leukocytes	0.12×10^{9}/l	$5.5–19.5 \times 10^{9}$/l
Neutrophils	0.08×10^{9}/l	$2.5–12.5 \times 10^{9}$/l
Lymphocytes	0.04×10^{9}/l	$0.4–6.8 \times 10^{9}$/l

Physical examination

Clinical examination reveals the following: body condition 3/5, weight 200 g (lower than that of his littermates), weakness, lethargy, poor coat, dehydration (approximately 8 %), excessive salivation, abdominal pain on palpation, rectal temperature of 41.2 °C, bradycardia (80 beats per minute), and a capillary refill time >2 seconds.

A complete blood count is performed (Table 2), and a faecal ELISA for the detection of canine parvovirus antigen produces a positive result.

What treatment options can be offered to *Ra*?

The appearance of hyperacute clinical signs, with a clear diagnosis of FPV and a state of shock, indicate that *Ra* needs to be hospitalised in isolation and that his two littermates need to be monitored and potentially undergo additional tests. In addition to fluid (Appendix 1) and antibiotic therapy, as recommended in Case Study 1, a blood transfusion (Appendix 4) and parenteral nutrition (Appendix 3) are proposed.

Evolution

Twenty-four hours after a blood transfusion and institution of parenteral nutrition, *Ra* begins receiving enteral nutrition.

The clinical picture is complicated by an upper airway respiratory process, which necessitates hospitalisation for longer than anticipated. After 7 days of hospitalisation with fluid and supportive therapy, *Ra*'s bodyweight is 270 g and his recovery is complete.

One of his littermates dies suddenly. Necropsy reveals intestinal lesions compatible with FPV (Fig. 4). The third littermate shows no signs of disease or haematological disorders.

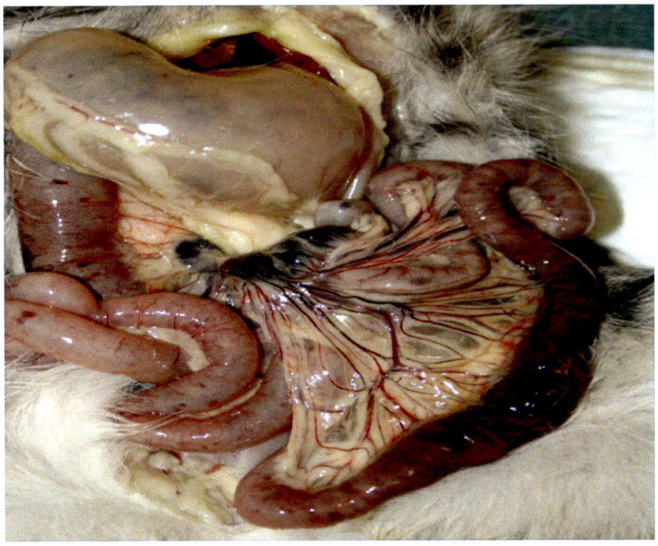

Figure 4. Intestinal lesions observed upon necropsy of one of *Ra*'s littermates.

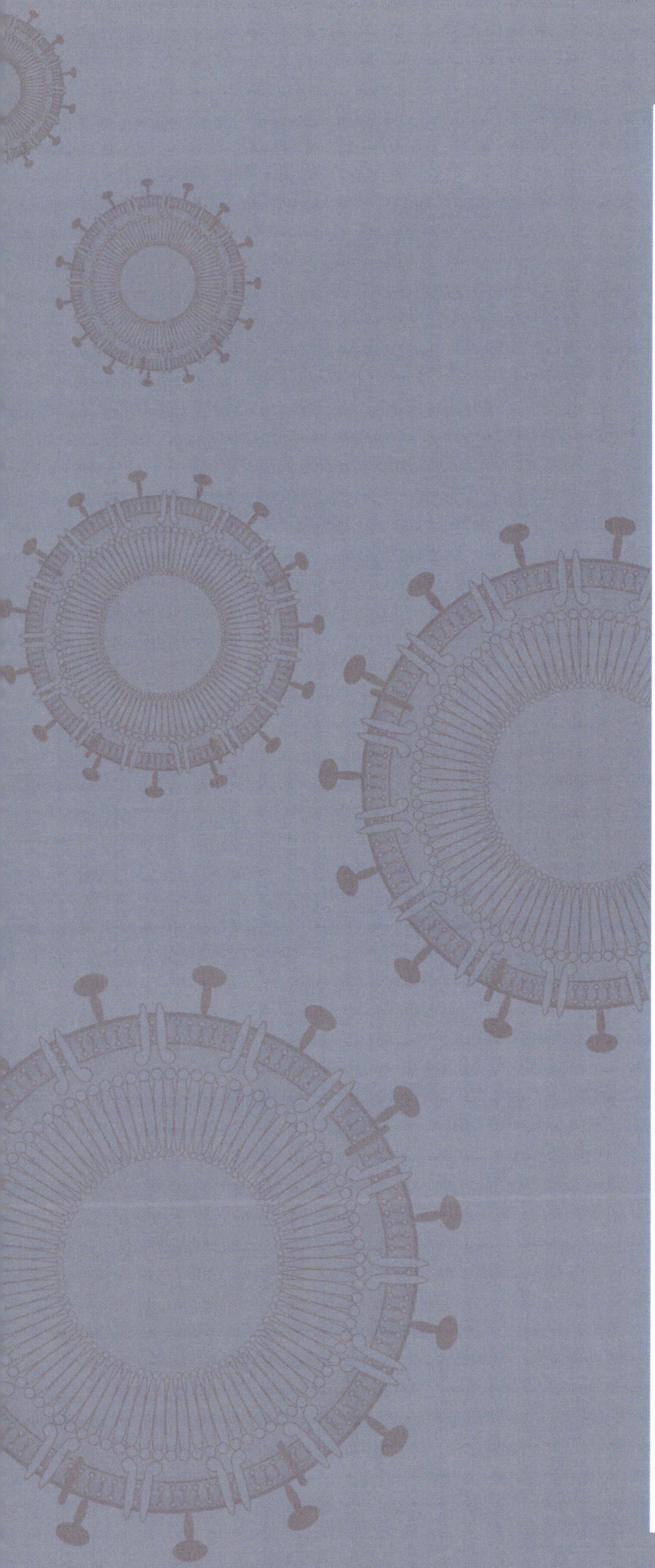

Feline infectious peritonitis

Feline infectious peritonitis

Aetiology and pathogenesis

Feline infectious peritonitis (FIP) is a disease caused by feline coronavirus (FCoV) that can affect cats of any age, but is most prevalent in cats of under 3 years of age and in particular those of 4 to 16 months of age (Pedersen, 2009). Although described as long ago as 1950, it is currently considered an emerging disease; FIP accounts for 1 in every 200 cases diagnosed in referral hospitals.

Mortality is extremely high when clinical signs appear, although some cats can live for weeks or months, in which case the quality of life of affected animals should be periodically assessed to ensure their well-being in their final days and weeks. Given the possibility of a fatal outcome and the lack of definitive diagnostic techniques and treatments, this disease has a great psychological impact on owners who have developed a bond with a new cat in their home (Fig. 1).

The objective of this chapter is to review direct and indirect tests for the diagnosis of FIP, with a particular emphasis on the limitations, sensitivity, and specificity thereof.

The FIP virus (FIPV) is the product of mutations in feline enteric coronavirus (FECV), which tends not to cause serious pathologies in cats. FECV is shed in the faeces of apparently healthy cats (Pedersen et al., 2004) and transmission occurs directly via the faecal-oral route or via fomites. Young cats are infected around nine weeks of age. At this moment, when levels of FECV replication are high, mutation can occur (Volgel et al., 2010), although only a small proportion of cats exposed to the mutated virus variant develop FIP.

Whether a cat develops FIP or not depends on genetic susceptibility, age at exposure, the type of viral mutation, and stress-related factors at the moment of infection.

The disease course, from the onset of clinical signs until death, is variable, and is shorter in young cats and those with the exudative form of the disease as compared with older cats and those with the non-exudative form.

FIP causes vasculitis mediated by the immune system, resulting in effusion in the abdomen, chest, or pericardium in the exudative form, or the appearance of pyogranulomatous lesions of varying severity in the non-exudative form. Exudative FIP can become non-exudative and vice versa (Fig. 2).

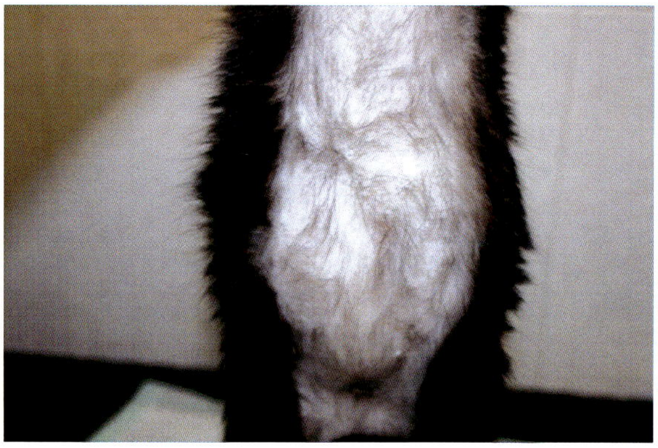

Figure 1. Cat with abdominal distension.

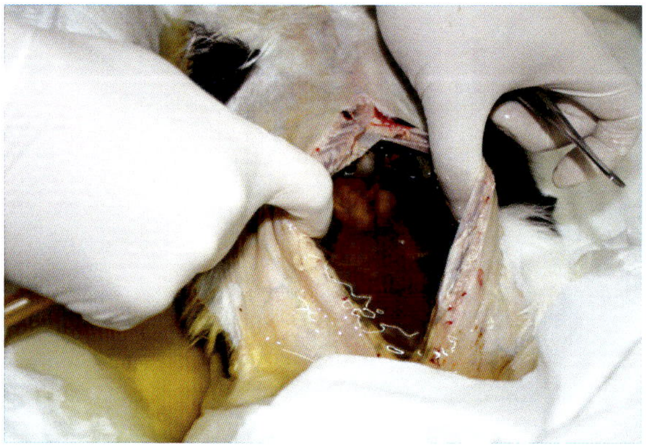

Figure 2. Necropsy of cat diagnosed with FIP, in which a large amount of abdominal effusion fluid is observed.

Diagnostic tests for FIP

Diagnosis should be based on the following parameters (Fig. 3):

- Age of cat.
- Origin of cat.
- Clinical signs.
- Physical examination.

Cats aged 4 to 36 months, living in environments with high densities of other cats, that present with remittent fever and are unresponsive to antibiotics, are highly likely to have FIP.

The most common **clinical signs** are abdominal distension with ascites, dyspnoea due to pleural effusion, jaundice, hyperbilirubinaemia, enlarged or irregular kidneys and mesenteric lymph nodes, uveitis, and neurological disorders.

The presentation of the exudative or wet form of FIP is more acute and occurs between 4 and 6 weeks after exposure to the stressor and to enteric coronavirus. The non-exudative or dry form can incubate for months. Non-exudative FIP is characterised by a more chronic response, with the formation of pyogranulomas in different locations (Figs. 4 and 5). The cat loses weight gradually, and becomes listless and anorexic. Clinical signs vary depending on the organ affected. Colloquially it is known as "purring disease", because affected cats maintain an appetite and are particularly affectionate.

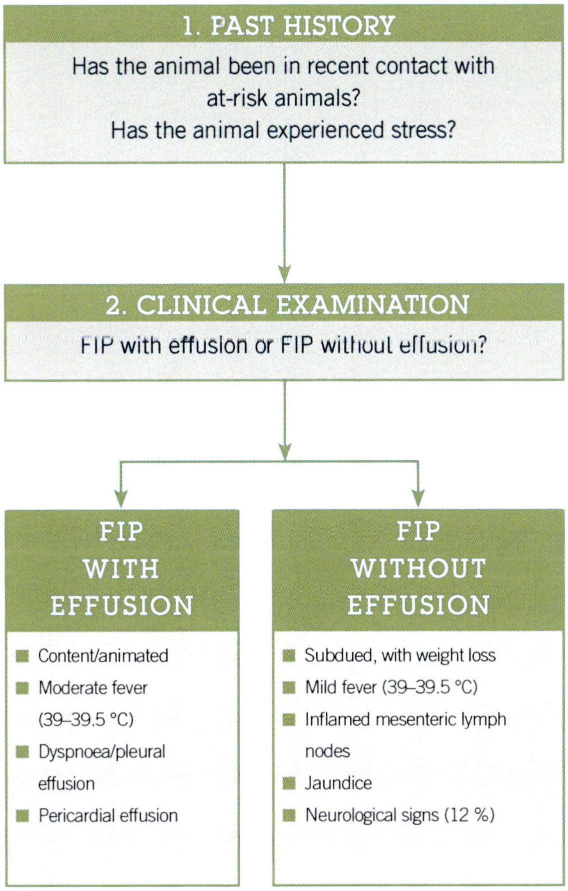

Figure 3. Clinical approach for patient with suspected FIP.

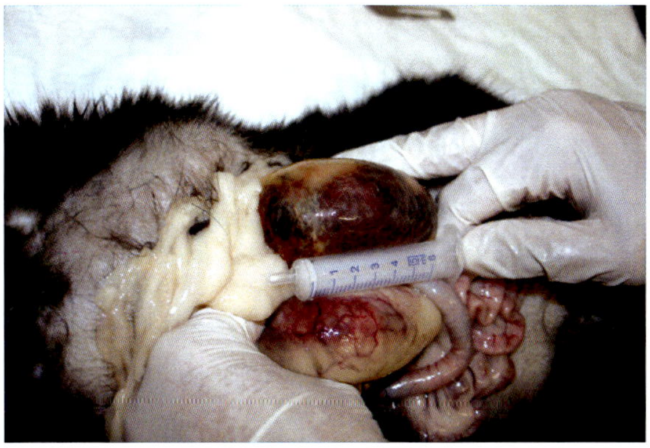

Figure 4. Pyogranulomatous lesions in different organs: kidneys, liver, and intestine.

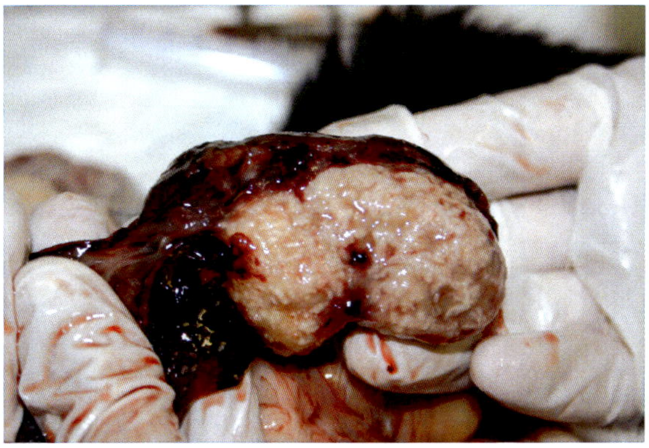

Figure 5. Detail of a pyogranulomatous lesion of the kidney.

At this point, a diagnosis of FIP can be established with reasonable certainty. However, due to high levels of mortality associated with this disease, many veterinary surgeons and carers feel the need for further diagnostic evidence.

The difficulty arises in choosing between tests that increase the diagnostic value of clinical signs caused by FIP (indirect evidence), and other definitive diagnostic tests that identify the specific causative agent of FIP (direct evidence). It is important to note that the sensitivity and specificity of any indirect test varies depending on the condition of the cat. Thus, the positive predictive value of the test (i.e. the probability of having the disease if the result of the diagnostic test is positive) is higher in cats that show compatible clinical signs, are young, and come from an environment of risk, as compared with cats that are unlikely to have been exposed to feline coronavirus and show no suspicious clinical signs compatible with FIP.

Indirect tests

Complete blood count, albumin, globulin, and bilirubin

Cats with FIP commonly present with chronic non-regenerative anaemia, leukocytosis with an increase in the total number of neutrophils, and a decrease in total lymphocyte number. An increase in levels of serum proteins may also be observed, associated with increased globulin (G) levels, decreased albumin (A) levels, and a low A/G ratio (Addie et al., 2009; Pedersen, 2009; Drechsler et al., 2011).

While hyperbilirubinaemia and hyperbilirubinuria are common in cats with FIP, particularly the exudative form, they are not associated with increased liver enzyme levels or cholangitis, but rather with increased destruction of red blood cells and impaired removal of waste products of haemoglobin (Addie et al., 2009).

While these findings can help establish a more accurate diagnosis, it is essential to consider the overall clinical picture, along with clinical signs and the results of the physical examination.

Effusion analysis

Damage associated with the wet form is due to the formation of immune complexes that cause vascular damage and effusion of fluid in both the pleural and abdominal cavities. Abdominal distension is not usually painful, and produces waves during palpation.

The analysis of peritoneal fluid, or less frequently pleural fluid, facilitates diagnosis of the exudative form of FIP.

The exudative form is the most common in purebred cats, except Birman breeds, in which the non-exudative presentation is more common. The fluid is usually yellow (due to the presence of bilirubin) or green (due to the presence of biliverdin), clear, viscous (with a density like that of egg white), and with a high protein concentration, similar to that of serum. It is classified as "modified transudate" due to its low cellularity, but more closely resembles inflammatory exudate.

In cases of effusion in which FIP is suspected, only by measuring total protein in the fluid can feline cardiomyopathy be ruled out, since the latter is generally

Characteristics of extracted fluid

- Colour: yellow, clear.
- Appearance: viscous and cloudy.
- Density: 1.017–1.047.
- Protein: concentration >3.5 g/dl, typically between 5 g/dl and 12 g/dl.
- Albumin/globulin ratio: <0.45.
- Cellularity: <5,000 cells/μl.

characterised by protein levels of less than 5 g/dl (Zoia et al., 2009).

Ultrasonography

Ultrasonography is useful to identify the presence of fluid and obtain a sample of peritoneal or pleural fluid. In a retrospective study of 16 cats diagnosed with exudative and non-exudative FIP, 11 showed normal hepatic echogenicity, 5 showed a hypoechoic subcapsular rim in one or both kidneys, and 9 showed signs of lymphadenopathy. The authors concluded that although there may be no specific sonographic finding of FIP, a compatible medical history and associated sonographic signs increases the level of certainty of a diagnosis of FIP (Lewis and O'Brien, 2010).

Albumin/globulin ratio

The albumin/globulin ratio is a good predictor of FIP infection when assessed in conjunction with medical history, clinical signs, physical examination, and the presence of abnormalities associated with the disease. When FIP prevalence is low, a high albumin/globulin ratio is useful to rule out the presence of FIP with almost 100 % certainty. Conversely, a low albumin/globulin ratio in the same circumstances is highly indicative of FIP, but does not constitute 100 % confirmation of the disease (Jeffery et al., 2012).

Ocular and neurological signs

Most young cats with ocular or neurological signs have the non-exudative form of FIP (Pedersen, 2009). Uveitis is the main ocular sign associated with FIP, and must be distinguished from idiopathic uveitis. Aqueous humour cytology is a useful means of making this distinction. In cases of uveitis associated with FIP, aqueous humour cytology reveals a predominance of neutrophils, whereas in idiopathic uveitis reactive lymphocytes and plasma cells predominate.

Neurological signs associated with FIP are more commonly seen in the non-exudative form and affect the central nervous system and spinal cord. FIP accounts for 50 % of cases of myelitis in cats (Marioni-Henry, 2010).

Antibody titre in feline coronavirus

Antibody screening tests do not differentiate between enteric coronavirus and FIP coronavirus. Although many healthy cats exposed to enteric coronavirus have antibody levels ranging from 1:100 to 1:400, as determined by indirect immunofluorescence, these levels are usually much higher in cats with FIP. Healthy cats rarely have titres of over 1:1600, while titres of over 1:3200 are indicative of the presence of the FIP virus (Hartmann et al., 2003).

Healthy cats with titres of less than 1:100 rarely shed enteric coronavirus in the faeces, whereas faecal analysis can be positive in cats with titres of 1:400 or higher.

Rivalta's test

Rivalta's test is an easy and inexpensive indirect analysis to increase the "reasonable certainty" of diagnosis of FIP (Fischer, 2012). It involves the addition of 2 or 3 drops of 8 % acetic acid (white vinegar) to a beaker of water at room temperature. A drop of effusion fluid is allowed to slowly fall into the solution. If it does not dissolve (and acquires a jellyfish-like appearance) the result is positive, whereas if it dissolves (acquiring a smoke-like appearance) the result is negative. This test has a sensitivity of 91 %, a specificity of 66 %, a negative predictive value (probability of not having the disease if the result of the diagnostic test is negative) of 93 %, and a positive predictive value of 58 %. These percentages increase further if cats with lymphoma and bacterial infections and those of over two years of age are excluded from the test. Interpretation of this test is subjective. It provides an additional datum that can further support reasonable suspicion of a possible case of FIP.

Acute phase proteins

The acute phase inflammatory reaction of the organism occurs in response to a potentially pathogenic stimulus. The process begins with the release by inflammatory cells of interleukins IL-1 and IL-6, as well as tumour necrosis factor (TNF). These interleukins produce fever, leukocytosis, and increased serum levels of acute phase proteins (APPs). The most important acute phase proteins in cats are serum amyloid A (SAA) and alpha-1 acid glycoprotein (AGP), levels of which increase within a few hours of the inflammatory stimulus and remain elevated as long as the stimulus persists (Cerón, 2012).

When the probability of FIP is high, based on medical history and clinical signs, moderate increases in AGP levels (1500–2000 µg/ml) aid the diagnosis of FIP. However, higher AGP levels (>3000 µg/ml) are required if the suspicion of FIP is low (Paltriniere et al., 2007).

These tests are easy to perform, and the results obtained can be added to the data included in the worksheet (see next page) to confirm a diagnosis of FIP (Table 1).

Direct tests

These appear to be the ideal tests required to establish a definitive diagnosis of FIP. However, we and many other veterinary surgeons believe that diagnosis of FIP can be made with reasonable certainty based on clinical signs, physical examination, and the results of indirect tests.

Definitive diagnosis of FIP requires identification of viral RNA or proteins in macrophages located in the tissues affected by FIP, i.e.:

- Identification of proteins by immunohistochemistry.
- Identification of viral RNA by PCR.

Immunohistochemistry

Immunohistochemistry of tissue or fluid affected by FIP is a reliable method, but requires a tissue sample, which must be handled properly to ensure accurate results are obtained. Immunohistochemistry can be

Table 1. Results of indirect tests that facilitate the diagnosis of FIP.

Laboratory results	Exudative or wet form	Non-exudative or dry form
Anti-FCoV antibodies	Frequent	>1:640
AGP	>1500 µg/ml	1000 µg/ml
Haematocrit <30 %	Possible	Yes
Neutrophilia	Probable	Probable
Effusion cytology	Neutrophils and macrophages	Not applicable
Increase in globulins	In effusion: total protein >3.5 g/dl	In plasma: globulins >4 g/dl
Albumin/globulin ratio	In effusion: • <0.4 → FIP very probable • >0.8 → FIP very improbable • 0.4–0.8 → FIP possible	Plasma: • <0.4 → FIP probable • >0.8 → FIP improbable • 0.4–0.8 → FIP possible
Rivalta's test	Negative (97 % negative predictive value)	Not applicable
Lymphopaenia	Possible	Yes

WORKSHEET FOR SUSPECTED CASE OF FIP

Medical history	
Cat name	
Clinical signs	
Breed	
Age	
Sex	
Cohabitates with other cats?	

Test	Blood	Effusion	Significance of results
Globulins			
Albumin			
Albumin/globulin ratio			
Bilirubin			
AGP			
Anti-FCoV antibody titre			
RT-PCR for FCoV			
Haematocrit			
Lymphocytes			
Cytology			
Other tests			

Differential diagnosis	Additional tests

Conclusion	
Diagnosis	
Treatment and monitoring	
Prognosis	
What follow-up tests can be performed?	

performed using samples of peritoneal, pleural or cerebrospinal fluid from cats with neurological signs (Ives et al., 2013). Immunohistochemistry tests have a sensitivity of 100 % and a specificity of 71.4 %.

Polymerase chain reaction (PCR)

Polymerase chain reaction using the enzyme reverse transcriptase (RT-PCR) can detect feline coronavirus RNA. The problem to date has been the differentiation of enteric coronavirus from FIP coronavirus.

A recently developed RT-PCR test enables analysis of fluid, blood, or tissue samples to distinguish between enteric coronavirus and systemic FIP caused by coronavirus mutations. This test evaluates only two FIP mutations: biotypes M1058L and S1060A. While mutations are detected in over 98 % of cases of FIP, the detection of these biotypes indicates the presence of a mutated and therefore systemic virus. Although a positive result increases the likelihood of diagnosis of FIP, it does not imply that the virus is the sole cause of the clinical signs observed. It is preferable to perform this test using fluid samples: despite its high sensitivity and specificity, blood or plasma levels of viral RNA may not be detectable (Porter et al., 2014).

Treatment

Various treatment approaches for FIP have been studied: some are designed to inhibit viral replication, some blunt the inflammatory response, and some stimulate the immune system.

The main problem with antiviral drugs is that they exert deleterious effects on the host cell machinery, resulting in undesirable toxicity.

Chloroquine, which is used in the treatment of malaria, inhibits replication of the FIP virus and has anti-inflammatory properties *in vitro* (Takano et al., 2013b). Studies of its effects on experimental FIP infection have demonstrated clinical improvements and increased ALT levels in treated animals.

Cyclosporine A inhibits replication of feline coronavirus *in vitro* but beneficial effects have not been demonstrated *in vivo* to date (Tanaka et al., 2013).

Other treatments trialed include feline **interferon** ω, which was found to be ineffective (evidence-based medicine [EBM] grade 1).

Evidence of the beneficial effects of corticosteroids is based on anecdotal reports, and is not supported by the findings of controlled studies (EBM grade 3).

Once a diagnosis of FIP has been confirmed, the role of the clinician is to try to relieve pain, suffering, and stress and provide the affected cat with a good quality of life. While tending to a terminally ill patient may sound like a frustrating task, it is anything but. Improving the cat's level of comfort, particularly in the case of a young, developing cat, can be highly rewarding. By evaluating quality of life through objective surveys, or surveys that are as objective as possible, the decision to euthanise the cat, when the time comes, will be easier to accept for both the clinician and the owner (see appendix on quality of life).

Immunity and prevention

After the death due to FIP of a cat that shares a home with other cats, coronavirus can remain active for 7 weeks. It is thus advisable to wait 2 months before introducing a new cat. The protocol applied to minimise the spread of coronavirus in an environment with multiple cats is shown below.

Protocol to minimise the spread of coronavirus

» Reduction of faecal contamination

- Sufficient number of litter boxes, proper hygiene, and separate materials for individual cats.
- Daily removal of faeces from litter box.
- Weekly removal of litter and disinfection of litter boxes.
- Keep litter boxes away from feeding bowls.
- Vacuum around litter boxes.

» Control the number of cats

- A normal home should not have more than 4 or 5 cats.
- In cases of larger numbers, stable groups of 3 or 4 cats should be established.
- In groups in which serological screening has been performed, positive and negative cats should be separated.

» Antibody test

- If a group of cats is demonstrated to be coronavirus-free, new cats should be screened for coronavirus antibodies before being introduced to the group.

» Vaccination (see appendix on vaccination)

- The cats that stand to gain the greatest preventive benefit from vaccination are those that have not been exposed to feline coronavirus, especially if they live in a contaminated environment and are at risk of contact.
- One of the major drawbacks of this vaccine is that vaccination begins at 16 weeks of age and in cats infections tend to occur much earlier.

References

ADDIE, D., BELÁK, S., BOUCRAUT-BARALON, C., EGBERINK, H., FRYMUS, T., GRUFFYDD-JONES, T., HARTMANN, K., HOSIE, M.J., LLORET, A., LUTZ, H. et al. Feline infectious peritonitis. ABCD guidelines on prevention and management. *Journal of Feline Medicine and Surgery*, 2009; 11:594-604.

CECILIANI, F., GROSSI, C., GIORDANO, A., POCACQUA, V., PALTRINIERI, S. Decreased sialylation of the acute phase protein α1-acid glycoprotein in feline infectious peritonitis (FIP). *Veterinary Immunology and Immunopathology*, 2004; 99:229-236.

CHANG, H.W., DE GROOT, R.J., EGBERINK, H.F., ROTTIER, P.J. Feline infectious peritonitis: insights into feline coronavirus pathobiogenesis and epidemiology based on genetic analysis of the viral 3c gene. *The Journal of General Virology*, 2010; 91:415-420.

CHANG, H.W., EGBERINK, H., HALPIN, R., SPIRO, D.J., ROTTIER, P.J. Spike protein fusion peptide and feline coronavirus virulence. *Emerging Infectious Diseases*, 2012; 18:1089-1095.

DRECHSLER, Y., ALCARAZ, A., BOSSONG, F.J., COLLISSON, E.W., DINIZ, P.P. FELINE coronavirus in multicat environments. *The Veterinary Clinics of North America. Small Animal Practice*, 2011; 41:1133-1169.

FISCHER, Y., SAUTER-LOUIS, C., HARTMANN, K. Diagnostic accuracy of the Rivalta test for feline infectious peritonitis. *Veterinary Clinical Pathology*, 2012; 41:558-567.

FISCHER, Y., WEBER, K., SAUTER-LOUIS, C., HARTMANN, K. The Rivalta's test as a diagnostic variable in feline effusions – evaluation of optimum reaction and storage conditions. *Tierärztliche Praxis*, 2013; 41:297-303.

GIORI, L., GIORDANO, A., GIUDICE, C., GRIECO, V., PALTRINIERI, S. Performances of different diagnostic tests for feline infectious peritonitis in challenging clinical cases. *The Journal of Small Animal Practice*, 2011; 52:152-157.

HARTMANN, K., RITZ, S. Treatment of cats with feline infectious peritonitis. *Veterinary Immunology and Immunopathology*, 2008; 123:172-175.

HARTMANN, K., BINDER, C., HIRSCHBERGER, J., COLE, D., REINACHER, M., SCHROO, S., FROST, J., EGBERINK, H., LUTZ, H., HERMANNS, W. Comparison of different tests to diagnose feline infectious peritonitis. *Journal of Veterinary Internal Medicine*, 2003; 17:781-790.

HORNYÁK, A., BÁLINT, A., FARSANG, A. Subgenomic mRNA of feline coronavirus by real time polymerase chain reaction based on primer-probe energy transfer (P-sg-QPCR). *Journal of Virological Methods*, 2012; 181:155-163.

IVES, E.J., VANHAESEBROUCK, A.E., CIAN, F. Immunocytochemical demonstration of feline infectious peritonitis virus within cerebrospinal fluid macrophages. *Journal of Feline Medicine and Surgery*, 2013; 15:1149-1153.

JEFFERY, U., DEITZ, K., HOSTETTER, S. Positive predictive value of albumin:globulin ratio for feline infectious peritonitis in a mid-western referral hospital population. *Journal of Feline Medicine and Surgery*, 2012; 14:903-905.

KIM, Y., MANDADAPU, S.R., GROUTAS, W.C., CHANG, K.O. Potent inhibition of feline coronaviruses with peptidyl compounds targeting coronavirus 3C-like protease. *Antiviral Research*, 2013; 97:161-168.

KIPAR, A., MELI, M.L., BAPTISTE, K.E., BOWKER, L.J., LUTZ, H. Sites of feline coronavirus persistence in healthy cats. *The Journal of General Virology*, 2010; 91:1698-1707.

LEGENDRE, A.M., BARTGES, J.W. Effect of Polyprenyl Immunostimulant on the survival times of three cats with the dry form of feline infectious peritonitis. *Journal of Feline Medicine and Surgery*, 2009; 11(8):624-6.

Lewis, K.M., O'Brien, R.T. Abdominal ultrasonographic findings associated with feline infectious peritonitis: A retrospective review of 16 cases. *Journal of the American Animal Hospital Association*, 2010; 46:152-160.

Paltrinieri, S., Giordano, A., Tranquillo, V., Guazzetti, S. Critical assessment of the diagnostic value of feline α1-acid glycoprotein for feline infectious peritonitis using the likelihood ratios approach. *Journal of Veterinary Diagnostic Investigation*, 2007; 19:266-272.

Pedersen, N.C. A review of feline infectious peritonitis virus infection: 1963-2008. *Journal of Feline Medicine and Surgery*, 2009; 11:225-258.

Pedersen, N.C., Sato, R., Foley, J.E., Poland, A.M. Common virus infections in cats, before and after being placed in shelters, with emphasis on feline enteric coronavirus. *Journal of Feline Medicine and Surgery*, 2004; 6:83-88.

Pedersen, N.C., Allen, C.E., Lyons, L.A. Pathogenesis of feline enteric coronavirus infection. *Journal of Feline Medicine and Surgery*, 2008; 10:529-541.

Pedersen, N.C., Liu, H., Dodd, K.A., Pesavento, P.A. Significance of coronavirus mutants in feces and diseased tissues of cats suffering from feline infectious peritonitis. *Viruses*, 2009; 1:166-184.

Pedersen, N.C., Liu, H., Scarlett, J., Leutenegger, C.M., Golovko, L., Kennedy, H., Kamal, F.M. Feline infectious peritonitis: Role of the feline coronavirus 3c gene in intestinal tropism and pathogenicity based upon isolates from resident and adopted shelter cats. *Virus Research*, 2012; 165:17-28.

Takano, T., Katoh, Y., Doki, T., Hohdatsu, T. Effect of chloroquine on feline infectious peritonitis virus infection in vitro and in vivo. *Antiviral Research*, 2013b; 99:100-107.

Tanaka, Y., Sato, Y., Sasaki, T. Suppression of coronavirus replication by cyclophilin inhibitors. *Viruses*, 2013; 5:1250-1260.

Taylor, S.S., Tappin, S.W., Dodkin, S.J., Papasouliotis, K., Casamian-Sorrosal, D., Tasker, S. Serum protein electrophoresis in 155 cats. *Journal of Feline Medicine and Surgery*, 2010; 12:643-653.

Terada, Y., Minami, S., Noguchi, K., Mahmoud, H.Y., Shimoda, H., Mochizuki, M., Une, Y., Maeda, K. Genetic characterization of coronaviruses from domestic ferrets, Japan. *Emerging Infectious Diseases*, 2014; 20:284-287.

Vogel, L., Van der Lubben, M., Te Lintelo, E.G., Bekker, C.P.J., Geerts, T., Schuijff, L.S., Grinwis, G.C.M., Egberink, H.F., Rottier, P.J.M. Pathogenic characteristics of persistent feline enteric coronavirus infection in cats. *Veterinary Research*, 2010; 41:71.

Wiggans, K.T., Vernau, W., Lappin, M.R., Thomasy, S.M., Maggs, D.J. Diagnostic utility of aqueocentesis and aqueous humor analysis in dogs and cats with anterior uveitis. *Veterinary Ophthalmology*, 2013; 17:212-220.

Zoia, A., Slater, L.A., Heller, J., Connolly, D.J., Church, D.B. A new approach to pleural effusion in cats: Markers for distinguishing transudates from exudates. *Journal of Feline Medicine and Surgery*, 2009; 11:847-855.

Information for cat guardians

Addie D.D. *My cat has feline infectious peritonitis-what now? A book for cat guardians*. Melchizedek Publications, 2006.

www.catvirus.com

ABCD: Comité asesor de enfermedades felinas europeo. www.abcd-vets.org.

CASE STUDIES

CASE STUDY 1: *Papillón*

Summary: young stray cat.

Reason for consultation: possible pregnancy.

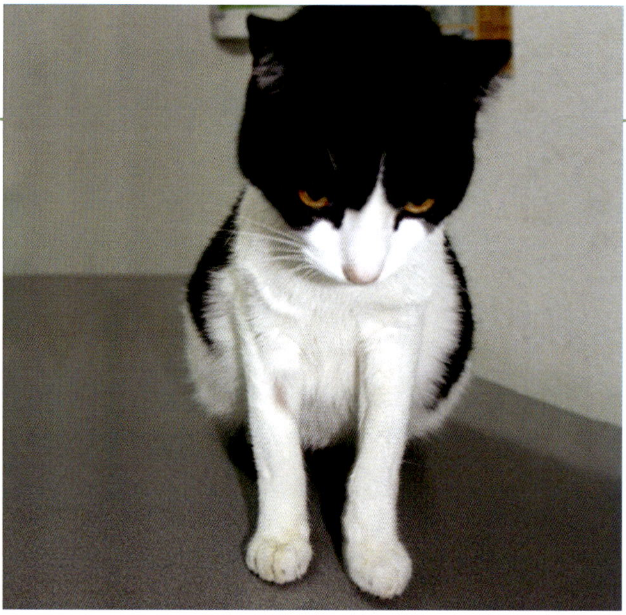

Figure 1. *Papillón* presents with malaise and muscle weakness.

Medical history

The subject is a young cat that had been found on the street (Fig. 1) and is suspected to be pregnant (Fig. 2).

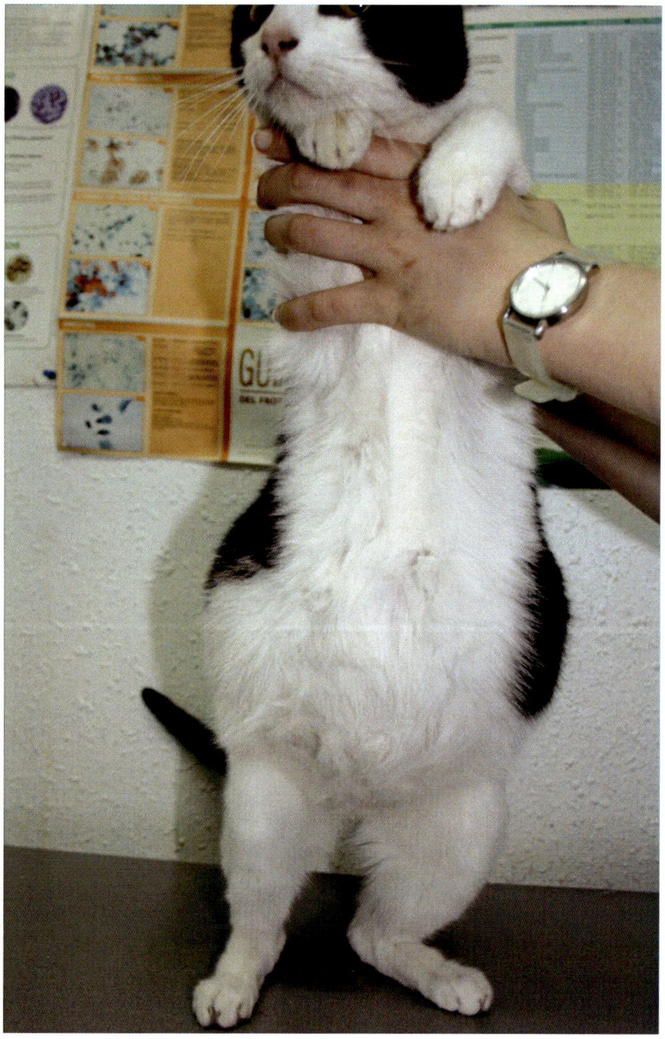

Figure 2. Abdominal distension, not painful on palpation.

Physical examination and diagnostic tests

On beginning the examination, the cat shows signs of restrictive dyspnoea with reduced cardiorespiratory sounds on auscultation (Fig. 3). It is decided to place the cat in an oxygenation chamber until her respiratory rate stabilises, and then continue the examination. While still in the oxygenation chamber a preliminary ultrasound is performed, revealing anechoic content in the abdomen, a sample of which is obtained by ultrasound-guided abdominocentesis. Chest ultrasound also reveals anechoic content (Fig. 4).

After stabilisation, the cat is sedated by intramuscular administration of dexmedetomidine (3 µg/kg), pethidine (3 mg/kg), and midazolam (0.2 mg/kg), followed by mask induction with 1.5 % isoflurane. Radiographs confirm the presence of pleural effusion (Figs. 5 and 6).

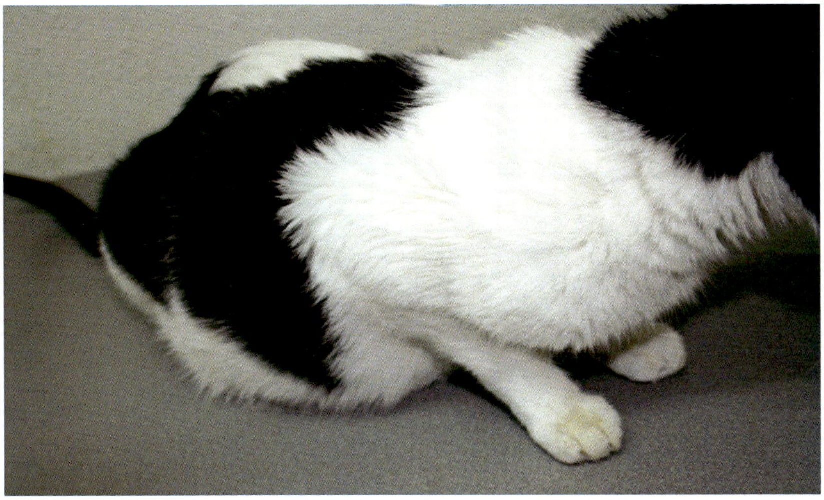

Figure 3. Orthopnoeic position due to dyspnoea.

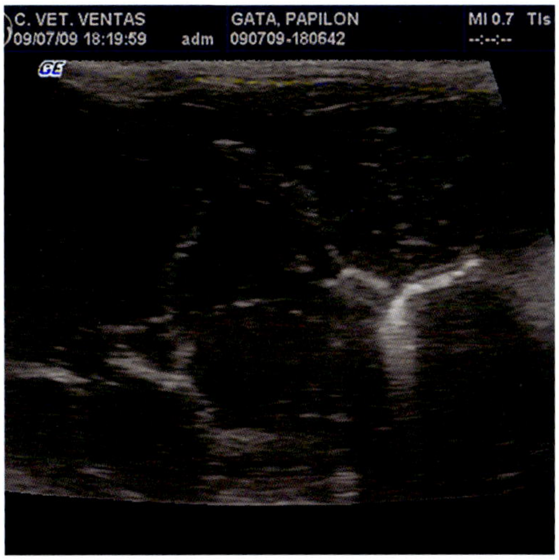

Figure 4. Ultrasound of the chest area showing presence of anechoic content.

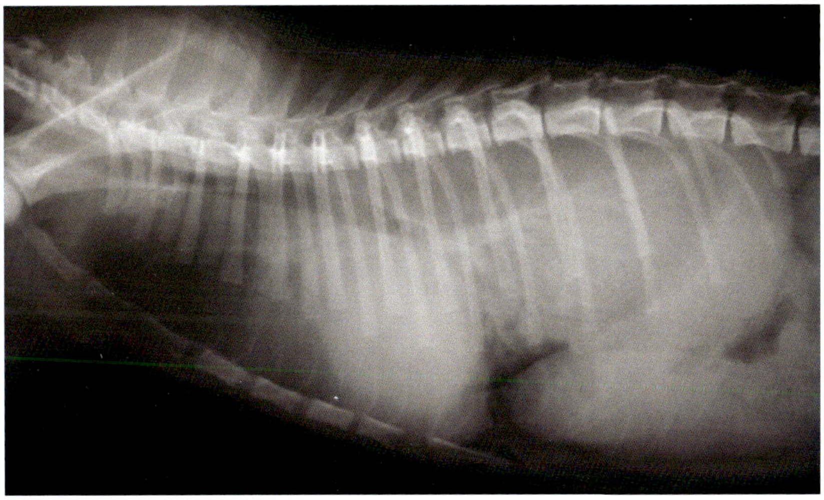

Figure 5. Laterolateral radiograph showing the presence of fluid in the abdominal and thoracic cavities.

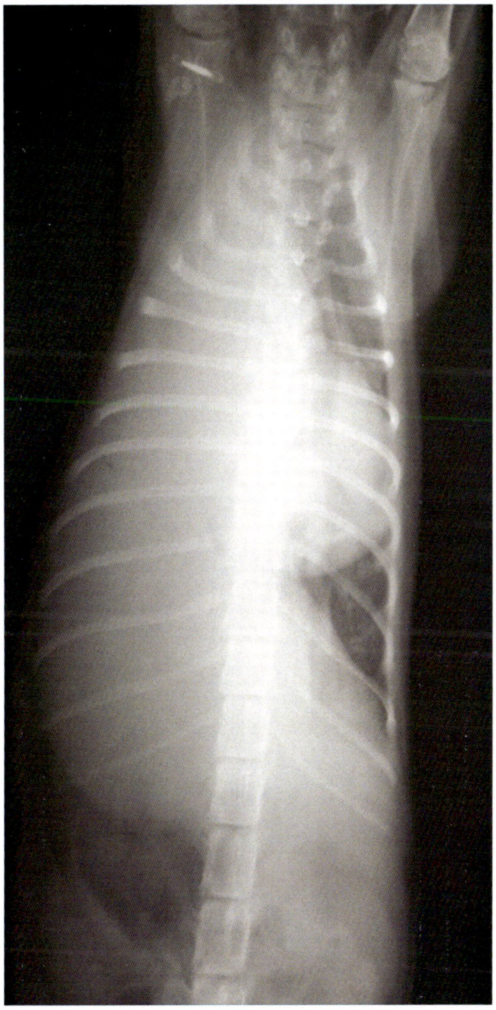

Figure 6. Ventrodorsal radiograph of *Papillón* revealing the presence of pleural and abdominal effusion.

A preliminary pleural puncture is performed to extract a fluid sample for analysis, and subsequently a permanent pleural drain is placed in each hemithorax (see appendix on pleural drainage).

Indirect tests are also conducted to orient the diagnosis and samples of abdominal and pleural effusion fluid are directly analysed by RT-PCR.

The worksheet for *Papillón* is shown below.

WORKSHEET

Medical history	
Cat Name	*Papillón*
Clinical signs	Dyspnoea, pleural effusion, abdominal distension
Breed	Domestic shorthair
Age	Approximately 8 months
Sex	Female
Cohabitates with other cats?	Yes

Test	Blood	Effusion	Significance of results
Globulins	7.1 mg/dl	7.2 mg/dl	See albumin/globulin ratio
Albumin	2 mg/dl	2.1 mg/dl	—
Albumin/globulin ratio	0.28	0.29	Possible FIP (<0.4)
Bilirubin	High	—	—
AGP	—	1950 µg/ml	Significantly elevated
Anti-FCoV antibody titre	—	>1:1,400	Very high
RT-PCR for FCoV	—	Positive	—
Haematocrit	29 %	—	—
Lymphocytes	—	—	—
Cytology	—	—	—
Other tests	—	Positive	—

Differential diagnosis	Additional tests
Thymic lymphoma	Effusion cytology, FeLV test
Bacterial pleuritis	Effusion cytology/culture
Virulent systemic infection (calicivirus)	Other signs of infection

Conclusion

Diagnosis	The virus is detected in the effusion fluid, the albumin/globulin ratio is low, and AGP levels are elevated, indicating a possible case of FIP. Furthermore, the result of RT-PCR for feline coronavirus is positive.
Treatment and monitoring	• Extraction of maximum volume of fluid possible: pleural catheters were left in place for two weeks. • Prednisolone: 2 mg/kg every 12 hours. • Analgesia. • Appetite stimulants. • Monitoring of quality of life (see appendix on quality of life).
Prognosis	Very bad. The patient lived for two months in a foster home until she stopped eating, and the decision to euthanise was made.
What follow-up tests can be done?	• Quality of life surveys. • Weekly telephone follow-up.

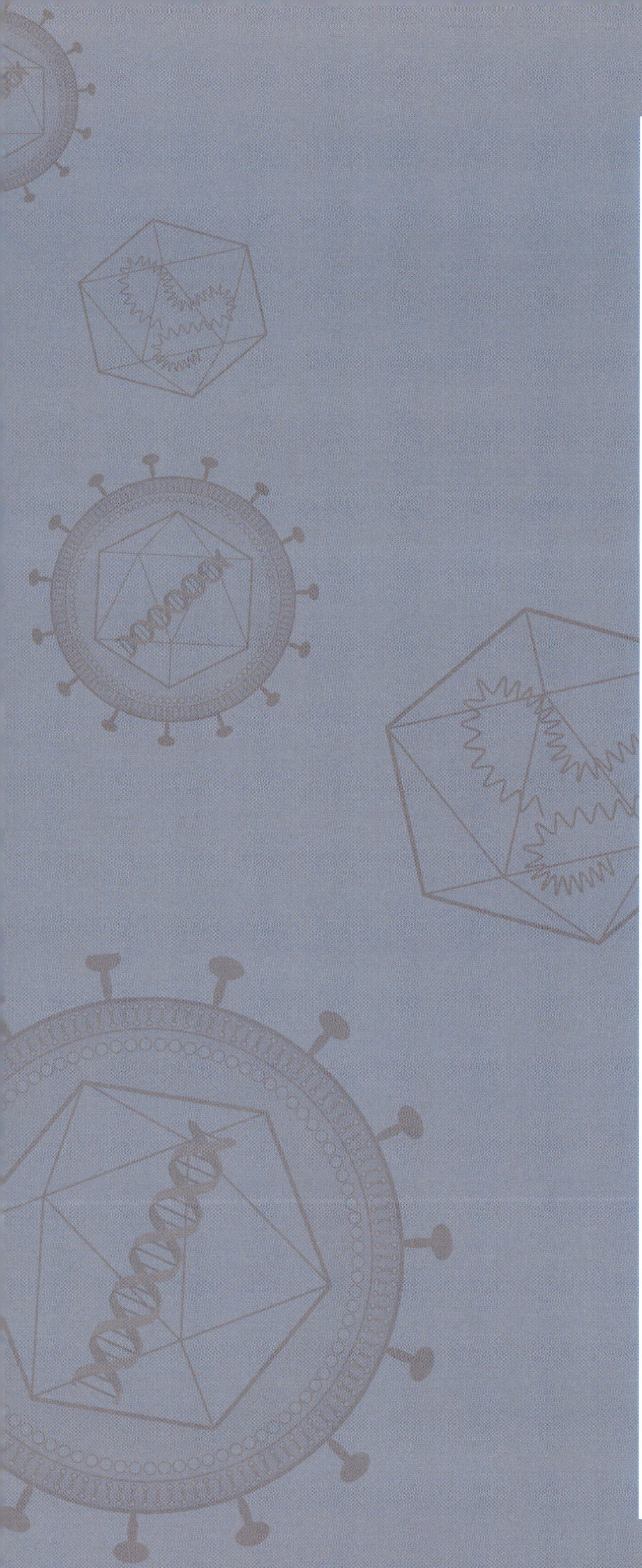

Upper respiratory tract infections

Upper respiratory tract infections

Upper respiratory tract infections (URTIs) in cats are caused by different pathogens and are characterised by the presence of acute respiratory and ocular signs, although affected animals may present with chronic infectious processes or an immune-mediated response to infection such as chronic feline gingivitis.

Because these infections are initially produced by the spread of pathogens, acute presentations are rare in cats living alone in a house, but constitute a major problem in shelters, communities, catteries, and homes with multiple cats.

The main infectious agents involved are listed in Box 1. *Bordetella bronchiseptica* is also a possible primary pathogen in URTIs of cats.

In addition to these agents or pathogens, environmental factors play a role in the development of infection. These include poor hygiene, inadequate ventilation, and poor immune status in the cat population. Another crucial factor is stress, to the extent that the incidence of URTI in a group of cats is considered an indicator of stress, and improving living conditions decreases the incidence of the disease.

Management and control of URTIs is a major challenge for veterinarians and those who care for or own cats. Although mortality is not high, except in kittens, morbidity is significant. URTI outbreaks reduce the likelihood that cats will be adopted from shelters and result in increased rates of euthanasia. Cat protection organisations spend much of their budget treating and preventing respiratory and eye processes of infectious origin. Vaccination against some of the infectious agents implicated in URTIs is effective, but does not prevent infection. As such, eradication in communities is not a realistic goal. However, this approach does help improve the management and quality of life of cats, reducing the morbidity and mortality associated with this disease (Helps et al., 2005) (Fig. 1).

Box 1. Main infectious agents that cause URTI.

- Feline herpesvirus type 1 (FHV-1).
- Feline calicivirus (FCV).
- *Chlamydophila felis.*
- *Mycoplasma felis.*
- *Bordetella bronchiseptica.*

Clinical signs

A systematic physical examination is essential. The general appearance of the cat will indicate the necessary therapeutic approach to take.

The most common clinical signs of URTI are:

- Nasal discharge: serous, mucous, or mucopurulent.
- Sneezing.
- Conjunctivitis.
- Ocular discharge: serous, mucous, mucopurulent, or serosanguinous.
- Ulcers on the tongue, gums, and nose.
- Hypersalivation.
- Cough.
- Fever.
- Lethargy.
- Loss of appetite.

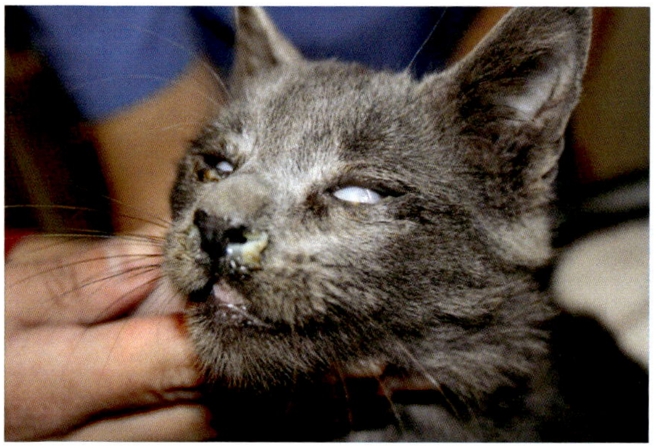

Figure 1. Kitten with signs of upper respiratory infection, conjunctivitis, and mucopurulent nasal discharge, clinical signs indicative of FHV-1 and secondary bacterial contamination.

Pathogenic agents

The following agents, alone or in combination, are detected in 80 % to 90 % of cats with URTI: feline herpesvirus type-1 (FHV-1), feline calicivirus (FCV) *Chlamydophila felis*, and *Mycoplasma felis*.

A recent extensive study examined the prevalence of URTI, conjunctivitis, and feline chronic gingivostomatitis in 358 cats in Spain, as well as associated risk factors (Fernández *et al.*, 2014). The results demonstrated a clear relationship between upper respiratory tract signs and the presence of FHV-1, FCV, and *Mycoplasma felis*, with increased prevalence in non-neutered male cats. Furthermore, ocular signs were associated with FHV-1 and *Chlamydophila felis*, and were more common in young non-sterilised cats, while feline chronic gingivostomatitis was associated with FCV, and was more common in older cats. Non-vaccination was a risk factor associated with the development of respiratory and ocular disease and gingivostomatitis. Vaccination does not prevent infection but does prevent the development of clinical signs.

Table 1. Main clinical signs associated with pathogens.

Clinical sign	Causal agent
Lameness	FCV
Oral ulcer	■ FCV ■ FHV-1
Keratitis, corneal ulcer	FHV-1
Conjunctivitis without rhinitis	■ *C. felis* ■ *Mycoplasma* spp.
Dermatitis, ulcerative dermatitis	■ Virulent systemic FCV ■ FHV-1
Cough	*B. bronchiseptica*

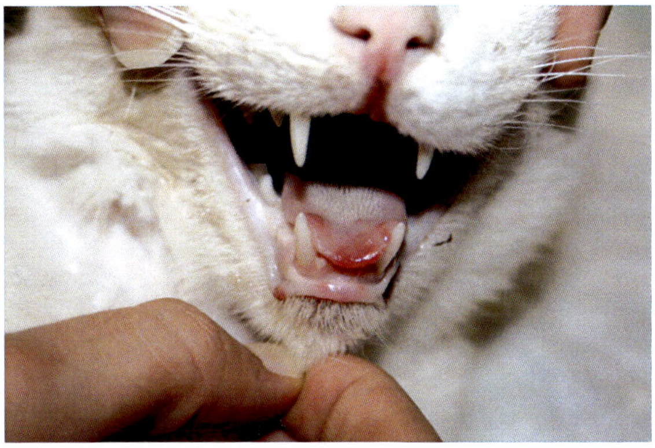

Figure 2. Cat with ulcers and necrosis of the epithelium of the tongue, clinical signs of FCV.

The role of *Mycoplasma felis* as a pathogenic agent requires further study, given that it is detected in 20 % of the population without clinical signs. These results are consistent with prevalence data reported for other countries.

Although extremely rare, the H5N1 virus can cause respiratory signs in cats, and has zoonotic potential.

Gram-positive or gram-negative bacterial infections can cause secondary complication of viral processes, and should be considered to ensure appropriate disease management.

Although there are no clinical signs that are truly pathognomonic of each pathogen, there are data that can help orient the clinical diagnosis and identify the potential causative agent of the URTI (Table 1).

Feline calicivirus (FCV)

This is a non-enveloped, single-stranded RNA virus, which displays large antigenic differences between serotypes. Because it lacks an envelope it is resistant in the environment and is transmitted on contaminated objects (feeders, trays, etc.) as well as in secretions. Cats that recover from acute infections can remain as carriers of the virus for long periods of time. Acute infection is more common in young cats than adults, and produces oral ulcers and blisters on the tongue with epithelial necrosis (Fig. 2). Pneumonia and lameness may be observed, but are less common clinical signs. FCV plays an important role in chronic feline gingivitis, as demonstrated in several studies.

There is a hyperacute form of FCV infection, known as virulent systemic (VS)-FCV. This systemic form occurs in outbreaks, most frequently affecting adult cats, and causes peripheral oedema, mucosal ulcers, and necrosis of the ears, legs and tail caused by vasculitis. Mortality due to VS-FCV is very high, and more than half of all infected cats die from hepatocellular necrosis, disseminated intravascular coagulation, and other complications (Radford *et al.*, 2009).

Feline herpesvirus type 1 (FHV-1)

FHV-1 is a double-stranded DNA virus and a member of the subfamily *Alphaherpesvirinae*. It is highly species-specific, i.e. no transmission occurs between different animal species. FHV-1 infection is very common, and the virus is widely distributed in cats worldwide (Gaskell *et al.*, 2007).

Some studies estimate that 90 % of cats are seropositive for this virus; 80 % can become carriers after first exposure, and remain latent for a period of time, with 45 % acting as carriers for their entire lives. Thus, in half of all cats that have had an FHV-1 infection, stress can induce a new round of viral replication and the reappearance of clinical signs.

The pathogenesis of the disease can help us to understand and manage the ocular and respiratory clinical signs associated with this disease (Figs. 3–5).

In many cats, after primary infection the virus remains latent, causing subclinical disease in some and clinical disease in others (Thiry *et al.*, 2009).

FHV-1 causes disease via two mechanisms:

- **A cytolytic process** affecting the cornea, conjunctiva, and respiratory epithelium, which causes ulcerative disease and dendritic ocular ulcers, rhinitis, dermatitis, and other systemic signs. This is the moment to apply antiviral agents, given that no active virus replication is occurring. All immunomodulatory drugs are contraindicated, as these promote viral replication. In the conjunctiva, the cytolytic effect of the virus induces serosanguinous secretions. Simultaneous ulceration of the conjunctival and corneal surfaces can result in adhesion of the two tissues (symblepharon).
- **An immune-mediated inflammatory process,** which can cause stromal keratitis. Stromal keratitis is a common response to FHV-1 infection, and is characterised by the infiltration of inflammatory cells, especially lymphocytes, via the stroma. Chronic inflammatory changes such as fibrosis and vascularisation can cause blindness. Viral replication is limited

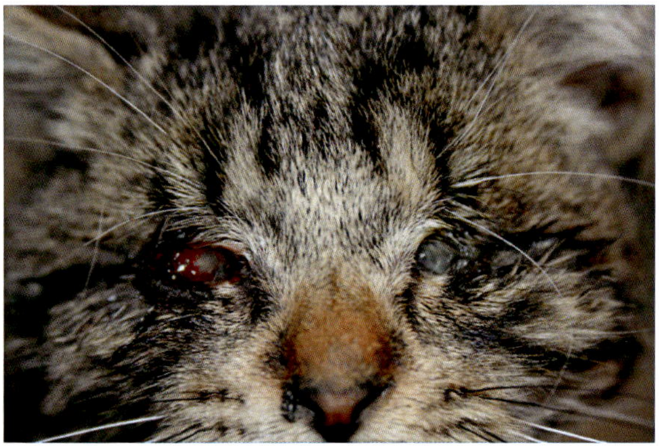

Figure 3. Keratitis in a cat with URTI.

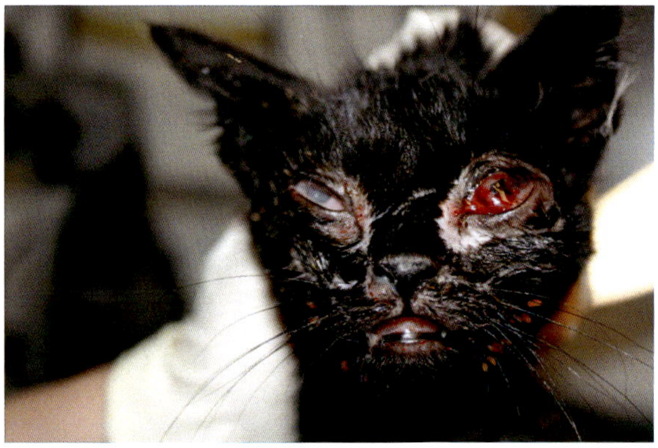

Figure 4. Conjunctivitis, keratitis, and dermatitis in a cat with URTI.

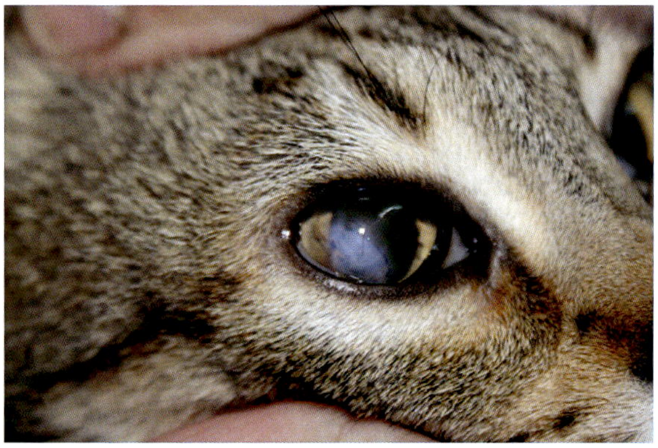

Figure 5. Corneal ulcer in a cat with signs of URTI caused by FHV-1 infection.

during the immune-mediated phase of the disease, making diagnosis and treatment challenging: antiviral agents are ineffective, and anti-inflammatory treatment may be indicated.

Chlamydophila felis

C. felis is an intracellular gram-negative bacteria, which does not survive long outside the host. It is transmitted by direct contact with an infected animal or via aerosols and fomites. The incubation period is 3 to 5 days (Gruffydd-Jones *et al.*, 2009).

C. felis is endemic in house cats around the world, and primarily causes acute and chronic conjunctivitis. It can also infect the respiratory tract causing mild respiratory signs. In experimentally infected cats, it has been associated with the development of lameness two weeks after the onset of conjunctivitis.

The following are the main ocular signs caused by this bacterium: conjunctival hyperaemia, chemosis, serous ocular discharge, and blepharospasm (Fig. 6). Mild nasal discharge and sneezing may also be observed. Conjunctivitis is usually unilateral, becoming bilateral after a few days. If left untreated it can progress to chronic conjunctivitis. *C. felis* is not associated with keratitis in cats.

Spread of the bacterium throughout the population is facilitated by an asymptomatic carrier state, and by the persistence of *C. felis* in the gastrointestinal and reproductive tracts.

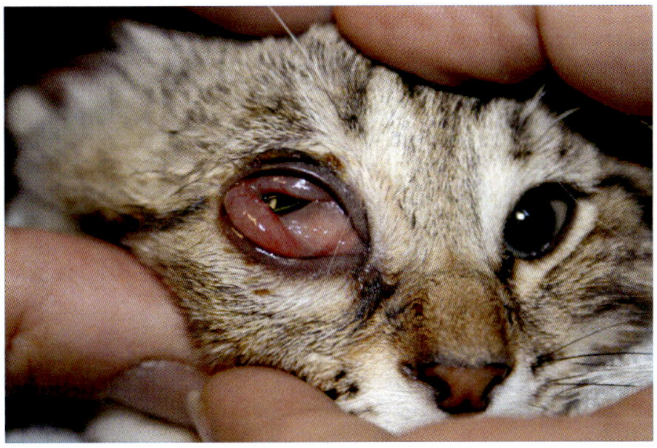

Figure 6. Unilateral conjunctivitis and chemosis in a cat with clinical signs of URTI attributable to *C. felis*.

Coinfection in cats with FIV can prolong the duration of clinical signs and lead to the development of chronic conjunctivitis (Sykes, 2005).

The prevalence of *C. felis* in asymptomatic cats is low. This disease has zoonotic potential (immunosuppressed individuals).

Diagnosis

URTI should be suspected in any cat with acute clinical signs of upper respiratory tract disease and/or conjunctivitis and a recent history of stress or contact with another at-risk cat. In the case of house cats, aetiological diagnosis is not necessary since the management approach will be the same, unless the cat presents secondary bacterial complications such as pneumonia.

In cases of increased incidence of URTI in shelters or groups of cats, diagnosis to identify the main pathogen involved can be useful to design prevention plans (Maggs, 2010).

Diagnosis of the specific agent causing URTI is not easy. The identification of clinical signs is the best diagnostic method. For example, the presence of ulcers of the oral mucosa indicates that FCV is likely the causative agent. PCR, bacterial cultures, viral isolation, and serologic tests can produce false negatives and false positives. In one study, analysis of the control group of 98 cats with no clinical signs of URTI revealed that 15 % were positive for FCV, 6 % for FHV, and 2 % for *C. felis* (Fernández et al., 2014).

In the case of an outbreak of URTI in a population, it is advisable to send samples taken from at least 30 % of the population and from cats that have recently developed acute signs. This reduces the possibility of diagnosing secondary pathogens.

Clinical diagnosis and veterinary experience are both central to identifying the causative agent.

Treatment

In everyday clinical practice, veterinary surgeons face doubts about when to treat, how to treat, whether the antibiotic should be administered topically or systemically, which antibiotics are best, when to switch antibiotics, treatment duration, and when to use antivirals.

The classification of cats according to their clinical signs allows us to establish a systematic approach to case management, facilitating clinical decision-making and ensuring adequate follow-up of patients. Table 2 shows the classification scheme for URTI according to clinical signs, and the corresponding diagnostic interpretations and potential treatments.

Supportive care

This is the most important part of treatment (Table 3). Adequate food should be provided and proper monitoring implemented to identify possible complications. Appetite can be decreased due to nasal congestion, pain caused by oral ulcers, and fever. Affected cats should thus be offered soft and very palatable food, which can be heated to enhance its

Table 2. Management scheme for upper respiratory tract infections.

Classification	Clinical signs	Interpretation	Treatment
1A: watery discharge	Watery eyes and nose or sneezing.	Mild URTI.	■ Isolation. ■ Monitoring of appetite. ■ Soft diet.
1B: watery discharge	1A + fever, dehydration, anorexia, oral ulcers, congestion, depression.	Moderate to severe URTI.	1A + supportive treatment (Table 3).
2A: non-watery discharge	1A + greenish, yellowish, or brown oculonasal discharge.	URTI + rhinitis and/or secondary bacterial eye infection.	**Doxycycline** ■ 10 mg/kg/day until resolution of clinical signs. ■ Re-evaluate after 3 days, consider switching antibiotic if no improvement observed. ■ Worsening of condition after withdrawal of treatment may be indicative of *C. felis*. A test should be conducted and antibiotic treatment continued for 4–6 weeks.
2B: URTI with non-watery discharge with NO response to treatment	1B + 2A with no response to doxycycline.	Moderate to severe URTI with secondary oculonasal infection.	**Fluoroquinolones (pradofloxacin or marbofloxacin)** ■ 5 mg/kg/day until resolution of clinical signs. ■ Re-evaluate after 3–5 days, and reconsider the diagnosis if no improvement observed.
3A: ocular signs	Unilateral or bilateral ocular discharge, conjunctivitis, chemosis.	Bacterial or viral eye infection.	**Gentamicin ophthalmic or tobramycin ophthalmic** ■ Reassess after 3–5 days, and consider administration of systemic antibiotics or antivirals if no improvement observed.
3B: ocular signs with NO response to treatment	3A + persistent ocular discharge, corneal oedema, corneal ulcer, blepharospasm.	Viral eye infection with or without bacterial component.	■ 3A + **famciclovir.** ■ 40 mg/cat every 8–12 hours.
4: systemic signs or no improvement	■ Fever, respiratory difficulties, coughing, vomiting, diarrhoea. ■ No response to treatment.	Complicated URTI or URTI associated with other problems.	■ Supportive treatment (Table 3). ■ Rethink the diagnosis.

odour. Analgesia is crucial when treating these processes. If anorexia persists, appetite stimulants such as mirtazapine (1/8–1/4 of a 15-mg tablet per cat every 3 days) can be administered. If these measures are not effective, placement of an oesophagostomy tube may be necessary.

Antibiotics

Antibiotic treatment should be considered, following the treatment and management scheme shown in Table 2. Doxycycline is the antibiotic of choice to treat *C. felis*, *B. bronchiseptica*, and *Mycoplasma* spp., and effectively penetrates the airways. Cats with clinical suspicion or diagnosis of *C. felis* should be treated for at least 4 weeks, and for 2 weeks after the remission of clinical signs. All cats living with the affected cat should also be treated. Long treatment durations (42 days +) are required for *Mycoplasma felis*. If antibiotic treatment is proposed to prevent secondary infections, the cat can be treated with beta-lactams (amoxicillin, amoxicillin-clavulanic acid) and azithromycin for 7 to 10 days (Ruch-Gallie et al., 2008).

Published studies have demonstrated the efficacy and safety of fluoroquinolones such as pradofloxacin and marbofloxacin, which are a good choice for cats that have responded poorly to doxycycline (Hartmann et al., 2008).

Antiviral treatments

Famciclovir is a safe and effective choice in cats displaying ocular and respiratory signs attributable to FHV (Malik *et al.*, 2009).

A clinical study conducted at our centre of 29 cats with severe ocular and cutaneous signs attributable to FHV-1 that were treated with famciclovir (40 mg/cat every 8 hours) revealed good tolerance and an improvement in clinical signs (Aybar, 2011) (Fig. 7).

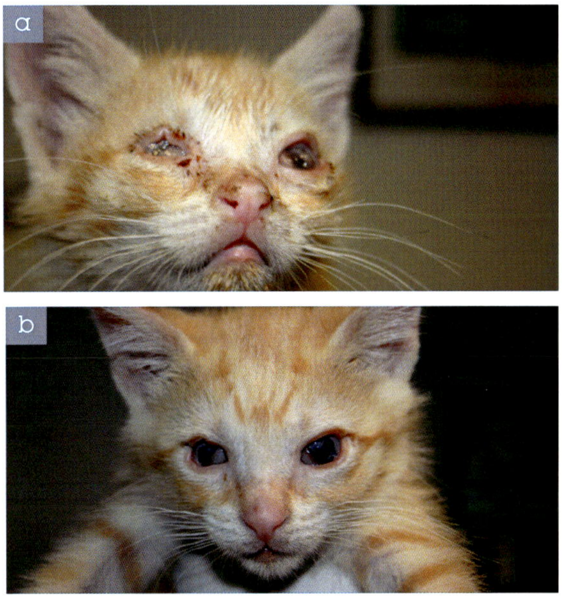

Figure 7. (a) Kitten with conjunctivitis, keratitis, and herpetic dermatitis upon starting famciclovir treatment. (b) Kitten after 2 weeks of treatment.

Table 3. Supportive treatment in upper respiratory tract infections.

Clinical signs	Treatment
Dehydration	■ Degree of dehydration >5 %: IV saline. ■ Vitamin B complex. ■ Add KCl to saline for anorexic cats.
Congestion	Flushing of nasal cavity with saline.
Anorexia	■ Hydration, analgesia, palatable food. ■ Comfortable environment in hospital. ■ Mirtazapine: 1/8 of a tablet (15 mg), every 3 days. ■ If anorexia persists for more than 5 days consider placement of an oesophagostomy tube.
Pain	■ Buprenorphine: 0.01–0.02 mg/kg every 4-6 hours, IM, SC, or intramucosal. ■ Meloxicam: 0.05 mg/kg every 24 hours, PO or SC.
Fever	■ IV saline administration. ■ External cooling systems. ■ Rule out lower respiratory tract problems.

Prevention

The goal is not to eradicate the signs of URTI, but to control and reduce the incidence and severity of the associated clinical signs. The most effective measures are vaccination (see appendix on vaccination) and improving the quality of life of affected cats. The incidence of URTI can be decreased by implementing environmental enrichment programs, providing the resources necessary to ensure that cats can live with minimal stress, including adequate diets, an optimal number of litter boxes, hideouts, scratching posts, and toys (Singer and Cohn, 2011).

Reducing the number of cats in a population by implementing sterilisation programs also helps reduce the incidence of URTI.

When a cat presents signs of URTI, it should be isolated to prevent transmission to other cats. When considering introducing a new cat into a house, it is important to be aware of its vaccination status and to wait 1 to 2 weeks before allowing it to join other cats in the house to ensure the absence of respiratory, ocular, or buccal signs.

When handling cats, it is critical to wash hands between one animal and the next. FCV is less easily inactivated with common disinfectants. Bleach at a dilution of 1/32 is a good choice.

References

Aybar, V. Congreso de Grupos de Trabajo AVEPA, 2011.

Fernández, M., Manzanilla, E.G., Lloret, A.M., *et al.* Prevalence of FHV-1, FCV, *Chlamydophila felis* in cats with URTD, conjuntivitis and chronic gingivostomatitis in Spain. ISFM Congress, 2014.

Gaskell, R., Dawson, S., Radford, A., *et al.* Feline herpesvirus. *Vet Res,* 2007; 38(2): 337-54.

Gruffydd-Jones, T., Addie, D., Belak, S., *et al. Chlamydophila felis* infection. ABCD guidelines on prevention and management. *J Feline Med Surg,* 2009; 11(7):605-9.

Helps, C.R., Lait, P., Damhuis, A., *et al.* Factors associated with upper respiratory tract disease caused by feline herpesvirus, feline calicivirus, *Chlamydophila felis* and *Bordetella bronchiseptica* in cats: experience from 218 European catteries. *Vet Rec,* 2005; 156(21):669-73.

Maggs, D.J. Antiviral therapy for feline herpesvirus infections. *Vet Clin North Am Small Anim Pract,* 2010; 40(6):1055-62.

Malik, R., Lessels, N.S., Webb, S., *et al.* Treatment of feline herpesvirus-1 associated disease in cats with famciclovir and related drugs. *J Feline Med Surg,* 2009; 11(1): 40-8.

Radford, A.D., Addie, D., Belak, S., *et al.* Feline calicivirus infection. ABCD guidelines on prevention and management. *J Feline Med Surg,* 2009; 11(7):556-64.

Sykes, J.E. Clamydophila felis. *Clin Tech Small Anim Pract,* 2005; 20(2):129-34.

Ruch-Gallie, R.A.,Veir, J.K., Spindel, M.E., Lappin, M.R. Efficacy of amoxycillin and azithromycin for the empirical treatment of shelter cats with suspected bacterial upper respiratory infections. *J Feline Med Surg,* 2008; 10(6):542-50.

Singer, L.M., Cohn, L.A. Immune deficiency, stress, and infection. In: Little, S. (Ed.). *The cat: clinical medicine and management,* Vol. 1. St. Louis (MO): Elsevier, 2011.

Thiry, E., Addie, D., Belak, S., *et al.* Feline herpesvirus infection. ABCD guidelines on prevention and management. *J Feline Med Surg,* 2009; 11(7):547-55.

Thiry, E., Addie, D., Belak, S., *et al.* H5N1 avian influenza in cats. ABCD guidelines on prevention and management. *J Feline Med Surg,* 2009; 11(7):615-18.

CASE STUDIES

CASE STUDY 1: *Nin*

Review: neutered male domestic shorthair cat, 11 months old.

Reason forconsultation: presents with inspiratory stridor, especially at rest, discomfort in one ear, and mild anisocoria.

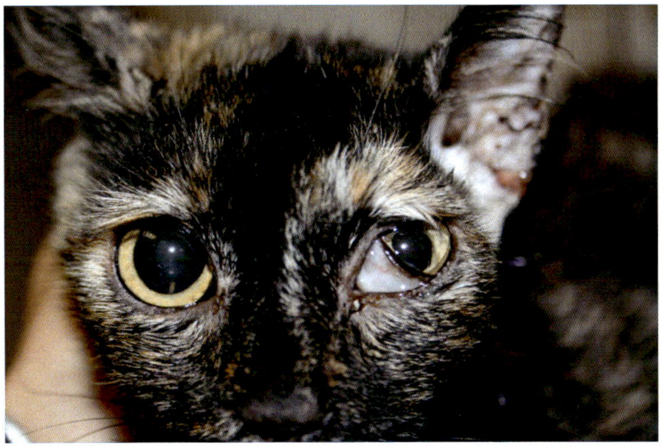

Figure 1. Patient with Horner syndrome.

Medical history

The patient is a neutered male domestic shorthair cat, of 11 months of age. He lives indoors and has been regularly vaccinated and dewormed.

Two months before the consultation, the patient had been treated for signs of inspiratory stridor. Under sedation, the animal had undergone an otoscopic examination of the nasopharynx, oropharynx, and larynx, and a radiological examination of the head including the nasal sinuses, nasal cavity, temporomandibular joint, and the tympanic cavity of the middle ear (tympanic bullae). The examinations revealed no observations that could explain the clinical signs. No treatment was administered.

When the cat was taken from the street at 1.5 to 2 months of age, he showed signs of upper respiratory tract disease, bilateral conjunctivitis, and uveitis affecting the left eye with hyphema and keratitis. ELISA for the detection of feline leukaemia virus (FeLV) and feline infectious immunodeficiency virus (FIV) was negative.

He was treated with amoxicillin and clavulanic acid, L-lysine, and chloramphenicol eye drops.

Physical examination

The patient presents clinical signs of inspiratory stridor, especially when asleep or at rest, and discomfort of the left ear that had begun several days beforehand. The cat has mild anisocoria of the left eye, with miosis (Fig. 1), and a slight head tilt to the left side (Fig. 2).

The **otoscopic examination** reveals swelling of the tympanic membrane of the left ear, with redness and pain on manipulation.

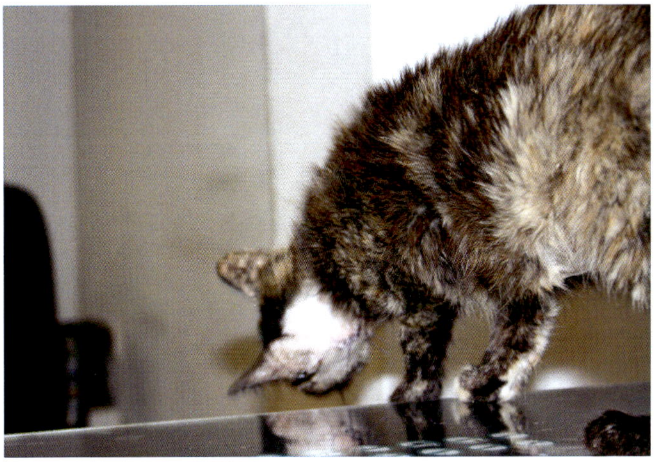

Figure 2. Patient displaying head tilt, indicative of vestibular syndrome.

During the **neurological examination** the cat is calm and alert, with normal gait and good posture. He shows no deficiencies in proprioception in any limb, the cranial nerves show no abnormalities (normal palpebral, threat, and photomotor reflexes, even in the left eye), spinal reflexes are normal, and both superficial and deep sensitivity are observed. Anal, perineal, and panniculus reflexes are also normal. No other abnormalities are detected in the general examination (Table 1).

Differential diagnosis

The differential diagnosis of nasal stridor is shown in Table 2, pharyngeal, laryngeal, and tracheal stridor in Table 3, anisocoria with miosis in Table 4, and head tilt in Table 5 (Rand, 2005).

Table 1. Results of general examination of the patient.

Parameter	Result	Normal values
Body weight	3.2 kg	—
Body condition and general appearance	■ 3/5 ■ Good general appearance	3/5
Auscultation	■ 30 breaths per minute (bpm) ■ Normal lung auscultation	20–40 bpm
Cardiac auscultation	■ 125 bpm ■ Normal auscultation, normal rhythm	120–200 bpm
Oral cavity	■ Teeth in good condition ■ No mucosal inflammation	—
Mucosae	■ Pink and moist ■ Capillary refill time (CRT) <2 seconds	■ Pink and moist ■ CRT <2 seconds
Abdominal palpation	■ No abdominal rigidity ■ Slightly distended bladder ■ No palpable abdominal mass or abnormal structures	—
Temperature	38.6 °C	38–39.5 °C

Table 2. Differential diagnosis of nasal stridor.

Origin	Process	Compatibility with case
Congenital	Stenosis of the external nares.	Unlikely: not brachycephalic and no compatible signs observed during examination.
Mechanical	Foreign body.	Unlikely: no nasal discharge.
	Nasopharyngeal polyp.	Unlikely: no sneezing or nasal discharge.
Inflammatory	Nasopharyngeal stenosis.	Unlikely: no obstruction, nasal discharge, or nausea.
Infectious	Bacterial.	Unlikely: no nasal discharge.
	Fungal.	Unlikely: no nasal discharge, deformation of the nose, or radiographic signs.
	Chlamydophila spp./*Mycoplasma* spp.	Unlikely: no conjunctivitis or ocular discharge.
Traumatic causes	Oronasal fistula.	Unlikely: not observed during examination.
	Fractured mandible.	Unlikely: no history of trauma and no radiographic evidence.
Neoplastic	Cancer.	Possible, although the cat is young.

Table 3. Differential diagnosis of laryngeal, pharyngeal, and tracheal stridor.

Origin	Process	Compatibility with case
Degenerative	Laryngeal paralysis.	Unlikely: no change in vocalisation.
	Tracheobronchial collapse.	Unlikely: not frequent and no radiographic evidence observed.
Congenital anomaly	Brachycephaly.	Unlikely: patient is a domestic shorthair cat.
Mechanical	Foreign body.	Unlikely: no nasal discharge.
Neoplastic	Lymphoma, lymphosarcoma, squamous cell carcinoma, adenocarcinoma.	Advanced diagnostic imaging tests are required.
Inflammatory	Laryngeal oedema, stenosis, laryngeal granuloma.	Advanced diagnostic imaging tests are required.

Table 4. Differential diagnosis of anisocoria with miosis.

Origin	Process	Compatibility with case
Neoplastic	Lymphoma.	Advanced diagnostic imaging tests are required.
Inflammatory	Uveitis.	Unlikely: no ocular discharge and no signs of blepharospasm or glaucoma.
	Spastic pupil syndrome.	Unlikely: associated with FeLV.
	Infections of the middle/inner ear.	Possible, but no exudate or alteration of tympanic membrane.
Idiopathic	Horner syndrome.	Unlikely: associated with enophthalmos, protrusion of the nictitating membrane, and palpebral ptosis.
Traumatic	Brachial plexus avulsion.	Unlikely: no alteration of the forelimb and no peripheral neurological deficit.
	Head trauma.	Unlikely: no compatible history or acute neurological signs.
Toxic	Organophosphates.	Unlikely: no digestive signs, salivation, or bilateral signs.
	Parasympathomimetic drugs.	Unlikely: no bilateral signs.

Table 5. Differential diagnosis of head tilt.

Origin	Process	Compatibility with case
Congenital anomaly	Chronic vestibular disease.	Unlikely: occurs from birth, typical in Siamese and Burmese breeds.
Neoplastic	Squamous cell tumour.	Unlikely: no alterations in mental status or cranial nerves.
Nutritional	Thiamine deficiency.	Unlikely: diet consists of commercial food, no signs of ataxia or ventroflexion of the neck.
Inflammatory/infectious	Otitis media/interna.	Unlikely: not observed with otoscope.
	FIP.	Unlikely: no fever or other cerebral signs.
	Cryptococcosis.	Unlikely: no cutaneous or respiratory signs.
	Inflammatory polyp of the middle ear.	Possible: presents with anisocoria, advanced diagnostic imaging tests required.
Idiopathic	Acute or hyperacute idiopathic vestibular syndrome.	Unlikely: other neurological abnormalities would be observed.
Iatrogenic	Aminoglycosides.	Unlikely: no recent history.
	Flushing.	Unlikely: no compatible history.

Additional tests

Blood tests (complete blood count and biochemistry) reveal no alterations (Tables 6 and 7).

The animal is sedated using a combination of medetomidine (0.01 mg/kg), pethidine (4 mg/kg), and midazolam (0.3 mg/kg). No lesions compatible with the patient's clinical signs are observed upon visual exploration of the nasopharynx, oropharynx, and trachea.

Table 6. Haematology: whole blood with EDTA (Idexx QBC Vet Autoreader).

Parameter	Value	Reference range
Haematocrit (%)	38.7	24–45
Haemoglobin (g/dl)	12.2	8–15
Mean corpuscular haemoglobin concentration (g/dl)	31.5	30–36.9
Platelets (× 10^9/l)	329	170–530
Leucocytes (× 10^9/l)	10.8	5–18.9
Neutrophils (× 10^9/l) *	6.2	3–13 *
Band neutrophils (× 10^9/l)*	0	0–0.2 *
Lymphocytes (× 10^9/l) *	4.3	0.9–7 *
Monocytes (× 10^9/l) *	0.3	0.1–0.6 *
Eosinophils (× 10^9/l)*	0	0.1–0.8 *

* Meyer and Hervey, 2007.

Table 7. Results of plasma biochemistry (Idexx VetTest 8008).

Parameter	Value	Reference range
Total protein (g/l) (refractometer)	70	57–79
Albumin (g/l)	34	23–39
Globulins (g/l) (calculation)	36	30-45
Alanine aminotransferase (ALT) (IU/l)	42	12–130
Alkaline phosphatase (AP) (IU/l)	48	14–111
Gamma-glutamyl transferase (GGT) (IU/l)	0	0–1
Urea (mmol/l)	9	5.7–12.9
Creatinine (mmol/l)	76	53–139 *
Glucose (mmol/l)	6.45	3.95–8.83
Phosphorus (mmol/l)	1.8	1–2.42

* Elliott, 2007.

Laterolateral and ventrodorsal radiographs of the chest and radiographs of the head, including the nasal sinuses, nasal cavity, and tympanic bullae show no detectable alterations.

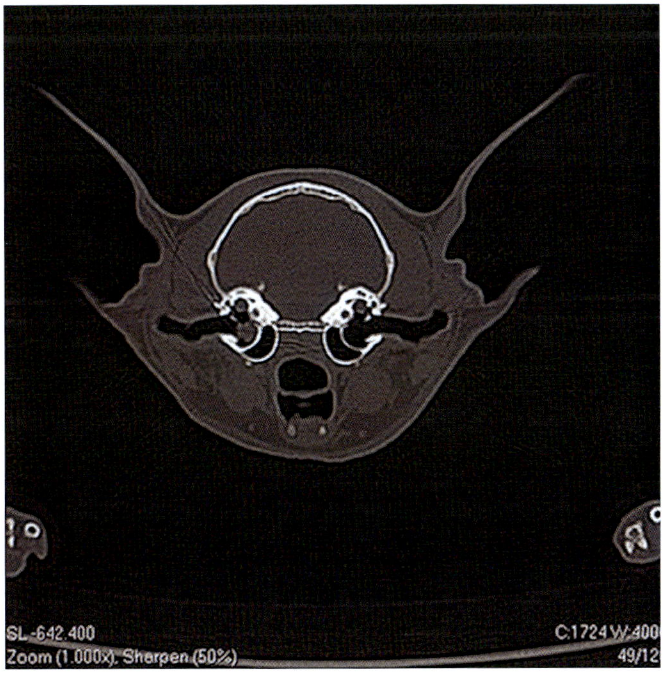

The results of serology for infectious feline leukaemia (FeLV), feline immunodeficiency virus (FIV), and *Dirofilaria immitis* (SNAP Feline Triple Test, Idexx) are as follows:

- FeLV antigen (ELISA): negative.
- FIV antibody (ELISA): negative.
- *Dirofilaria immitis* antigen (ELISA): negative.

Serological tests for the detection of toxoplasmosis and coronavirus reveal the following:

- IgG and IgM against *Toxoplasma gondii* (indirect immunofluorescence): negative.
- Anti-feline coronavirus (FCoV) IgG (ELISA): negative.

Computerised axial tomography (CAT) is proposed to the owners, given the sensitivity of this technique for the study of the nasal cavity and middle ear. This approach reveals the presence of a soft tissue mass of 0.4 × 0.6 cm within the dorsolateral compartment of the left tympanic bulla, protruding into the tympanic membrane and causing thickening of the bony septum separating the ventromedial and dorsolateral compartments (Fig. 3).

Figure 3. Computed axial tomography (CAT) revealing a mass in the tympanic bulla.

Slight inflammation of the nasopharyngeal orifice, which may explain the inspiratory stridor, is also observed.

Treatment

Based on these findings, it is decided to perform middle ear surgery (**ventral bulla osteotomy**) to remove the tissue mass observed in the CAT scan.

The anaesthetic premedication protocol used is identical to that used for sedation: medetomidine (0.01 mg/kg), pethidine (4 mg/kg), and midazolam (0.3 mg/kg). Induction of anaesthesia is achieved using propofol, administered at a starting dose of 1 mg/kg, and fentanyl (0.02 mg/kg). Anaesthesia is maintained with isoflurane, with an initial oxygen flow of 2 l/min, decreasing to 0.6 l/min, isoflurane concentration ranging from an initial 3 % to 0.5 %, and continuous infusion of fentanyl (0.005 mg/kg/min). Antibiotic treatment consists of intravenously administered cefadroxil (22 mg/kg).

Immediately after the operation the patient is treated with buprenorphine (0.01 mg/kg, SC), cefadroxil (22 mg/kg, IV), and oral meloxicam (0.1 mg/kg), the administration which is continued indefinitely (0.05 mg/kg every 24 hours). Amoxicillin and clavulanic acid (15 mg/kg every 12 hours, PO) are prescribed until confirmation of the results of bacterial cultures.

Ventral tympanic bulla osteotomy

- The patient is placed in dorsal decubitus with the head extended and the forelimbs directed towards the rear. A towel is used to elevate the neck, thus maintaining the head in the appropriate position for access to the tympanic bulla.
- The tympanic bulla is located by palpation of the area caudomedial to the temporomandibular joint. An incision is made in the skin covering the bulla and the platysma muscle.
- This is followed by blunt dissection of the lateral digastric muscle, the mylohyoid and hypoglossal muscles, and the hypoglossal nerve. The ventromedial portion of the bulla bone is exposed and is carefully debrided using a periosteal elevator. Proper visualisation of the field is achieved using blunt Gelpi retractors positioned at different angles and two Farabeuf retractors.
- Next, drilling at low speed, a 2-mm Steinmann pin is used to open the ventromedial compartment (Fig. 4). The opening is widened with a small rongeurs to enable exploration of the entire compartment (Fig. 5).
- A sample is collected for microbiological culture to check for growth of specific microorganisms.
- The lateral-most part of the bony septum separating this compartment from the dorsolateral compartment is removed, taking care to avoid damaging the parasympathetic preganglionic fibres that run over the oval promontory.
- The tissue is then extracted and kept for subsequent histopathologic analysis.
- Another sample is collected for microbiological culture and curettage of the epithelium of the dorsolateral cavity is performed using a Volkmann curette. This is followed by lavage with copious amounts of saline.
- Placement of a drain is not usually necessary. The muscle planes are closed separately, followed by the subcutaneous tissue. Wound closure is completed by subcuticular suture using a simple continuous pattern with a synthetic absorbable monofilament (glyconate) of 3/0 diameter (all layers).

Follow-up

The removed tissue is a bright red, oval-shaped dense mass, consisting of a vascularised mass of fibrous connective tissue covered by stratified squamous epithelium, containing inflammatory cells including macrophages, lymphocytes, and plasma cells. **Diagnosis: inflammatory polypoid mass.**

No complications are observed during the first few hours after surgery. However, over the following days the patient develops ptosis of the left eye, with protrusion of the nictitating membrane and enophthalmos. These clinical signs are compatible with Horner's syndrome, but do not interfere with normal daily activities. These clinical signs disappear completely within five weeks without the need for additional treatment.

Microbiological culture results in the growth of a small number of *Pseudomonas* spp. colonies that are sensitive to cefovecin, marbofloxacin, ciprofloxacin, orbifloxacin, and neomycin. Amoxicillin and clavulanic acid are withdrawn and marbofloxacin (2 mg/kg) administered for 14 days.

Discussion

Otic and nasopharyngeal polyps are masses formed by benign nodular tissue originating from the mucosa of the middle ear or the transition between the middle ear and the Eustachian tube, and can expand into the nasopharynx or towards the external horizontal ear canal (Anderson et al., 2000). While

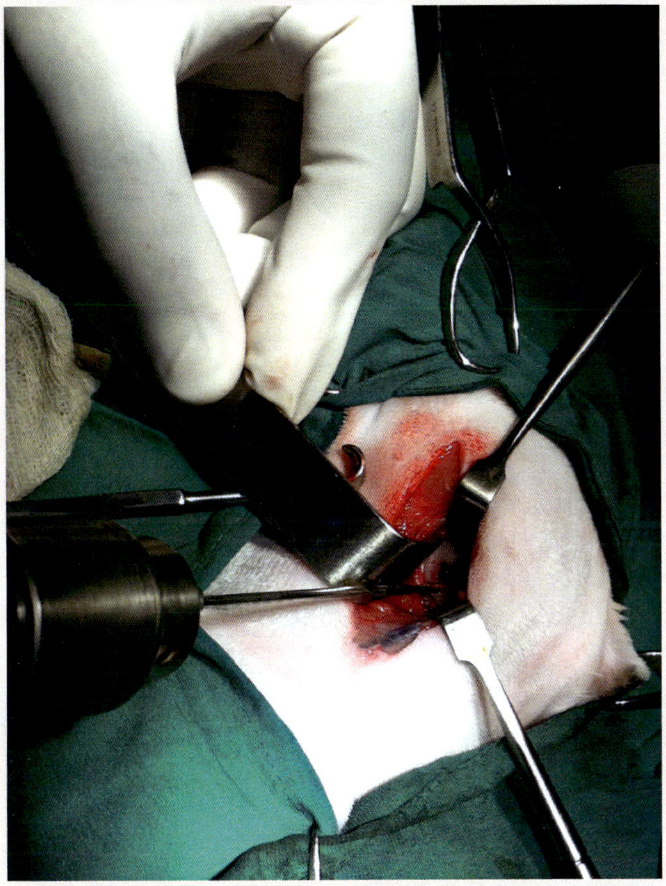

Figure 4. Surgical approach and tympanic bulla osteotomy.

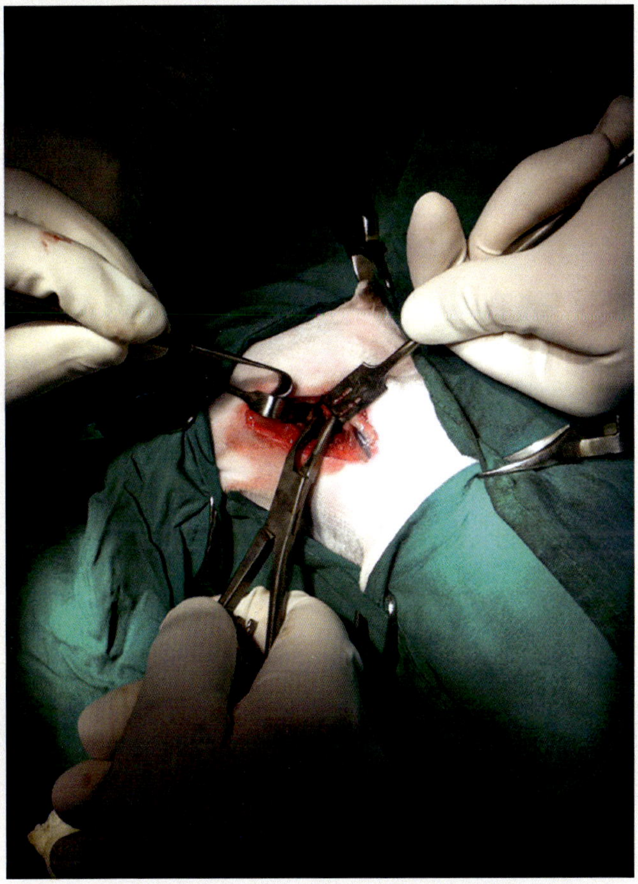

Figure 5. Removal of the ventromedial wall of the tympanic bulla using a rongeurs to extract all material.

usually described in young animals, they have also been documented in cats of over 15 years of age (Muileburg and Fry, 2002).

The aetiology is unknown. It is thought that these inflammatory masses develop in response to inflammatory processes of the middle ear, as they consist of vascularised fibrous connective tissue covered by a squamous stratified epithelium, with an internal core of inflammatory cells. Several studies have investigated the role of feline calicivirus and herpesvirus, *Mycoplasma*, *Bordetella*, and *Chlamydophila* as causative agents of polyps. While these organisms have been shown to cause respiratory processes of the upper respiratory tract and alterations of the middle ear, they have not to date been isolated from polypoid tissues extracted from affected animals (Veir et al., 2002; Klose et al., 2007 and 2010).

Clinical signs depend on the location of the polyp. Cats with polypoid masses in the ear canal show signs of otitis externa with head shaking, scratching the ear area, and otic discharge. Masses affecting the middle ear produce clinical signs of otitis media or interna with Horner syndrome (miosis, ptosis, protrusion of the nictitating membrane and enophthalmos – ipsilateral) or vestibular syndrome (head tilt, nystagmus, and ataxia – also ipsilateral). Cats with nasopharyngeal polyps present with nasal discharge, sneezing, respiratory stridor, difficulty eating, nausea, and altered vocalisations (Muileburg and Fry, 2002; Tobias and Morris, 2009).

Diagnosis is established through otoscopic and nasopharyngeal examination, direct examination of the external auditory canal, or by retracting the soft palate with atraumatic forceps or traction sutures, for which sedation is required (Muileburg and Fry, 2002; Forster-van Hijfte et al., 2011). Imaging studies, including conventional head radiographs, are required to evaluate the nasal sinuses, nasal cavity, nasopharynx, and tympanic bullae. More advanced methods such as CAT and magnetic resonance imaging (MRI) offer greater sensitivity in cases in which polyps cannot be directly observed, particularly those that exclusively affect the middle ear, as in the present case (Lamb et al., 2003).

Histological evaluation of the mass is necessary to rule out other processes, such as cancer.

The management of polyps depends on their location. The objective is to remove inflamed tissue and avoid recurrence of the process. In the case of nasopharyngeal polyps or polyps protruding from the horizontal external ear canal, in the absence of radiological changes in the tympanic bullae, careful traction/avulsion of the polyp using the appropriate forceps is advisable. Moreover, the rate of recurrence can be markedly reduced by administering oral prednisolone at an anti-inflammatory dose of 1 mg/kg daily for 2 weeks during the immediate postoperative period, applying a subsequent withdrawal protocol.

The recurrence rate is also reduced if otic polyps are removed via the middle ear, either by myringotomy or ventral bulla osteotomy (Anderson et al., 2000; Tobias and Morris, 2009; MacPhail, 2009). Other proposed methods include endoscopy via the stomach, passing through the oesophagus to reach the nasopharynx and remove the polyp (Esterline et al., 2005).

If radiographs of the head reveal compatible alterations, ventral bulla osteotomy is the best treatment option. In cats, ventral osteotomy is preferable, given the much lower morbidity associated with this approach as compared with lateral osteotomy (Faulkner and Budsberg, 1990; Anderson et al., 2000; Tobias and Morris, 2009).

In the present case, no polyps were found in the nasopharynx or the external ear canal: the polyp was restricted to the laterodorsal compartment of the middle ear, limiting the available surgical options to bulla osteotomy. The surgeon selected the ventral approach, which produced a satisfactory result.

Complications range from recurrence of the process, depending on the presentation and treatment approach used, to neurological complications such as Horner syndrome (miosis, ptosis, prolapse of the third eyelid) in the case of ventral bulla osteotomy, although these complications can also be observed following traction/avulsion. Depending on the damage to the ganglion fibres of the oval promontory, this may be a temporary, disappearing within a few weeks, or permanent. Vestibular syndrome, with ataxia, head tilt, and paralysis of the temporal facial nerve, is another possible complication, as are episodes of otitis interna and externa, scar formation problems with tissue dehiscence, bacterial contamination of the wound, seroma, and abscesses (Muileburg and Fry, 2002; Tobias and Morris, 2009).

Conclusion

Inflammatory polyps in feline species usually affect the nasopharynx or middle ear. These are non-tumoural inflammatory masses that respond well to normal management techniques, depending on tumour location.

References

Anderson, D.M., Robinson, R.K., White, R.A. Management of inflammatory polyps in 37 cats. *Veterinary Record*, 2000; 147:684-87.

Elliott, J. Staging chronic kidney disease. Capítulo 11. En: *BSAVA Manual of Canine and Feline Nephrology and Urology*, 2ª ed. Elliott, J., Grauer, G.F. (eds.). British Small Animal Veterinary Association, UK, 2007; pp. 159-166.

Esterline, M.L., Radlinsky, M.A., Schermerhorn, T. Endoscopic removal of nasal polyps in a cat using a novel surgical approach. *Journal of Feline Medicine and Surgery*, 2005; 7:121-124.

Forster-Van Hijfte, M.A., Groth, A.M., Emmerson, T.D. Expansile, inflammatory middle disease causing nasopharyngeal obstruction in a cat. *Journal of Feline Medicine and Surgery*, 2011 Jun; 13(6):451-453.

Faulkner, J.E., Budsberg, S.C. Results of ventral bulla osteotomy for treatment of middle ear polyps in cats. *Journal of the American Animal Hospital Association*, 1990; 26:496-499.

Klose, T.C., Rosychulk, R.A., MacPhail, C.M., Hawley, J.R., Veir, J., Schultheis, P., Lappin, M.R. Association between upper respiratory tract infections and inflammatory aural and nasopharyngeal polyps in cats. *Journal of Veterinary Internal Medicine*, 2007; 21:628.

Klose, T.C., Rosychulk, R.A., MacPhail, C.M., Hawley, J.R., Veir, J., Schultheis, P., Lappin, M.R. Prevalence of select infectious agents in inflammatory aural and nasopharyngeal polyps from clients-owned cats. *Journal of Feline Medicine and Surgery*, 2010; 12:769-774.

Lamb, C.R., Richbell, S., Mantis, P. Radiographic signs in cats with nasal disease. *Journal of Feline Medicine and Surgery*, 2003; 5:227-237.

MacPhail, C.M. Examining options to treat feline inflamatory polyps. *DVM Surgery Stat,* American College of Veterinary Surgeons, 2009; pp. 31-32.

Meyer, D.J., Hervey, J.W. Intervalos de referencia y tablas de conversión. Apéndice 4 en *Medicina Laboratorial Veterinaria. Interpretación y Diagnosis*. 3ª ed. Meyer, D.J., Hervey, J.W. (eds.). Barcelona: Multimédica Ediciones Veterinarias, 2007; pp. 423-437.

Muileburg, R.K., Fry, T.R. Feline nasopharingeal polyps. *The Vetererinary Clinics Small Animal Practice*, 2002; 32:839-849.

Rand, J.S. *Problem-based feline medicine*. Elsevier Saunders, 2006.

Tobias, K.M., Morris, D. Cirugía del oído. En: *BSAVA Manual de cirugía de cabeza, cuello y tórax de pequeños animales*. Edición española. Brockman, D.J., Holt, D.E. (eds.). Gloucester: British Small Animal Veterinary Association (BSAVA), 2009; pp. 83-106.

Veir, J.K., Lappin, M.R., Folley, J.E., Gezy, D.M. Feline inflammatory polyps: historical, clinical and PCR findings for feline calicivirus and feline herpesvirus-1 in 28 cases. *Journal of Feline Medicine and Surgery*, 2002; 4:195-199.

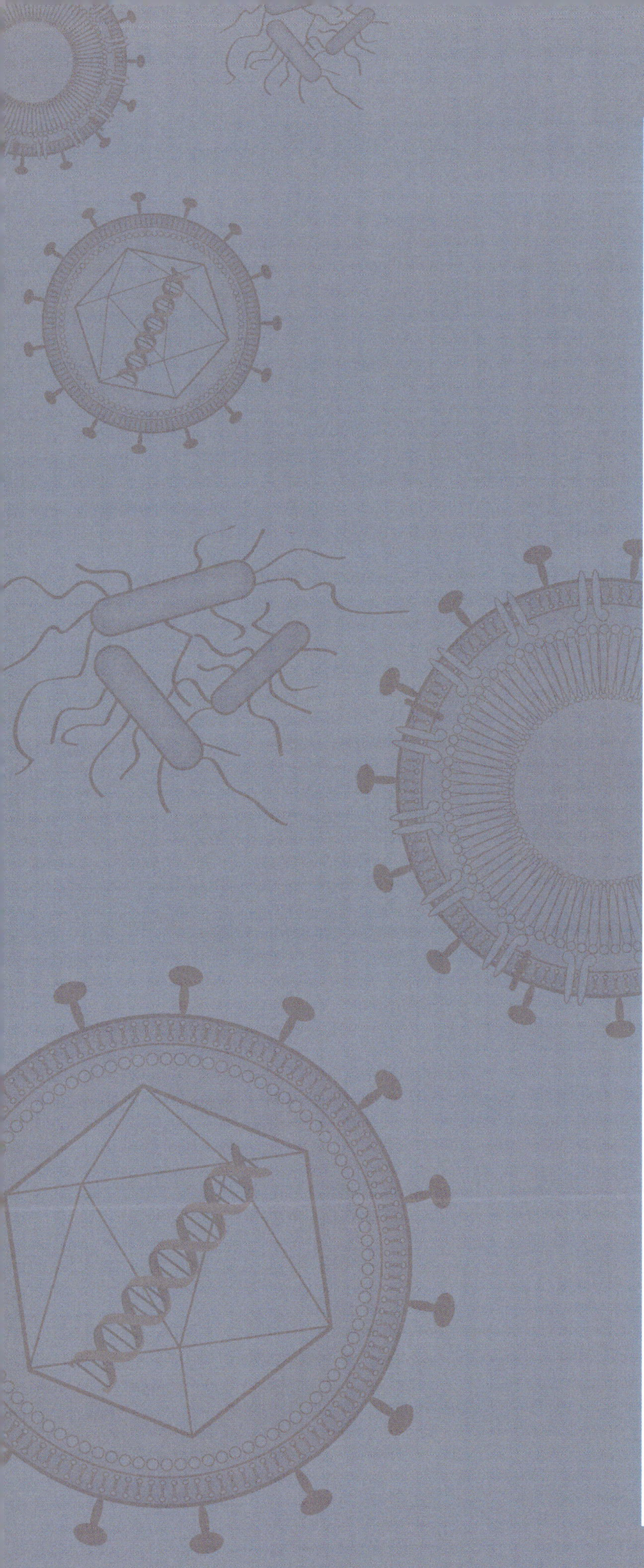

Lower respiratory tract infections

Lower respiratory tract infections

In cats, lower respiratory tract infections (LRTIs) can be caused by bacteria, viruses, fungi, or parasites. Most cause inflammation of the lung parenchyma (pneumonia).

Complex tests including histopathology and specific viral detection are required to detect pneumonia-causing viruses. However, routine tests can be used to diagnose parasites, bacteria, or fungi.

Medical history, haematology, and radiology can help identify the clinical process. Bronchoalveolar lavage (BAL) or fine-needle aspiration cytology and microbiology of the lung allow establishment of a probable diagnosis in most situations.

Clinical signs

The following are the most common clinical signs (Cohn, 2010; Foster et al., 2004a; Foster and Martin, 2011; Gaskell et al., 2006; McDonald et al., 2003; Miller, 2007; Swift et al., 2009):

- Tachypnoea, dyspnoea (49 %).
- Nasal discharge (21 %).
- Fever (15–24 %).

The physical examination is extremely important. Careful observation of the animal's breathing can be extremely useful when assessing the clinical presentation. Certain abnormalities in breathing patterns can help identify the process in question. When at rest, cats display very little movement of the thoracic wall while breathing. When breathing becomes more difficult, the ribs are displaced caudolaterally by the diaphragm, and the muscles of the thoracic wall and abdomen are moved slightly outward.

Contraction of the abdominal muscles is indicative of a significant respiratory effort. The breathing pattern therefore facilitates specific identification of the respiratory problem.

Very shallow and short breaths with a small tidal volume are indicative of a lung that fails to inflate normally or a problem known as pleural or thoracic wall restriction.

Narrowing of the airway results in inspiratory rather than expiratory alterations.

Auscultation using a stethoscope also provides information useful for the detection of LRTI. This approach often detects wheezing (rhythmic, non-strident musical sounds) generated by stenosis or obstruction of the airways. Other potential findings include crepitation, which are short, explosive sounds associated with the presence of fluid in the lower airways, as occurs in pneumonia, pulmonary oedema, or complicated bronchitis (Miller, 2007).

Diagnostic tests

Haematology

The results of haematological analyses can vary greatly. Leukocytosis and neutrophilia are commonly observed (Foster and Martin, 2011; Miller, 2007). Leukopaenia and neutropaenia are less common. One study (Foster et al., 2004a) detected eosinophilia in 4 out of 18 affected cats.

In general, haematology is considered to be of little assistance in establishing diagnosis.

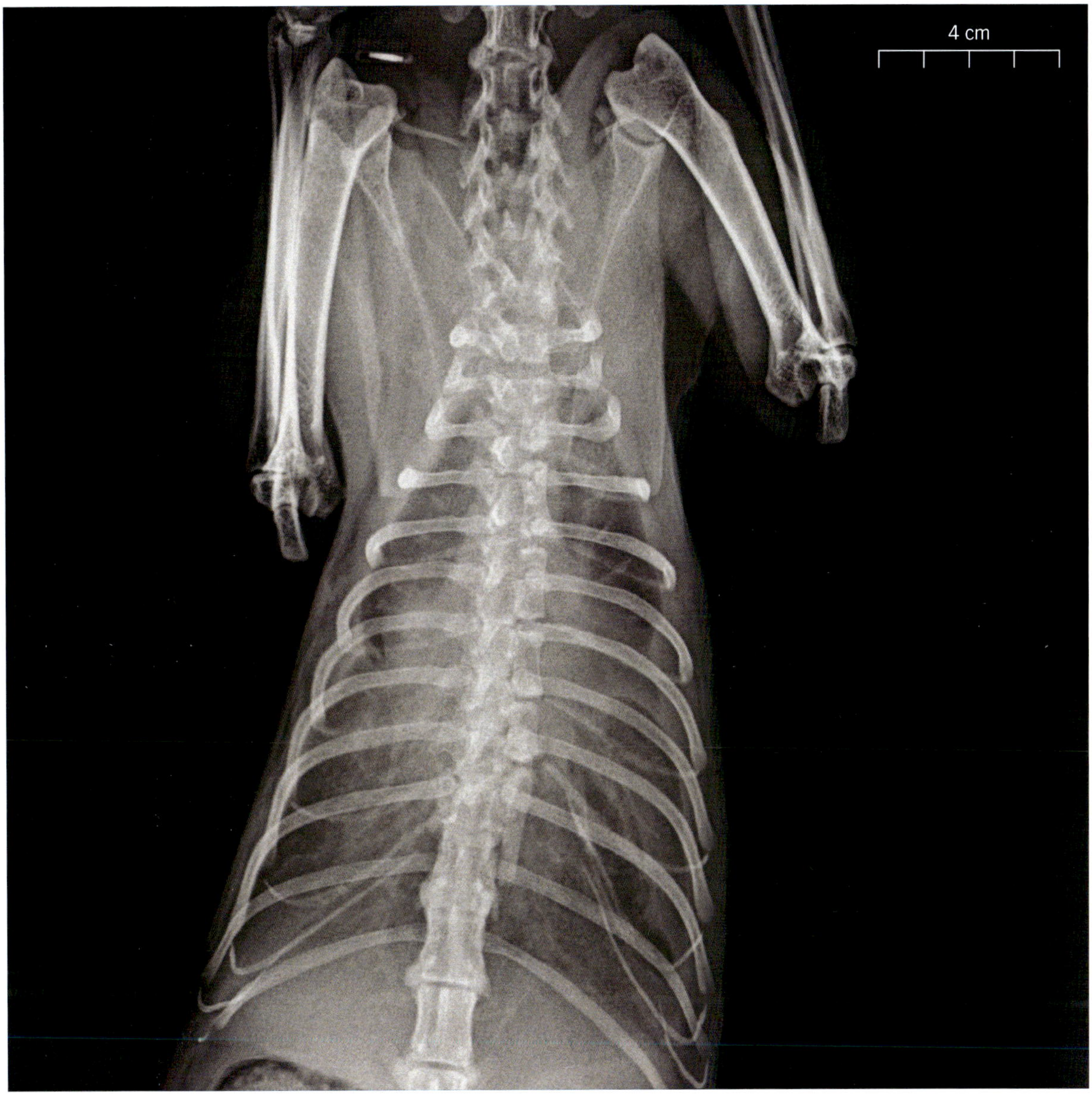

Figure 1. Ventrodorsal radiograph of a cat with a mixed alveolar and bronchial pattern caused by bronchopneumonia.

Biochemistry

The most important findings are increases in total protein and globulin levels (Foster and Martin, 2011).

Radiology

Radiographs can reveal different types of patterns (Foster et al., 2004a; Foster and Martin, 2011; McDonald et al., 2003). An alveolar radiographic pattern is observed in 65 % of cats with LRTI, of which 81 % have a mixed alveolar and bronchial pattern (Fig. 1).

Nodular patterns have been described in cases of cryptococcosis, toxoplasmosis, and mycoplasmosis.

These processes can also occur in the absence of any radiological alteration.

Bronchoalveolar lavage

This is the gold standard technique for the collection of samples for the diagnosis of LRTI (Foster ***et al.***, 2004b; Foster and Martin, 2011; Hamilton ***et al.***, 1991; Hawkins, 2004; Johnson and Drazenovich, 2007; Norris et al., 2002; Sparkes et al., 1997). It can be performed with or without bronchoscopy. When performed in conjunction with bronchoscopy this technique is associated with very few complications, and fewer still if performed after premedication with terbutaline.

Bronchoscopy is not always an option. If technical or economic constraints do not allow the use this method, bronchoalveolar lavage can be performed without an endoscope.

Transtracheal aspiration

This is rarely the first choice of technique in cats, as it can exacerbate respiratory signs, and leaves no means of quick access to the airway if bronchospasm occurs (Syring, 2004).

This technique is indicated in cases in which general anaesthesia is contraindicated. Local anaesthesia in the region of the cricothyroid ligament is induced using 2 % lidocaine or bupivacaine. An intravenous catheter (18–22 G) is introduced, and once the interior of the trachea is reached, the needle is removed.

Warm sterile saline (0.5 ml/kg) is infused and aspirated as quickly as possible. Compared with bronchoalveolar lavage less material is collected using this procedure, which may need to be repeated.

Non-bronchoscopic lavage technique

» This is generally performed using a short-duration anaesthetic that induces deep anaesthesia. This allows endotracheal intubation, which in turn is used to guide the technique.

» The animal is intubated with a sterile endotracheal tube, which is introduced very carefully through the oropharynx to prevent contamination that could alter the results of subsequent analyses (Fig. 2).

» The cat is placed on one side with the affected lung facing down; this allows collection of a greater amount of material, which will be used for subsequent analyses (Foster and Martin, 2011).

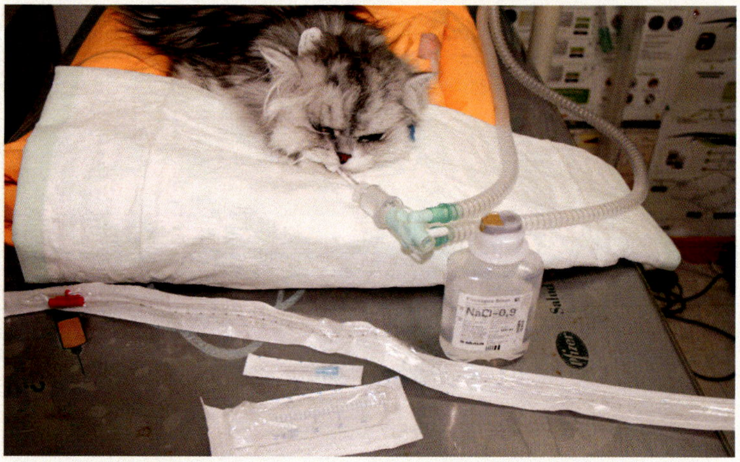

Figure 2. Cat on operating table prior to undergoing bronchoalveolar lavage (BAL). The patient is in sternal decubitus and has been intubated. The equipment necessary for BAL has been prepared: syringes, saline, and urinary catheter, which will be introduced into the endotracheal tube.

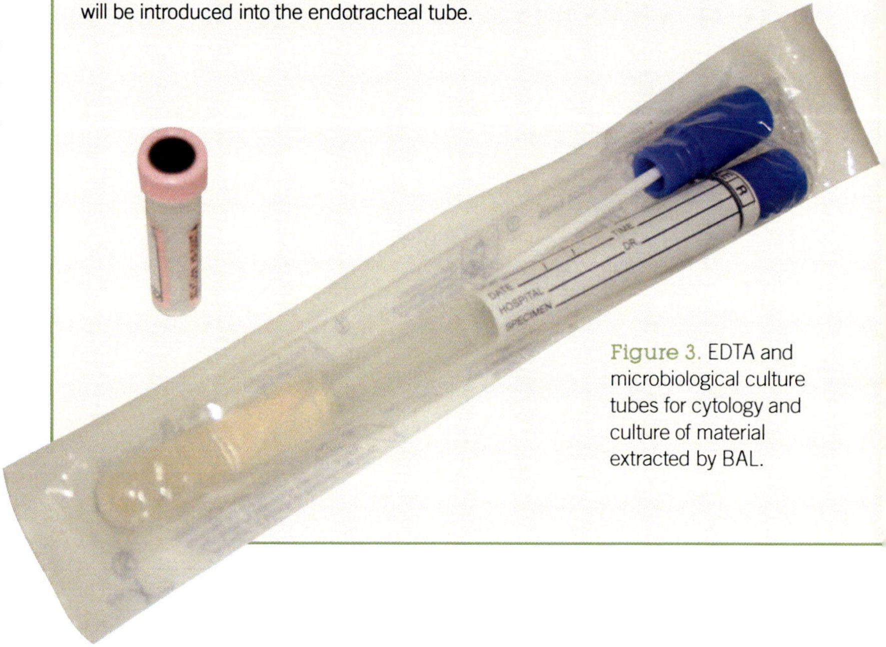

Figure 3. EDTA and microbiological culture tubes for cytology and culture of material extracted by BAL.

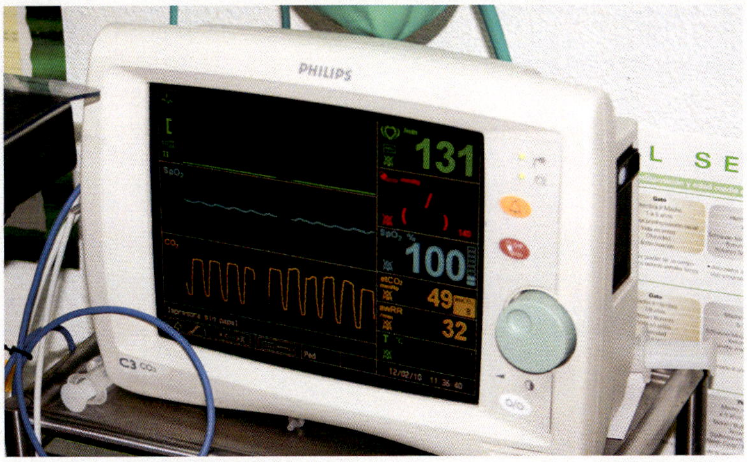

Figure 4. Capnography monitoring during BAL procedure.

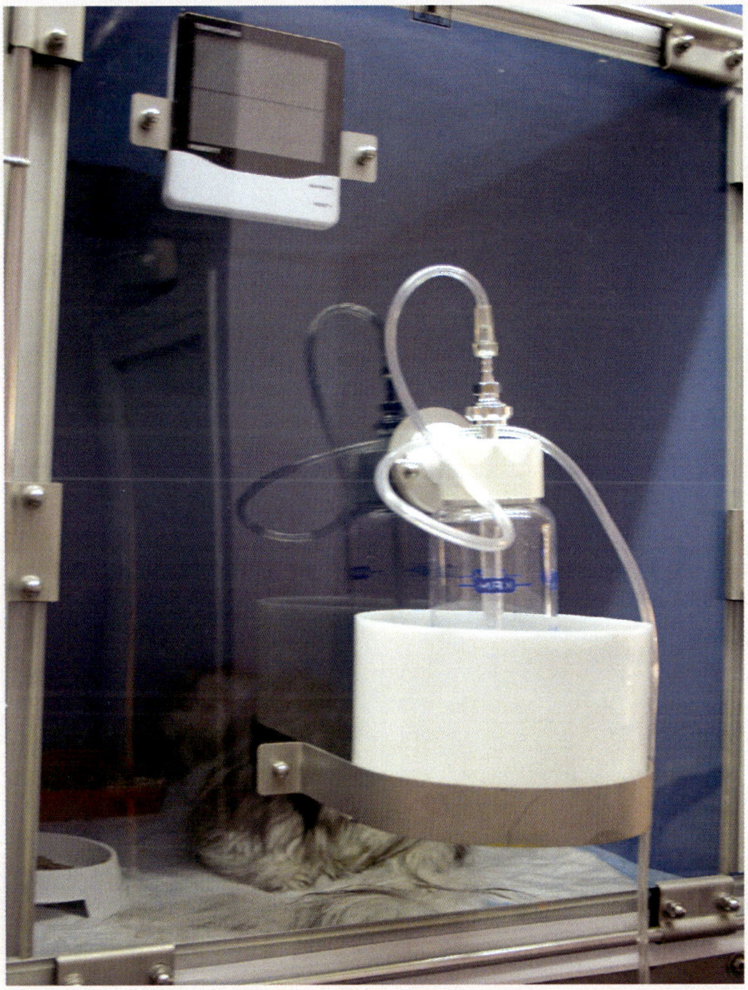

Figure 5. Patient recovering in oxygenation chamber after BAL.

» A catheter of a smaller diameter than the endotracheal tube or of the same diameter as the primary bronchus (measured on the radiograph) is introduced into the endotracheal tube. This catheter should be semi-rigid, to ensure proper passage and correct positioning. A dog urinary catheter can be used for this purpose. The catheter is introduced into the endotracheal tube as far as the bifurcation of the trachea or the distal-most region possible, taking great care not to pierce the bronchus.

» Between 5 ml and 10 ml of warm sterile saline is injected via the catheter. The thoracic wall is tapped several times (*coupage*) to facilitate detachment of all material from the bronchi. The lavage fluid is collected into a syringe and prepared for cytology and microbiological culture (Fig. 3).

» It is advisable to have terbutaline available in case acute bronchospasm occurs following the procedure. If required, it can be administered at a dose of 0.01 mg/kg IV, IM, or SC (Foster and Martin, 2011) (Figs. 4 and 5).

Fine-needle aspiration

This helps determine the nature of the lesions observed by radiography or ultrasound (DeBerry et al., 2002; Foster and Martin, 2011; Norris et al., 2002; Zekas ***et al.***, 2005). The procedure depends on the lesion type (mass or diffuse) and location (central or peripheral) and the patient's clinical status.

Needle aspiration can be performed blindly or guided by ultrasound, fluoroscopy, or computed tomography (CT).

In theory, this technique can cause more potential lesions than BAL, although studies have shown that 22–27-G needles caused few complications, while 18–22-G needles caused pneumothorax, pulmonary haemorrhage, or both in 43 % of cats (DeBerry et al., 2002; Foster and Martin, 2011).

Cytology

Cytology can be performed on samples obtained by BAL, transtracheal aspiration, or fine-needle aspiration (Foster and Martin, 2011; Padrid et al., 1991).

One problem is that the material obtained is mixed with bronchial mucus, which may hinder interpretation of the analysis. It can be difficult to assess the presence of *Aelurostrongylus abstrusus*.

Some laboratories use cytospin preparations (Dehard et al., 2008), which help to improve visualisation of the samples by centrifugation, especially samples with low cellularity. Samples should be prepared as quickly as possible to ensure optimal results. Box 1 shows the cellular characteristics of normal samples.

Box 1. Cell count in normal samples.

» 60–90 % macrophages.

» <7 % neutrophils.

» 10–20 % eosinophils.

Eosinophil counts exceeding 20 % and neutrophil counts exceeding 7 % are indicative of an inflammatory phenomenon.

If cytology reveals the presence of bacteria, culture of the material obtained is recommended, except in cases of mycoplasmosis (mycoplasmas are difficult to detect by cytology as they respond poorly to Diff-Quik and Gram staining).

There is little overlap between the results of histopathology of samples obtained by puncture/aspiration and cytology of BAL samples.

Microbiological tests

In principle, the airways of healthy animals are not sterile. Thus, when performing microbiological analysis of the material obtained, it is important to obtain bacterial counts to ensure correct interpretation of cytology and microbiology results.

The most common bacteria found in the airways of healthy animals, at less than 2×10^3 CFU/ml, include *Escherichia coli, Pasteurella* spp., *Pseudomonas* spp., *Staphylococcus* spp., *Streptococcus* spp., *and Micrococcus* spp. (Foster and Martin, 2011; Padrid et al., 1991).

Anaerobes and mycoplasmas have not been isolated from the lower airways of healthy animals.

Box 2 lists the main causative agents of LRTIs in cats.

Faecal floatation tests and other parasite detection methods should be performed routinely to detect parasites that may be present in feline LRTIs (Lacorcia ***et al.***, 2009).

Box 2. IRTI-causing agents.

Most common bacteria:

- *Bordetella bronchiseptica*.
- *Pasteurella* spp.
- *Mycoplasma* spp.
- *Streptococcus* spp.
- *Escherichia coli*.

Other bacteria that cause pneumonia:

- *Salmonella typhimurium*.
- *Pseudomonas* spp.

Viruses:

- Herpesvirus.
- Coronavirus.

Parasites of the lungs:

- *Aelurostrongylus abstrusus*.
- *Eucoleus aerophilus*.

Protozoa:

- *Toxoplasma gondii*.

Fungi:

- *Cryptococcus* spp.
- *Candida albicans*.
- *Mucor* spp.
- *Aspergillus* spp.

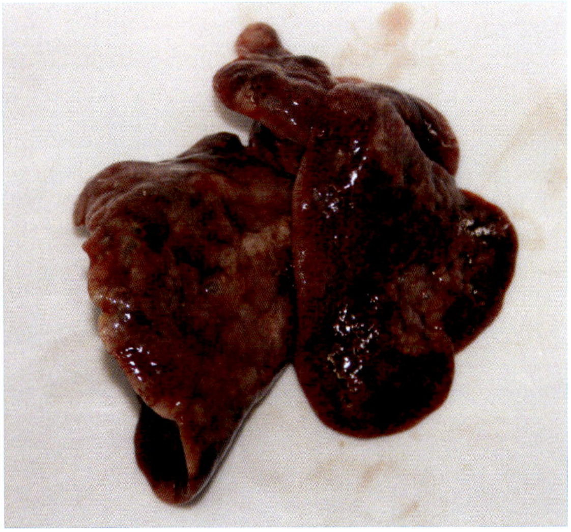

Figure 6. Lung of cat in which histology identified bronchopneumonia caused by *Mycoplasma*.

LRTI-causing bacteria

Mycoplasmas

These are the smallest forms of life: self-replicating cells that lack a cellular wall. Although commonly present in many mucosa, they are not usually found in the lower respiratory tract (Chandler and Lappin, 2002; Foster and Martin, 2011; Pedersen, 1987; Trow et al., 2008; Waites et al., 2004 and 2008).

Mycoplasmas have long been known to cause LRTIs in other species, as well as other processes including pyothorax, pneumonia, and pulmonary abscesses in cats. They have also been implicated in chronic bronchial disease in cats (as causal more so than secondary agents), producing an exacerbated inflammatory response in the airways that results in an inflammatory bronchial process similar to that caused by *Mycoplasma pneumoniae* in humans (Foster and Martin, 2011; Rollins et al., 2010) (Fig. 6).

Diagnosis

Mycoplasma spp. cannot be stained using Diff-Quik or Gram stains. Moreover, culture of this bacteria is very difficult due to changes that can occur during transport to the laboratory and the need for special media such as peptone-enriched blood agar.

Polymerase chain reaction (PCR) is probably the best method for diagnosis of mycoplasma, but is not a routine test. Consequently, clinical veterinary surgeons often prefer a therapeutic trial as an alternative diagnostic method (Foster and Martin, 2011).

Treatment

Treatment is often empirical due to the difficulty in establishing diagnosis.

Because culture is difficult, it is not possible to establish the antibiotic sensitivity of the microorganism. Therefore, antibiotics with documented efficacy against mycoplasma are used.

Mycoplasmas are sensitive to the following antibiotics:

- Macrolides: erythromycin, clarithromycin, tylosin.
- Fluoroquinolones: enrofloxacin, ciprofloxacin, pradofloxacin.
- Tetracyclines: doxycycline.
- Chloramphenicol.
- Gentamicin.

Mycoplasmas are more sensitive to doxycycline than enrofloxacin (Foster and Martin, 2011), but pradofloxacin has shown similar efficacy for the management of mycoplasmas that cause respiratory disease in the upper airways, and tends to be preferred as an empirical treatment (Hartmann et al., 2008) over doxycycline, the potential side effects of which can include oesophageal stricture (German et al., 2005).

If LRTI is also associated with chronic bronchitis/feline asthma, anti-inflammatory or immunosuppressive treatment should be added to the patient's regimen, clinical situation permitting (Foster and Martin, 2011).

Treatment duration is variable, but is generally prolonged. In human medicine chronic mycoplasma infections have been described, requiring treatment for up to 5 or 6 weeks.

Therefore, one treatment recommendation is to administer a dose of 5 mg/kg doxycycline PO every 12 hours, for a minimum of 6 weeks.

Bordetella bronchiseptica

Bordetella bronchiseptica is a primary pathogen of the respiratory tract of cats (Foley et al., 2002, Foster and Martin, 2011; Little, 2000). It can cause infections of the upper respiratory tract with clinical signs including sneezing and oculonasal discharge, as well as LRTI with signs including cough, dyspnoea, and cyanosis, and potential complications caused by the development of bronchopneumonia.

Young cats are highly susceptible to respiratory problems caused by *B. bronchiseptica*, and can easily develop bronchopneumonia. However, this bacterium has also been detected in adult cats with clinical signs of severe bronchopneumonia.

Failure of bronchopneumonia to respond adequately to intensive therapy is usually indicative of the presence of viruses such as feline calicivirus (FCV) and feline herpesvirus (FHV) in addition to *B. bronchiseptica*.

Treatment

It is advisable to start antibiotic therapy quickly to avoid major complications.

B. bronchiseptica is usually resistant to beta-lactam antibiotics such as amoxicillin, ampicillin and various cephalosporins. Conversely, it is very sensitive to tetracycline, enrofloxacin, amoxicillin-clavulanic acid, chloramphenicol, and gentamicin.

Currently, the most commonly recommended treatment for bronchopneumonia caused by *B. bronchiseptica* is doxycycline and fluoroquinolones such as pradofloxacin (Foster and Martin, 2011; Hartmann et al., 2008).

Streptococcus spp.

Beta-haemolytic streptococci are very common components of the normal microflora of the pharynx, skin, upper respiratory tract, and genital tract of cats (Greene and Prescott, 2006; Sura et al., 2008; Thaillefer et al., 2004; Zhang et al., 2006).

Infection caused by group G *Streptococcus* species in kittens and adults occasionally manifest as pneumonia associated with pleural effusion and cervical lymphadenopathy, fasciitis, myositis, and endotoxic shock.

Most infections in cats caused by beta-haemolytic streptococci are caused by group G species, usually *S. canis*, although *S. equi* infections, which can cause mortality rates of up to 10 % in shelters, have also been documented (Blum et al., 2010).

The most common clinical signs of the disease are purulent nasal discharge and coughing, progressing to rhinosinusitis, dyspnoea, and ultimately death in cases of complications (e.g. bacteraemia).

S. pneumoniae (group C) has been associated with interstitial pneumonia in kittens that die due to myositis and fasciitis.

Group G streptococci are sensitive to penicillins, which are the antibiotics of choice. Clindamycin is the antibiotic of choice for necrotising fasciitis and toxic shock caused by group G streptococci in humans. It has also been used for the treatment of group G streptococci infections in cats. Fluoroquinolones are not recommended for the treatment of streptococcal infections (Foster and Martin, 2011).

Escherichia coli

Although rare, this bacterium causes high mortality in kittens when it coexists with other LRTI-causing microorganisms (Highland et al., 2009; Sura et al., 2008).

Pasteurella spp.

This bacteria is part of the normal microflora of the nasopharynx and airways of healthy animals. It is associated with the presence of viruses and other pathogens, greatly complicating respiratory processes. It is sensitive to beta-lactam antibiotics.

Salmonella spp.

Causes pneumonia of varying severity, in addition to systemic salmonellosis.

Can cause concomitant infections with *Aelurostrongylus abstrusus* and *Pseudomonas* spp., producing clinical signs similar to those of feline bronchial disease/asthma, including chronic cough, dyspnoea, and tachypnoea.

Mycobacterium spp.

M. tuberculosis, *M. bovis*, and *M. thermoresistibile* have been isolated from LRTIs in cats. Abyssinian and Siamese cats are highly sensitive to mycobacteriosis.

Diagnosis requires techniques such as cytology, histopathology, and bacterial culture. BAL is of little diagnostic use.

Management of infections caused by mycobacteria depends on the specific microorganism isolated. Mycobacteria often develop resistance to common antibiotics, complicating their management.

Other bacteria

The following bacteria have also been isolated from cats with LRTI, but are of less clinical relevance or lower prevalence than those described above (Foster and Martin, 2011):

- *Neisseria* spp.
- *Rhodococcus equi*.
- *Yersinia pestis*.

LRTI-causing parasites

Aelurostrongylus abstrusus

In general, there is a tendency to under-diagnose this parasite as a cause of LRTI (Gaglio et al., 2008; Lacorcia et al., 2009; Traversa et al., 2008 and 2009). It has been associated with feline bronchial disease/asthma and in some cases symptomatic treatments with anti-inflammatories, bronchodilators, and immunomodulators are so effective that *A. abstrusus* goes unnoticed (Fig. 7).

It is associated with dyspnoea and coughing. It may predispose animals to infections caused by enteric bacteria such as *Salmonella* spp. or *E. coli* as a result of migration of larvae, which act as a vehicle for intestinal bacteria.

Diagnosis

Diagnosis is achieved using BAL and fine-needle aspiration of the lung parenchyma, but is not easy to establish. The Baermann faecal flotation technique is the most sensitive test for identification of the parasite, but takes a long time to perform (24–36 hours). Other faecal flotation methods can also be used, but are less sensitive than the Baermann technique.

A recently developed approach involves PCR analysis of a sample of pharyngeal mucosa, and offers a sensitivity of 96.6 % and a specificity of 100 %. This is now the reference diagnostic technique.

Treatment

A single dose of ivermectin (400 µg/kg) administered subcutaneously is effective, while a single dose administered orally (300 µg/kg) is less so.

Doses of 200 µg/kg SC can also be used. This dose initially proved ineffective when administered as a single dose, but retreatment 2.5 weeks later can provide complete control of parasitosis, as evidenced by the absence of the parasite in multiple faecal analyses using the Baermann method.

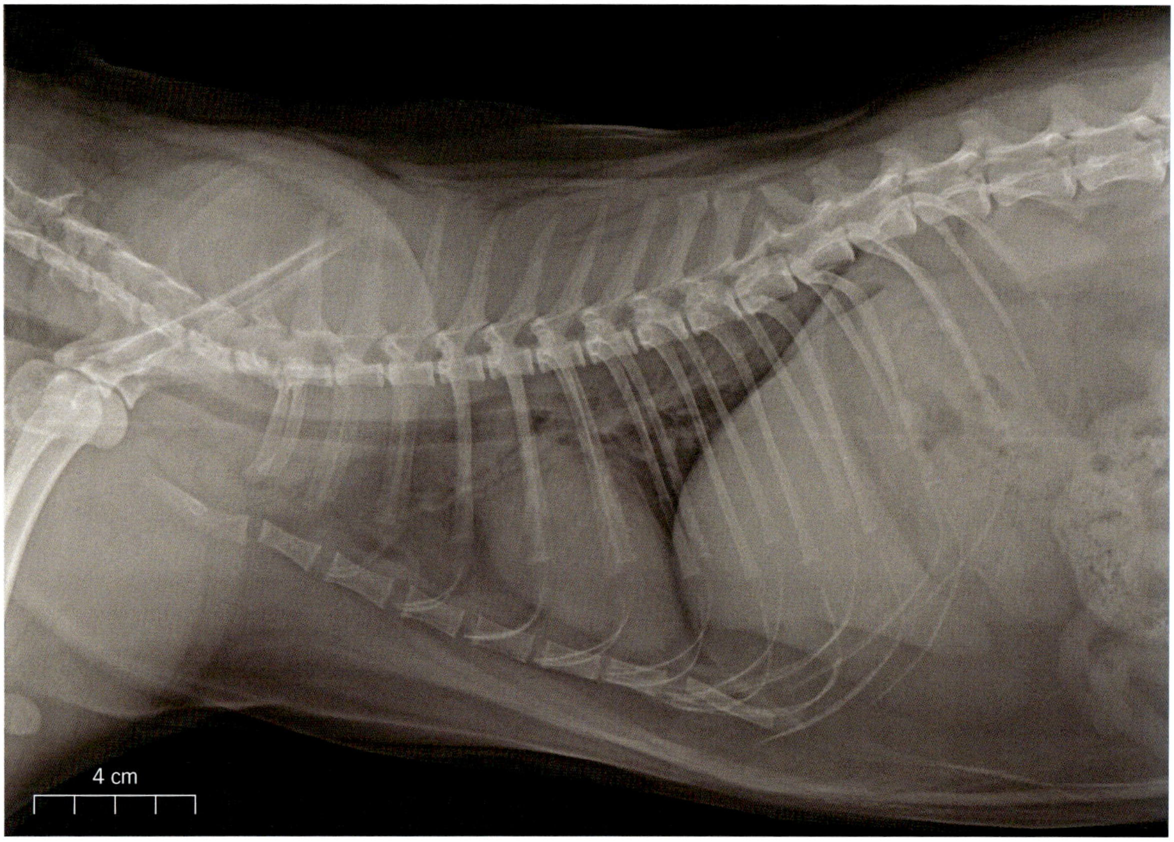

Figure 7. Laterolateral chest radiograph showing a bronchial pattern in a cat with *Aelurostrongylus abstrusus*.

Abamectin has also proven effective when administered subcutaneously in 2 doses of 300 µg/kg, separated by 2 weeks (Foster and Martin, 2011).

Oral fenbendazole (50 mg/kg) for 10 to 20 days is also highly effective.

The combination of imidacloprid and moxidectin administered topically as a single dose is 100 % effective, and is the treatment of choice in many countries. Topical application of the combination of emodepside and praziquantel has an efficacy of 99 %, whereas topical selamectin is effective in only 50 % of cats (Foster and Martin, 2011).

Eucoleus aerophilus

This parasitic species, formerly known as *Capillaria aerophila*, has a worldwide distribution (Lalosevic et al., 2008). While its prevalence in LRTI is thought to be low, it should be considered as a possible cause during the diagnostic process, particularly given the potential risk of zoonosis. In humans it can cause severe bronchial signs, and even induce bronchial carcinoma.

Diagnosis is usually established using routine faecal flotation tests. This parasite can be mistaken for *Trichuris* spp., as both produce operculate eggs.

Treatment involves the same drugs and doses as used for *A. abstrusus*; abamectin administered twice, separated by a 2-week interval, and oral fenbendazole administered for 10 to 14 days, in addition to topical treatments.

Toxoplasma gondii

The cat is the definitive host of this protozoan parasite. The lung is the target organ in cases of both primary toxoplasmosis and reactivation of a previous process (Foster and Martin, 2011; Last et al., 2004).

The risk of infection is greater in immunodeficient cats. Accordingly, episodes of toxoplasmosis are significantly more common in cats that receive immunomodulatory treatment with cyclosporine A for certain pathologies.

Diagnosis

Diagnosis of LRTI caused by *T. gondii* is very difficult. Radiological and cytological findings are similar to those observed for neoplasms. While BAL and fine-needle aspiration can be useful, demonstrating the presence of the bacterium can be difficult in some cases.

In human medicine immunohistochemistry and culture of lung biopsy samples have been proposed as diagnostic tests in patients with acquired immunodeficiency syndrome (AIDS). These same approaches may also be useful in feline medicine.

Treatment

Few published studies have examined the effectiveness of toxoplasmosis treatments (Beaty et al., 2006). Studies have shown that oral clindamycin (11 mg/kg every 24 hours or 12.5 mg/kg every 12 hours) acts to suppress rather than cure toxoplasmosis.

Clindamycin alone appears to be insufficient for the management of LRTI caused by toxoplasmosis, and should be administered in conjunction with another drug such as pyrimethamine (0.25–0.5 mg/kg PO every 12 hours), especially in cases of immunosuppressed cats that have developed pulmonary toxoplasmosis after cyclosporine A administration.

LRTI-causing fungi

Although many fungi are implicated in the development of LRTI, the most representative are those of the genus *Cryptococcus* (Foster and Martin, 2011; Norris, 2004).

The lungs are the typical site of cryptococcal infections in humans. This is less common in cats, although pulmonary affectation may be underdiagnosed if BAL or fine-needle aspiration cytology and histopathology are not performed.

Itraconazole has been used to successfully treat pulmonary cryptococcosis.

Some considerations regarding LRTI in cats (Foster and Martin, 2011)

1» Empirical treatment is not recommended in cases of LRTI given the many and varied causes. A more specific diagnostic approach is required.

2» When bacteria are involved it is important to remember that several types may coexist, thus requiring antibiotics with different characteristics and different serum concentrations. It should be borne in mind that the concentration of antimicrobials in the airway may be decreased due to the presence of bronchial secretions.

3» Non-specific supportive therapy may be required. Intravenous hydration helps maintain blood volume and hydration of the airway. However, care should be taken with the rate of fluid administration in cats with severe pneumonia, in which the alveolar barrier may be compromised.

4» Oxygen should be administered if the SpO_2 is less than 94 % or the PaO_2 is less than 80 mmHg. In cases of severe hypoxaemia intubation with mechanical ventilation may be required.

5» A pulmonary lobectomy may be necessary if antimicrobial treatment fails to resolve the clinical signs of LRTI and residual pneumonia of the pulmonary lobe is observed.

LRTI-causing viruses

Ante-mortem diagnosis of viral processes that cause LRTI is rare in daily practice, as this requires histopathological analysis and specific viral detection using various methods.

Feline calicivirus

This virus has been shown to cause interstitial pneumonia in experimental conditions, and can produce multifocal interstitial bronchopneumonia in combination with other microorganisms such as *B. bronchiseptica.* Interstitial bronchopneumonia can also be observed in virulent systemic calicivirus infections (Telm et al., 2004).

Feline herpesvirus

This is an uncommon cause of LRTI. While always considered possible in debilitated kittens, a recent study revealed the presence of the virus in cases of necrotising fibrinous pneumonia, with severe necrosis of the bronchial and alveolar epithelia, in young adult and older cats. This suggests that herpesviruses may be underdiagnosed as a cause of pneumonia in adult or older cats that experience sudden death and in those in which post mortem histopathology confirms the presence of feline herpesvirus (Chvala-Mannsberger et al., 2009; Malik et al., 2009).

Pyothorax

Infectious alterations of the pleural space deserve a special mention in this chapter on LRTIs.

The pleural or chest cavity is the space between the lungs, mediastinum, diaphragm, and thoracic wall. The pleura coats all of these structures and is divided into the parietal pleura and the visceral pleura, depending on whether it makes contact with the thoracic wall or coats the viscera and organs of the chest, respectively.

The accumulation of a small amount of transudate fluid in the pleural space is normal; this fluid facilitates movement of the various thoracic structures against one another during respiration.

The generation and absorption of this lubricating fluid is a continuous process, which is controlled by the so-called Starling forces. There is a relationship between the hydrostatic pressure of extravascular fluid, the oncotic pressure of intravascular fluid, and the relative impermeability of the vascular membrane. Pleural effusion develops when any process, such as a disease, alters the normal fluid dynamics of the pleural space.

Pyothorax is an inflammatory condition that results in increased permeability and obstruction of lymphatic drainage, giving rise to the accumulation within the pleural cavity of fluid containing a large amount of protein and cells. Bacteria from the lung parenchyma, trachea, bronchus, oesophagus, and thoracic wall then come into contact with this pleural fluid (McPhail, 2007; Wong and Noor, 1984).

Causes

The origin of pyothorax cannot always be identified. Of the possible causes of pyothorax in cats, the most common include extension of pneumonia, rupture of lung abscesses, parasitic migration, and foreign bodies penetrating from the oesophagus or lung parenchyma. Another cause includes bites from other cats that penetrate the thoracic wall (from which microorganisms of the normal flora of the oral cavity have been isolated). Seasonality has been observed, with infections more frequent in spring and summer owing to an increase in fighting during periods of oestrus.

The risk is greater in households with several cats; larger populations imply a greater incidence of upper respiratory tract infections that predispose cats to bacterial pneumonias and the subsequent development of pyothorax.

The most common organisms are anaerobic bacteria or a mixture of anaerobic and facultative anaerobic bacteria (Box 3).

Clinical signs

While the age range of presentation of pyothorax is very broad, young adult cats are most commonly affected. No breed disposition has been described.

Affected cats present with rapid shallow breathing indicating a restricted respiratory capacity attributable to the presence of fluid in the pleural space.

Box 3. Microorganisms associated with pyothorax.

- *Pasteurella* spp.
- *Escherichia coli*.
- *Actinomyces* spp.
- *Nocardia* spp.
- *Bacteroides* spp.
- *Fusobacterium* spp.
- *Peptostreptococcus* spp.
- *Clostridium* spp.
- *Porphyromonas* spp.
- *Enterobacter* spp.
- *Klebsiella* spp.
- *Staphylococcus* spp.
- *Streptococcus* spp.

Clinical signs are usually very non-specific, and include lethargy, anorexia, weight loss, and cough. About one third of cats show signs of sepsis or systemic inflammatory disease. Bradycardia and salivation may also be observed.

The duration of clinical signs varies widely, from days to months. The presentation can range from subacute dyspnoea to a very slow, insidious process.

Diagnostic tests

Haematology and biochemistry

Common findings include anaemia or stress leukogram. Biochemical alterations are non-specific and include the following:

- Hypoalbuminaemia.
- Hyperglobulinaemia
- Hyper- or hypoglycaemia.
- Electrolyte disturbances.

Radiology

In cases of cats that are highly compromised, with severe dyspnoea, it is necessary to wait before performing diagnostic radiography. In some cases pleural drainage by thoracentesis may be necessary.

Radiographs provide an indication of the extent of pleural effusion (uni- or bilateral) and facilitate assessment of the presence or absence of mediastinal or pulmonary masses.

Visualisation of a pyothorax by radiography reveals a loss of the cardiac silhouette and diaphragmatic border, a widened mediastinum, and collapsed pulmonary lobes (Fig. 8). This collapse manifests as an alveolar pattern that can indicate pulmonary atelectasis or pneumonia.

Radiographs can aid selection of the specific location in which to perform thoracentesis or place a pleural drain.

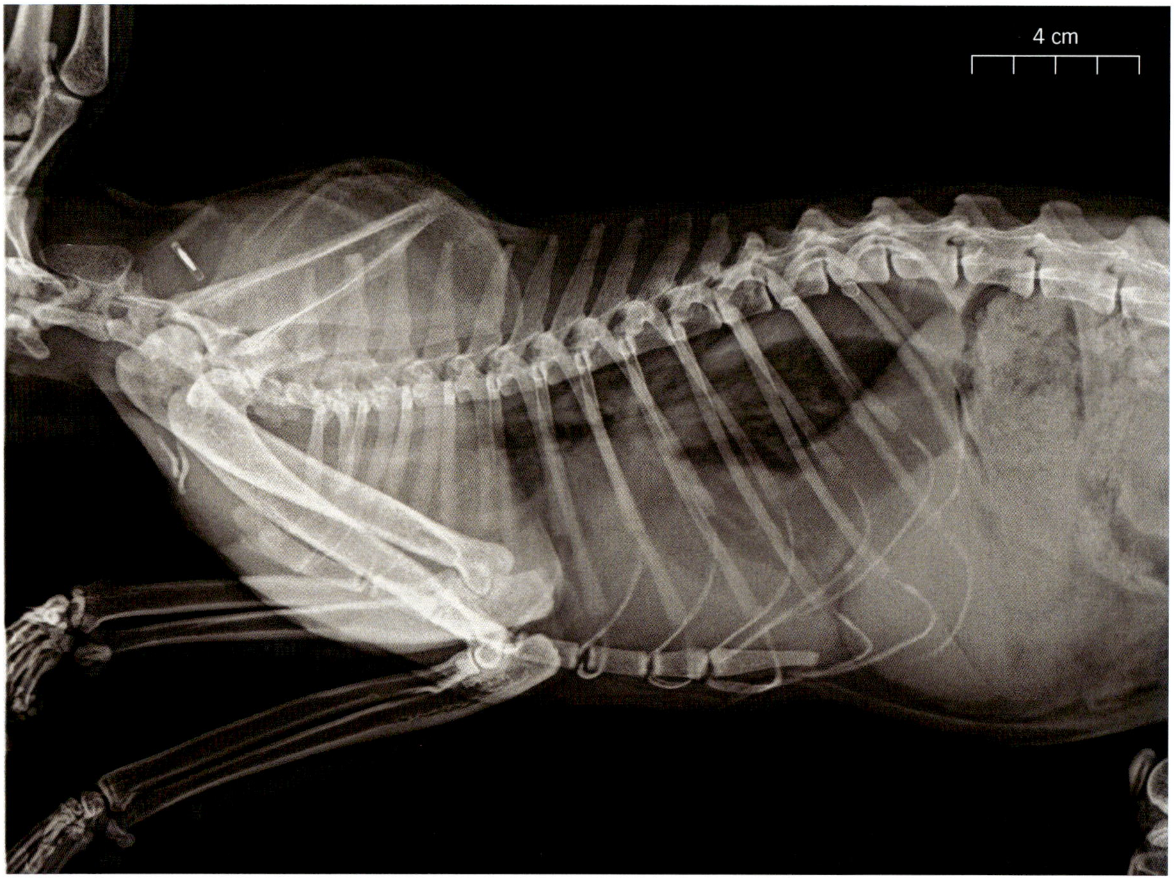

Figure 8. Laterolateral radiograph of a cat with pyothorax.

Analysis of pleural fluid

The pleural fluid typically observed in pyothorax is opaque and haemorrhagic, and in some cases foul smelling (Fig. 9). The protein concentration is greater than 3.0 g/dl, the relative density greater than 1.025, and the cell count greater than 3000 cells/µl, with degenerate neutrophils and bacteria among the most common cell types found. The extracted fluid can also be used for culture and antibiogram.

Based on human medicine protocols, a pleural fluid analysis protocol has been developed. This involves measuring pH and the levels of glucose and the enzyme lactate dehydrogenase (LDH). The results of these measurements help categorise the severity of the process.

A pH of less than 7.2, a glucose concentration of less than 60 mg/dl, and an LDH concentration three times higher than the upper limit in serum (about 200 IU/l) are indicative of a very serious process, with a guarded to poor prognosis, that requires intensive therapy.

Other diagnostic imaging tests

Ultrasound can be of great help in identifying collapsed lungs, mediastinal masses, abscesses, and tumours. It is also used to increase accuracy when performing a puncture to obtain pleural fluid samples in cases of small pleural effusions.

The use of more advanced imaging techniques, such as computed axial tomography (CAT) and magnetic resonance imaging (MRI) is also helpful in diagnosing pyothorax to determine the extent of the process, find small areas of fluid that are inaccessible or insensitive to other diagnostic approaches, or to identify causes that may otherwise go unnoticed.

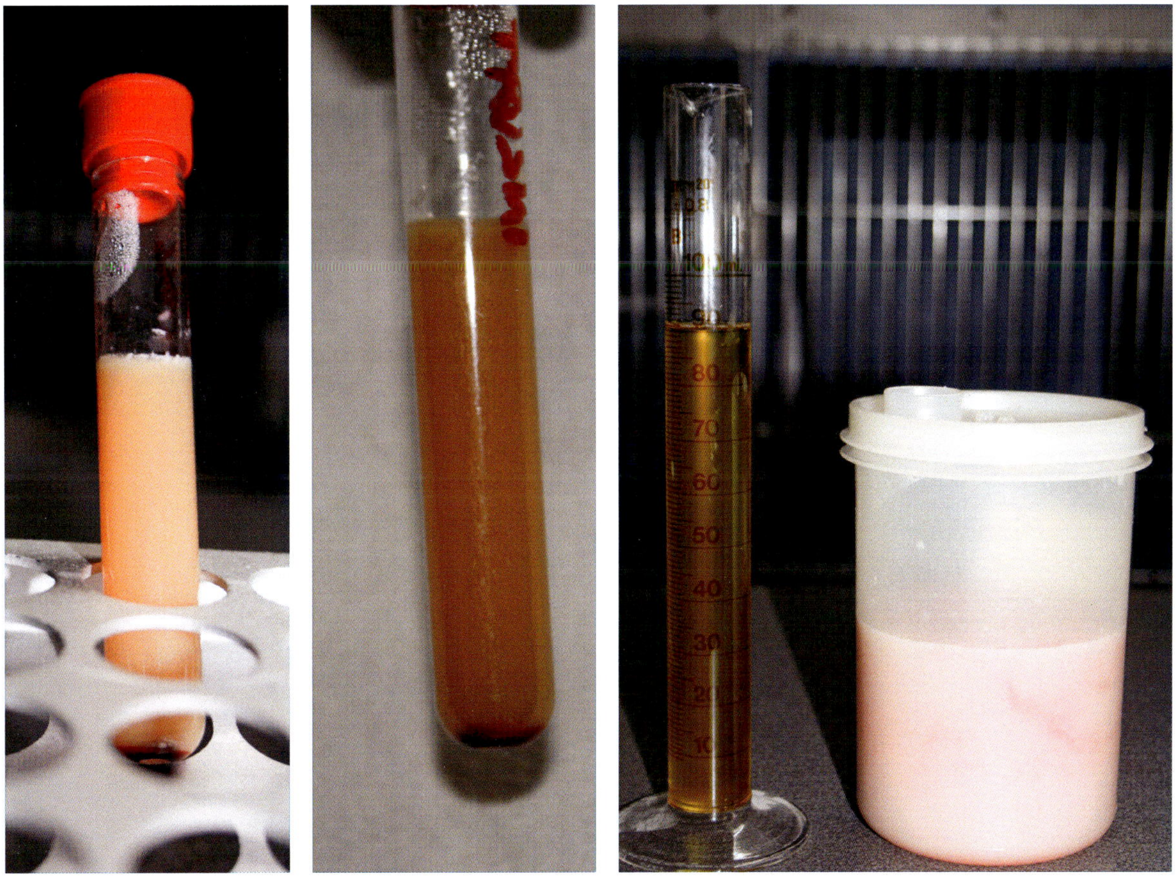

Figure 9. Fluids extracted by thoracocentesis from patients with pyothorax.

Diagnosis

Diagnosis is based on medical history and clinical findings obtained by physical examination, chest radiography, and in the pleural fluid examination.

Treatment

There are many possible treatment options, none of which is ideal. The results of recent studies indicate that basic antimicrobial treatment should first be instituted, while maintaining the necessary care depending on the animal's clinical situation (maintaining fluid therapy, respiratory function, etc.).

Removal of pleural fluid with a drainage needle, placement of a permanent tube, and even exploration of the chest and pleural cavity may be necessary if less invasive procedures are ineffective.

Systemic antimicrobial treatment

A broad-spectrum antibiotic should be initially administered to cover all possible microorganisms that may be involved. Penicillins and their derivatives, which are widely used for this purpose, may be sufficient.

Cefoxitin, enrofloxacin, and sulfamethoxazole + trimethoprim are also a good choices for initial treatment.

If signs of sepsis are observed, administration of antibiotics that cover gram-positive, gram-negative, aerobic, and anaerobic bacteria is necessary.

Once culture results are obtained and the antibiotic to which the microorganism is sensitive is identified, this product should be administered until complete resolution of all signs is observed.

Thoracentesis

Aseptic aspiration using a fine-needle or a butterfly needle coupled to an extension serves as an initial diagnostic method as well as a form of treatment, since this reduces the amount of fluid in the pleural cavity, improving the animal's ventilatory capacity (see appendix on punctures and drainage devices).

> Thoracentesis should be bilateral given that this process usually affects both pleural cavities, regardless of the cause.

Pleural drainage tube or thoracostomy

If the process continues despite aspiration, a thoracostomy tube is inserted to ensure more long-term drainage (see appendix on punctures and drainage devices). When performing aspiration using a fine-needle or butterfly needle, one tube should be placed in each hemithorax.

Washing of the pleural cavity is indicated in human medicine and in dogs, but is controversial in cats, as it can further compromise ventilation and harm the animal.

In human medicine, in addition to washing, fibrinolytic solutions (mainly streptokinase) are infused to disintegrate the fibrosis generated by the presence of fluid in the pleural cavity, thereby facilitating drainage by decreasing the density of the fluid. However, because less fibrin is formed in cats than in humans, this procedure is not as useful in the former.

Thoracotomy

If the situation does not improve after several days of drainage and the amount of fluid in the pleural cavity has not noticeably decreased, it becomes necessary to open the chest to investigate other possible causes that have not been identified using non-invasive techniques.

It is advisable to perform a median sternotomy to allow exploration of both hemithoraces (Fig. 10).

The objectives of this surgery are to evaluate the entire thorax and its contents, identify, remove, and debride all necrotic tissue, and place or replace thoracostomy

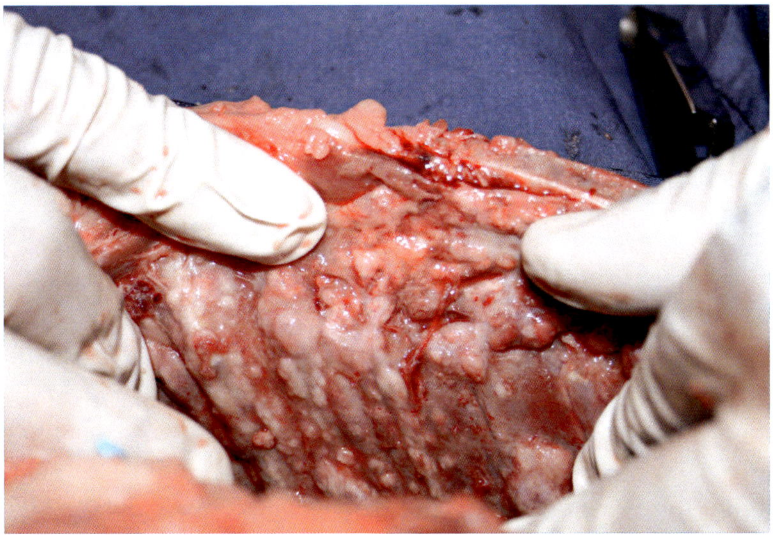

Figure 10. Thoracic wall with multiple granulomas, a consequence of pyothorax.

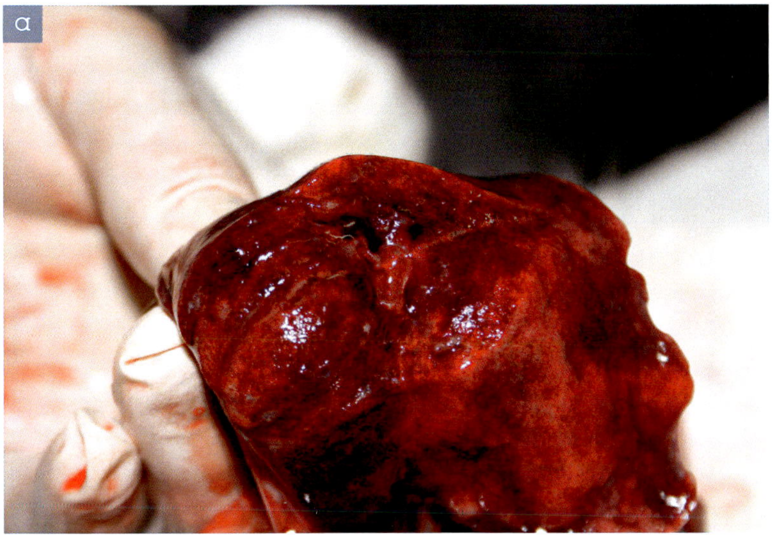

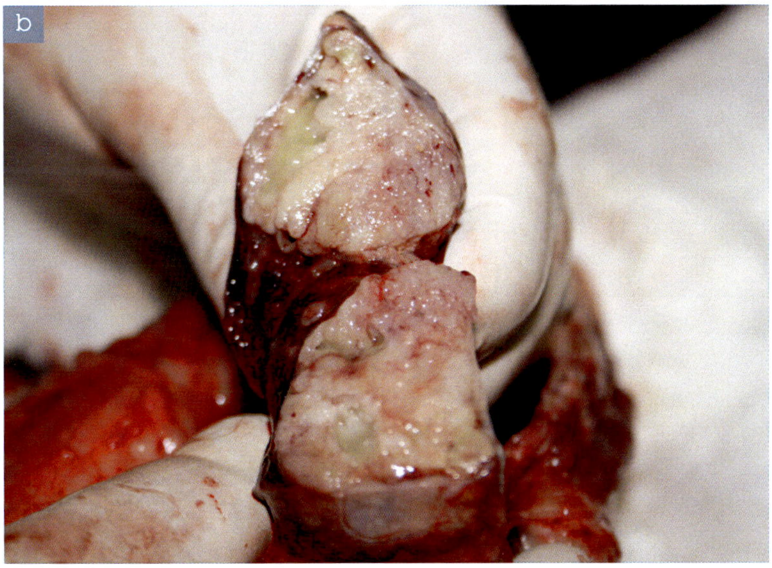

Figure 11. Pulmonary hepatisation (a) and abscess of a lung lobe (b) in a cat with bronchopneumonia caused by pyothorax. In this case a lobectomy was required.

tubes in locations that will ensure optimal drainage of the pleural cavity.

Some cases may require partial or complete removal of a lung lobe or, in cases in which the pericardium is affected, a pericardiectomy (Fig. 11). Culture and histopathology of the extracted material should be performed.

Thoracoscopy

This is a less invasive technique than thoracotomy, somewhere between conservative management and surgery. It is used to study and explore the pleural cavity.

It is a common and first-choice technique in human medicine in cases of pyothorax, but not yet in veterinary medicine.

It is used as a diagnostic technique, to help reduce fibrosis of the pleural cavity, and to ensure proper placement of pleural drainage tubes, thereby ensuring optimal drainage.

Prognosis

The prognosis of pyothorax is highly variable. Mortality rates range from 0 % to 42 %.

The rate of recurrence is also variable, and is higher in cases of pyothorax caused by or involving *Actinomyces* spp. or *Nocardia* spp.

References

BEATTY, J.A., SWIFT, N., FOSTER, D.J., BARRS, V.R. Suspected clindamycin-associated oesophageal injury in cats: five cases. *J Feline Med Surg*, 2006; 8:412–419.

BLUM, S., ELAD, D., ZUKIN, N., et al. Outbreak of *Streptococcus equi* subsp. *zooepidemicus* infections in cats. *Vet Microbiol*, 2010; 144:236–39.

CHANDLER, J.C., LAPPIN, M.R. Mycoplasmal respiratory infections in small animals: 17 cases (1988–1999). *J Am Anim Hosp Assoc*, 2002; 38:111–19.

CHVALA-MANNSBERGER, S., BAGÓ, Z., WEISSENBÖCK, H. Occurrence, morphological characterization and antigen localization of feline herpesvirus-induced pneumonia in cats: a retrospective study (2000–2006). *J Comp Pathol*, 2009; 141:163–69.

COHN, LA. Pulmonary parenchymal disease. En: Ettinger, S.J., Feldman, E.C. (eds.). *Textbook of veterinary internal medicine*. 7th ed. St Louis: Saunders Elsevier, 2010; pp. 1096–119.

DEBERRY, J.D., NORRIS, C.R., SAMII, V.F., GRIFFEY, S.M., ALMY, F.S. Correlation between fine-needle aspiration cytopathology and histopathology of the lung in dogs and cats. *J Am Anim Hosp Assoc*, 2002; 38:327–36.

DEHARD, S., BERNAERTS, F., PEETERS, D., et al. Comparison of bronchoalveolar lavage cytospins and smears in dogs and cats. *J Am Anim Hosp Assoc*, 2008; 44:285–94.

FOLEY, J.E., RAND, C., BANNASCH, M.J., NORRIS, C.R., MILAN, J. Molecular epidemiology of feline bordetellosis in two animal shelters in California, USA. *Prev Vet Med*, 2002; 54:141–56.

FOSTER, S.F., MARTIN, P. Lower respiratory tract infections in cats: Reaching beyond empirical therapy. *J Fel Med Surg*, 2011; 13(5):313-332.

FOSTER, S.F., MARTIN, P., ALLAN, G.S., BARRS, V.R., MALIK, R. Lower respiratory tract infections in cats: 21 cases (1995–2000). *J Feline Med Surg*, 2004a; 6:167–80.

FOSTER, S.F., MARTIN, P., BRADDOCK, J.A., MALIK, R. A retrospective analysis of feline bronchoalveolar lavage cytology and microbiology (1995–2000). *J Feline Med Surg*, 2004b; 6:189–98.

GAGLIO, G., CRINGOLI, G., RINALDI, L., BRIANTI, E., GIANNETTO, S. Use of the FLOTAC technique for the diagnosis of *Aelurostrongylus abstrusus* in the cat. *Parasitol Res*, 2008; 103:1055–57.

GASKELL, R.M., DAWSON, S., RADFORD, A. Feline respiratory disease. En: Green, C.E., (ed.). *Infectious diseases of the dog and cat*. St Louis: Saunders Elsevier, 2006; pp. 145-54.

GERMAN, A.J., CANNON, M.J., DYE, C., et al. Oesophageal strictures in cats associated with doxycycline therapy. *J Feline Med Surg*, 2005; 7:33–41.

GREENE, C.E., PRESCOTT, J.F. Streptococcal and other Gram-positive bacterial infections. En: Greene, C.E. (ed.). *Infectious diseases of the dog and cat*. 3rd ed. St Louis: Saunders Elsevier, 2006; pp. 302–16.

HAMILTON, T.A., HAWKINS, E.C., DENICOLA, D.B. Bronchoalveolar lavage and tracheal wash to determine lung involvement in a cat with cryptococcosis. *J Am Vet Med Assoc*, 1991; 198:655–56.

HARTMANN, A.D., HELPS, C.R., LAPPIN, M.R., WERCKENTHIN, C., HARTMANN, K. Efficacy of pradofloxacin in cats with feline upper respiratory tract disease due to Chlamydophila felis or Mycoplasma infections. *J Vet Intern Med*, 2008; 22:44–52.

HAWKINS, E.C. Bronchoalveolar lavage. En: King, L.G. (ed.). *Textbook of respiratory disease in dogs and cats*. St Louis: Saunders, 2004; pp. 118–28.

HIGHLAND, M.A., BYRNE, B.A., DEBROY, C., SAMITZ, E.M., PETERSON, T.S., OSLUND, K.L. Extraintestinal pathogenic *Escherichia coli*-induced pneumonia in three kittens and fecal prevalence in a clinically healthy cohort population. *J Vet Diagn Invest*, 2009; 21:609–15.

JOHNSON, L.R., DRAZENOVICH, T.L. Flexible bronchoscopy and bronchoalveolar lavage in 68 cats (2001–2006). *J Vet Intern Med*, 2007; 21:219–225.

JOHNSTON, S.L., MARTIN, R.J. Chlamydophila pneumoniae and Mycoplasma pneumoniae: a role in asthma pathogenesis? *Am J Respir Crit Care Med*, 2005; 172:1078–89.

LACORCIA, L., GASSER, R.B., ANDERSON, G.A., BEVERIDGE, I. Comparison of bronchoalveolar lavage fluid examination and other diagnostic techniques with the Baermann technique for detection of naturally occurring Aelurostrongylus abstrusus infection in cats. *J Am Vet Med Assoc*, 2009; 235:43–49.

LALOSEVIC, D., LALOSEVIC, V., KLEM, I., STANOJEV-JOVANOVIC, D., POZIO, E. PULMONARY capillariasis miming bronchial carcinoma. *Am J Trop Med Hyg*, 2008; 78:14–16.

LAST, R.D., SUZUKI, Y., MANNING, T., LINDSAY, D., GALIPEAU, L., WHITBREAD, T.J. A case of fatal systemic toxoplasmosis in a cat being treated with cyclosporin A for feline atopy. *Vet Dermatol*, 2004; 15:194–98.

Little, S. Bordetella bronchiseptica infection in a cat. *Fel Pract*, 2000; 28:12–15.

Macdonald, E.S., Norris, C.R., Berghaus, R.B., Griffey, S.M. Clinicopathologic and radiographic features and etiologic agents in cats with histologically confirmed infectious pneumonia: 39cases (1991–2000). *J Am Vet Med Assoc*, 2003; 223:1142–50.

Malik, R., Lessels, N.S., Webb, S., et al. Treatment of feline herpes-virus-1 associated disease in cats with famciclovir and related drugs. *J Feline Med Surg*, 2009; 11:40–48.

Mc Phail, C.M. Medical and surgical management of piotorax. *Vet Clin Small Anim* 2007; 37:975-988.

Miller, C.J. Approach to the respiratory patient. *Vet Clin Smal Anim*, 2007; 37 861-878.

Norris, C.R. Fungal pneumonia. En: King, L.G. (ed.). *Textbook of respiratory disease in dogs and cats.* St Louis: Saunders, 2004; pp. 446–56.

Norris, C.R., Griffey, S.M., Samii, V.F., Christopher, M.M., Mellema, M.S. Thoracic radiography, bronchoalveolar lavage cytopathology, and pulmonary parenchymal histopathology: a comparison of diagnostic results in 11 cats. *J Am Anim Hosp Assoc*, 2002; 38:337–45.

Padrid, P.A., Feldman, B.F., Funk, K., Samitz, E.M., Reil, D., Cross, C.E. Cytologic, microbiologic, and biochemical analysis of bronchoalveolar lavage fluid obtained from 24 healthy cats. *Am J Vet Res*, 1991; 52:1300–7.

Pedersen, N.C. Mycoplasmal infections. En: Holzworth, J. (ed.). *Diseases of the cat.* Philadelphia: Saunders, 1987; pp. 308–19.

Rollins, D.R., Beuther, D.A., Martin, R.J. Update on infection and antibiotics in asthma. *Curr Allergy Asthma Rep*, 2010; 10:67–73.

Sparkes, A., Wotton, P., Brown, P. Tracheobronchial washing in the dog and cat. *In Practice*, 1997; 19:257–59.

Sura, R., Hinckley, L.S., Risatti, G.R., Smyth, J.A. Fatal necrotising fascitis and myositis in a cat associated with *Streptococcus canis. Vet Rec*, 2008; 162:450–53.

Sura, R., Van Kruiningen, H.J., DebRoy, C., et al. Extraintestinal pathogenic *Escherichia coli*-induced acute necrotizing pneumonia in cats. *Zoonoses Public Health*, 2007; 54:307–13.

Swift, S., Dukes-McEwan, J., Fonfara, S., Loureiro, J.F., Burrow, R. Aetiology and outcome in 90 cats presenting with dyspnoea in a referral population. *J Small Anim Pract*, 2009; 50:466–73.

Syring, R.S. Tracheal washes. En: King, L.G. (ed.). *Textbook of respiratory disease in dogs and cats.* St Louis: Saunders, 2004: 128–34.

Taillefer, M., Dunn, M. Group G streptococcal toxic shock-like syndrome in three cats. *J Am Anim Hosp Assoc*, 2004; 40:418–22.

Telm, L., Grant, C.K., Hurley, K.F. Pathologic, immunohistochemical, and electron microscopic findings in naturally occurring virulent systemic feline calicivirus infection in cats. *Vet Pathol*, 2004; 41:257–63.

Traversa, D., Iorio, R., Otranto, D. Diagnostic and clinical implications of a nested PCR specific for ribosomal DNA of the feline lungworm *Aelurostronglus abstrusus* (Nematoda, Strongylida). *J Clin Microbiol*, 2008; 46:1811–17.

Traversa, D., Milillo, P., Di Cesare, A., et al. Efficacy and safety of emodepside 2.1%/praziquantel 8.6% spot-on formulation in the treatment of feline aelurostrongylosis. *Parasitol Res*, 2009; 105(suppl 1):S83–S89.

Trow, A.V., Rozanski, E.A., Tidwell, A.S. Primary mycoplasma pneumonia associated with reversible respiratory failure in a cat. *J Feline Med Surg*, 2008; 10:398–402.

Waites, K.B., Balish, M.F., Atkinson, T.P. New insights into the pathogenesis and detection of Mycoplasma pneumoniae infections. *Future Microbiol*, 2008; 3:635–48.

Waites, K.B., Talkington, D.F. Mycoplasma pneumoniae and its role as a human pathogen. *Clin Microbiol Rev*, 2004; 17:697–728.

Wong, W.T., Noor, F. Pyothorax in the cat: a report of two cases. *Kajian Vetrinar*, 1984; 16:15–17.

Zekas, L.J., Crawford, J.T., O'Brien, R.T. Computed tomography-guided fine-needle aspirate and tissue-core biopsy of intrathoracic lesions in thirty dogs and cats. *Vet Radiol Ultrasound*, 2005; 46:200–4.

Zhang, S., Wilson, F., Pace, L. *Streptococcus pneumoniae*-associated cellulitis in a two-month-old domestic short hair kitten. *J Vet Diagn Invest*, 2006; 18:221–24.

Zoia, A., Slater, L., Heller, J., Connolly, D., Church, D. A new approach to pleural effusion in cats: markes of distinguising transudates from exudates. *J Feline Med Surg*, 2009; 11(10):847-55.

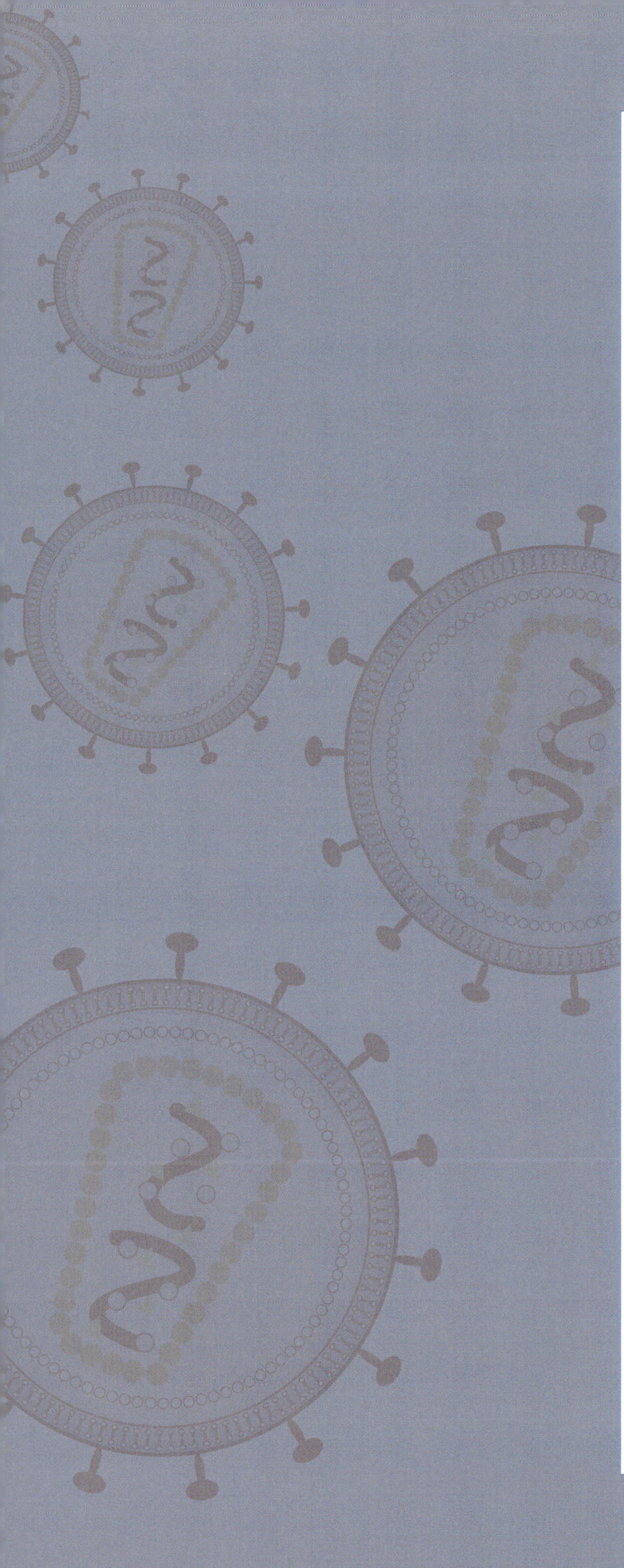

Feline immunodeficiency virus

Feline immunodeficiency virus

Feline immunodeficiency virus (FIV) is a retrovirus of the genus *Lentivirus* that closely resembles HIV, but is species-specific and does not cross-infect humans. It has been isolated from several non-domestic feline species including the puma, leopard, and lion.

The structure of the virus is complex. It possesses accessory genes including *gag*, *pol*, and *env*, which encode various features by which the virus can be distinguished:

- The *gag* gene encodes p24 capsid protein, the identification of which facilitates diagnosis.
- The *pol* gene encodes the protease, integrase, and reverse transcriptase enzymes that account for the virulence of FIV.
- The *env* gene encodes the glycoproteins gp120 and gp41, which are determinants of diversity among isolates (Hartmann, 1998).

Five genetic subtypes have been identified, designated A, B, C, D, and E (Bienzelle et al., 2004; Hosie et al., 2009). The virus is distributed worldwide, with distinct subtypes found in different regions. Most viruses belong to subtypes A and B. In some countries, such as the UK, only group A viruses have been isolated. In others such as Switzerland, Australia, parts of the United States, Japan, Germany and South Africa, type A viruses predominate but other subtypes are also found. Subtype B has been isolated in Spain. Subtype C is less common and subtype D has been isolated only in Japan.

This genetic diversity poses difficulties for those attempting standardise PCR viral identification tests.

The virus is highly labile in the environment; it survives for only a few minutes and is sensitive to any type of disinfectant (Levy et al., 2008; Most et al., 2013).

Epidemiology

FIV has a global distribution in domestic cats. The prevalence of serologically positive animals ranges from 1 % to 14 % in cats without clinical signs and exceeds 44 % in sick cats. It is more common in non-neutered adult male cats (Fig. 1).

The main route of transmission is through bites, resulting in inoculation with the virus itself or with infected cells from the saliva of a persistently infected animal.

Vertical transmission from mother to offspring is possible, although only a small percentage of infected offspring remain infected. This percentage depends on the viral load of the mother during gestation or at birth. If the mother is in a state of active immunodeficiency, over 70 % of kittens will become persistently infected, whereas if the mother is clinically asymptomatic almost no kittens will be infected (MacDonald, 2004; Horzinek, 2013).

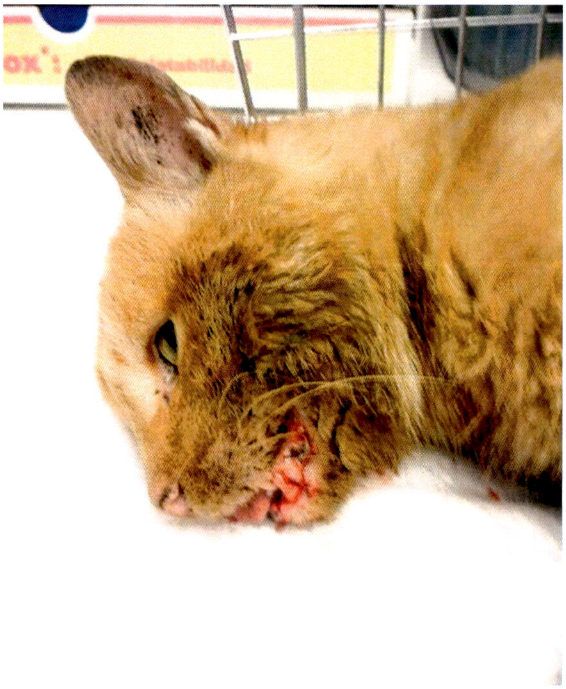

Figure 1. FIV-infected cat taken from a colony.

Pathogenesis

FIV targets CD4+ lymphocytes, which play an important role in the development of cellular and humoural immunity, resulting in destruction and decreased production of these cells, and, consequently, immunodeficiency (MacDonald, 2004; Hosie et al., 2009).

After initial inoculation with FIV, the virus replicates in T and B lymphocytes and macrophages in the lymph nodes, and in lymphoid tissue in other organs such as the spleen and thymus, giving rise to an **acute viraemia phase** that can last for 6 to 10 weeks after infection.

The clinical signs are non-specific:

- Anorexia.
- Lethargy.
- Lymphadenopathy.
- Leukopaenia.

This initial viraemia causes the virus to spread to other lymph tissues in the bone marrow, intestine, lung, kidney, and nervous system.

After dissemination of the virus, viraemia decreases due to the development of cellular and humoural immunity, although this response is insufficient to inactivate the virus.

The next stage is the **lag phase**, an asymptomatic period that can last from months to the entire lifetime of the animal. In this phase, despite the absence of clinical signs, the immune system is gradually weakened, with decreases in the population of CD4+ T lymphocytes and in the CD4+/CD8+ ratio. This period is thus a phase of clinical latency but not viral activity. During the latency phase in a normal viral infection, the virus that has become integrated into the host genome is not expressed in any way, meaning that neither the virus, its genetic material, nor corresponding proteins can be detected.

When the CD4+/CD8+ ratio is so low as to indicate the death of CD4+ lymphocytes the **immunodeficiency phase** begins. This is the period during which opportunistic infections develop. The immune system

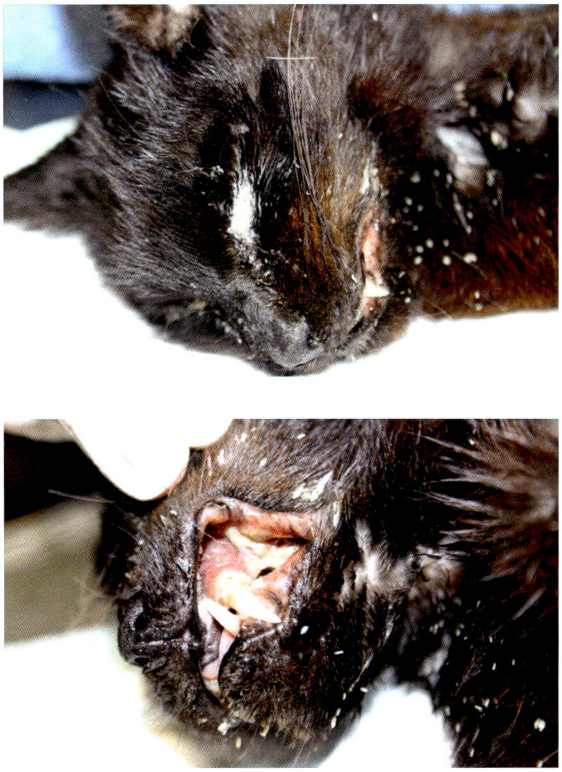

Figures 2 and 3. FIV-infected cat in the immunodeficiency phase with severe myiasis (larval parasitosis).

is unable to develop an effective response (Figs. 2 and 3).

Cats remain infected for life due to the integration of FIV into the host cell genome.

In FIV, the role of passive immunity, whereby an animal acquires antibodies (Ab) through colostrum from vaccinated or FIV-infected mothers, remains unclear. It has been proposed that passive immunity may provide protection against FIV (Hohdatsu, 1993; MacDonald, 2004).

FIV-infected cats are persistently infected, despite all the animal's immunological mechanisms to combat the infection.

CD8+ cells are detected in blood within one week of infection. Infected animals produce anti-FIV antibodies, which are detected between 2 and 4 weeks post-infection, although seroconversion can be delayed if the viral load at the time of exposure is low.

Clinical signs

Non-specific signs produced during the initial viraemia phase can include fever, anorexia, lack of energy, and lymphadenopathy (Levi et al., 2008; Hosie et al., 2009; Horzinek, 2013).

In the immunodeficiency phase clinical signs are the result of infections secondary to this immunodeficiency. It is therefore essential to identify the root cause of these opportunistic infections. Common clinical signs during this period include chronic gingivitis (see appendix on feline oral diseases) (Figs. 4 and 5), chronic rhinitis, dermatological disorders, reproductive disorders, lymphadenopathy, immune-mediated tubulointerstitial glomerulonephritis with proteinuria of variable severity, and tumoural processes such as squamous cell carcinoma and B-cell lymphosarcoma. In general, this period is characterised by weight loss.

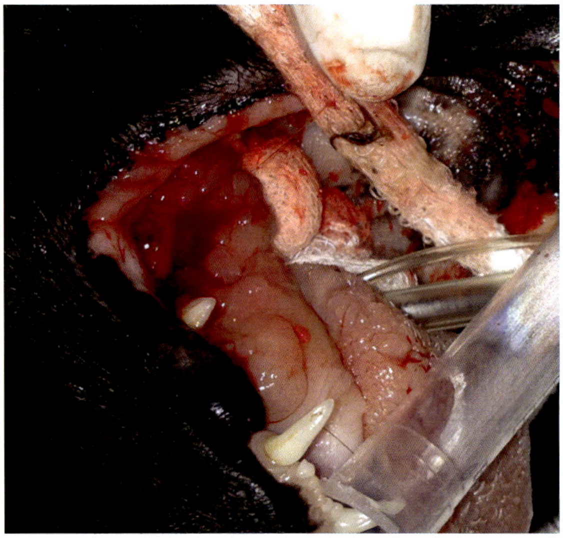

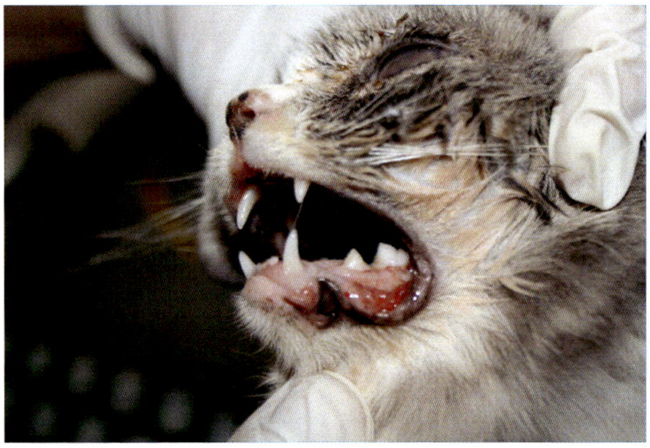

Figures 4 and 5. Chronic gingivitis in FIV-positive cats.

The presence of the virus itself can also cause neurological alterations with peripheral and cerebral neuropathies (with behavioural changes), seizures, alterations in the sleep-wake cycle, and paresis.

As in human medicine, FIV can result in the appearance of amyloid protein in multiple organs including the liver and kidney, impairing organ function due to the replacement of functional organ tissue with amyloid material (Asproni et al., 2013).

Diagnosis

Virus isolation

This is the method of choice for diagnosis. It is a laborious procedure that is not usually used routinely. Samples of peripheral blood or other fluids are cultured.

Polymerase chain reaction

This technique involves the detection of proviral DNA (Crawford, 2005 and 2007). Due to the high genetic variability of the virus, the specificity and sensitivity of the test range from 40 % to 100 %. Consequently, serology is the preferred diagnostic technique. PCR accurately detects subtype A, but results are much more variable for other subtypes, and thus it is not the test of choice in areas in which this subtype is less prevalent (e.g. Spain). Moreover, this technique entails very strict sample handling and transport conditions (Horzinek et al., 2013).

Serology

This is the most widely used test in routine clinical practice. It identifies antibodies through recognition of structural proteins such as membrane protein p24 and the peptide gp41.

The most commonly used techniques are enzyme-linked immunoassay (ELISA) and immunochromatography.

However, in case of doubt, the gold standard test is the Western blot. ELISA detects anti-FIV antibodies based on the presence of p24 protein and membrane antigens (Fig. 6). Immunochromatography detects only membrane protein antibodies. Western blot involves the purification of proteins by electrophoresis and the detection of antibodies corresponding to each FIV subtype.

The sensitivity and specificity of ELISA and immunochromatography are high, approaching 100 %, but depend largely on the predictive value of the test performed, which takes into account the prevalence of the disease in a particular area (Hosie et al., 2009).

Kittens born to FIV-infected mothers can be seropositive as a result of acquired immunity transferred from the mother via maternal antibodies. These cats should be tested at 16 weeks of life, at which point levels of maternal antibodies are thought to decline. However, sometimes these antibodies persist beyond six months of age, and another test should be performed to determine whether levels have decreased (Fig. 7).

In Europe, where no FIV vaccine is available (unlike the United States), serology is a good alternative for the diagnosis of FIV viraemia. Because these tests do not differentiate between vaccinated and infected animals, the vaccination status of any animals that come from the United States should be confirmed.

Discrepancies between the results of serology and PCR are sometimes observed (Bienzele et al., 2004; Horzinek et al., 2013). Negative PCR results may be obtained for seropositive animals if the specific FIV subtype is not recognised by the PCR. Positive PCR results may be obtained for seronegative cats living with other FIV-infected cats, as they may have formed provirus without generating detectable levels of antibody. These animals ultimately become seropositive weeks or months later (Fig. 8).

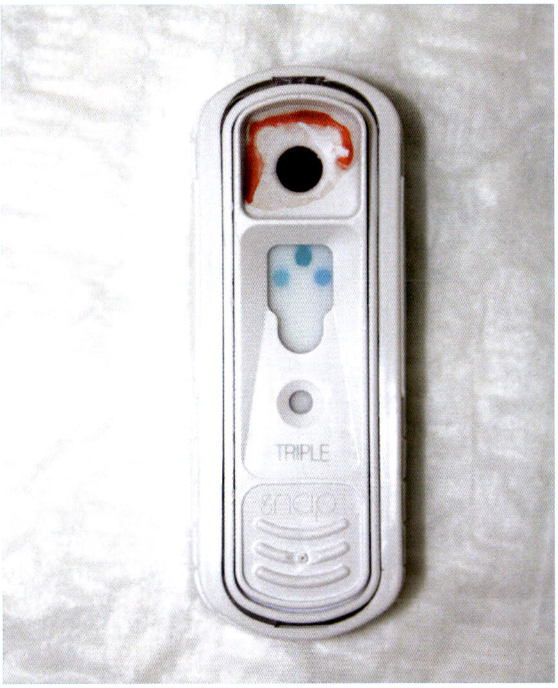

Figure 7. Rapid ELISA serological test showing positive result for FIV and feline infectious leukaemia.

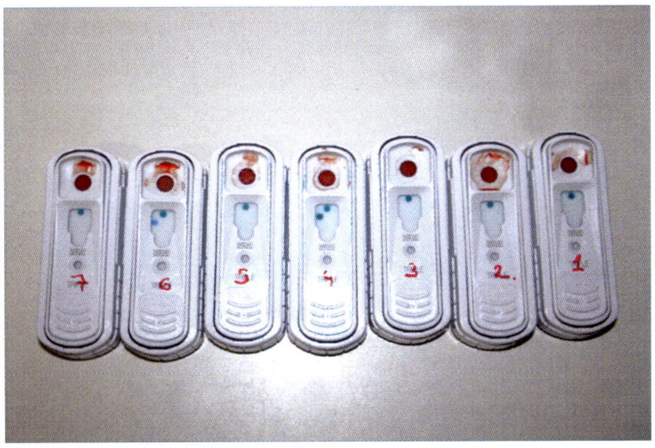

Figure 6. Rapid ELISA serological test for FIV showing 2 positive results out of a population of 7.

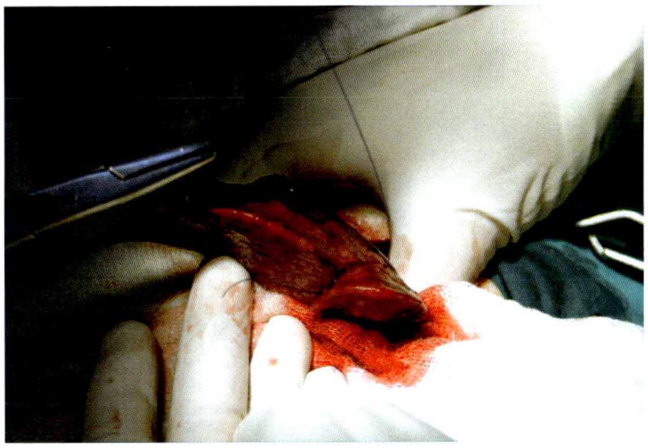

Figure 8. Liver biopsy of an FIV-positive animal that has developed a hepatic lymphosarcoma.

Treatment

In the case of a positive result in an FIV test, current guidelines do not recommend euthanasia, as infected animals can live just as long as uninfected animals. It is estimated that the younger animals are when infected, the more likely they are to progress to the immunodeficiency phase (Levy et al., 2008; Horzinek, 2013).

Initial management of FIV-infected cats seeks to protect against other infectious processes and prevent the progression of FIV infection. It is recommended to keep affected cats indoors. This also limits their capacity to infect other animals. In homes with multiple cats, affected cats should be isolated. Infected animals should be sterilised to limit aggression and attacks. Routine veterinary checks, including weight monitoring, should be conducted approximately every 6 months. Special care should be taken to avoid any situations of stress, such as unnecessary travel. Extra care is also needed during surgical procedures.

Supportive care

Cats that develop clinical signs compatible with the disease should receive supportive treatment as soon as possible to ensure that their immunodeficient state does not result in rapid deterioration.

Some cats require antibiotic treatment for opportunistic infections. The use of corticosteroids or immunomodulators in cats with FIV that develop signs of chronic gingivitis should be approached with care, as these drugs can increase the rate of viral replication.

Human recombinant erythropoietin (EPO) is a safe and effective treatment choice in animals that develop non-regenerative anaemia as a result of myelosuppression caused by concomitant diseases.

Antiviral treatment

Most antiviral drugs used in cats are substances used in human medicine for the treatment of HIV. While some have been used for the management of FIV in cats, certain drugs have proven toxic or ineffective.

Zidovudine or azidothymidine (AZT)

AZT (3-azido-2',3'-dideoxythymidine) is a nucleoside derivative that blocks the reverse transcriptase of retroviruses, inhibiting replication of FIV both *in vitro* and *in vivo*, and enhancing the immune system and therefore the cat's quality of life. A 1995 study (Hartmann et al., 1995) in cats with chronic gingivitis investigated the effects in AZT, administered at doses of 5–10 mg/kg every 12 hours either orally or subcutaneously (diluted in saline to avoid local irritation). Treatment resulted in a marked reduction in inflammation of the oral mucosa, improved appetite, an increase in body weight, and a considerable reduction in viral load.

High doses should be used with caution as they can produce more adverse effects, including reduced bone marrow activity. Therefore, high-dose treatment should be avoided in animals that are already immunosuppressed and should be discontinued when haematocrit levels fall below 20 %.

Plerixafor (AMD3100)

This drug belongs to a new class of selective CXCR4 receptor antagonists, which prevent FIV penetration of the host cell. It is effective *in vitro*, and in a double-blind controlled study of 40 cats naturally infected with FIV it resulted in a dramatic improvement in clinical signs, a reduction in viral load, and no side effects when administered subcutaneously at 0.5 mg/kg every 12 hours for 6 weeks (Hartmann et al., 2002).

(R)-PMPDAP

This is another retroviral drug that has been evaluated in two studies (Tafin et al., 2014; Hartmann et al.,

2014) with promising results; it reduced viral load, but was associated with significant side effects, including a marked reduction in red blood cell count.

Human interferon α

Human interferon α has been tested at different doses, from 1–50 IU/kg PO every 24 hours to 10^4–10^6 IU/kg SC every 24 hours, resulting in improved survival of CD4+ lymphocytes (Pedretti, 2006; EBM grade 3). However, high doses eventually become ineffective as cats develop neutralising antibodies directed against the heterologous interferon.

Feline interferon ω

Feline interferon ω is licensed for use in some European countries and in Japan. It is active against FIV *in vitro*, but has shown no significant effect with respect to placebo in naturally infected animals (De Mari, 2004; EBM grade 1).

Many immunomodulators have been tested in cats with FIV, with a view to activating the immune system in order to improve quality of life and life expectancy. However, the results of all studies conducted provide no evidence to support such an effect, both in animals with and without clinical signs (Crawford, 2007).

Vaccination

Whether or not to vaccinate animals infected with FIV remains a controversial issue. In asymptomatic animals in the early stages of FIV infection, vaccination against other diseases induces a strong immune system response, generating effective neutralising antibodies against these diseases. However, it is unknown whether this same immune response is induced following vaccination of infected animals that already present clinical signs of FIV. Moreover, there is a risk that vaccination will accelerate the progression of the state of immunodeficiency in these animals.

In vivo, vaccination of animals infected with FIV decreases the CD4+/CD8+ ratio. It is therefore important to assess the risks and benefits of vaccination in each animal, depending on the risk of becoming infected in a given area (Most et al., 2013; Levy et al., 2008; Horzinek, 2013).

Currently, no vaccine against FIV is available in Europe. An inactivated virus vaccine has been available in the United States since 2002 and in Australia and New Zealand since 2004. Because these vaccines have not been tested against FIV subtypes found in Europe, current guidelines recommend not vaccinating animals in Europe with FIV vaccines marketed in the aforementioned countries (Horzinek et al ., 2013).

Special considerations

» The risk of transmission of FIV in homes in which several cats live is generally low. However, transmission is a possibility, and should be considered.

» When the population of cats in a house is stable and there is no territory-related stress, the risk of bites and fights, and hence contagion, is low. It is important not to introduce more cats that could alter the balance between individuals in the group.

» In shelters for abandoned cats, it is important to consider the possibility of FIV contagion. It is recommended to analyse all new animals that enter the shelter. Positive FIV test results in cats of less than 6 months of age should be interpreted with caution, and these animals should be retested shortly afterwards.

» FIV is generally not a problem in catteries, in which cats live indoors. However, all new arrivals should be tested.

References

Asproni, P., Abramo, F., Millantra, D., Poli, A. Amyloidosis in association with spontaneus feline inmunodeficiency virus infection. *Jour Fel Med Surg*, 2013; 15:300-306.

Bienzle, D., Reggeti, F., Wen, X., Little, S., Hobson, J., Kruth, S. The variability of serological and molecular diagnosis of feline immunodeficiency virus infection. *Canadian Vet J*, 2004; 45:753-757.

Crawford, P.C., Slater, M.R., Levy, J.K. Accuracy of polymerase chain reaction assays for diagnosis of feline immunodeficiency virus infection in cats. *J Am Vet Med Assoc*, 2005; 226(9):1503-7.

Crawford, P.C., Levy, J.K. New challenges for the diagnosis of feline immunodeficiency virus infection. *Vet Clin North Am Small Anim Pract*, 2007; 37(2):335-50.

De Mari, K., Maynard, L., Sanquer, A., Lebreux, B., Eun, H.M. Therapeutic effects of recombinant feline interferon-omega on feline leukemia virus (FeLV)-infected and FeLV/feline immunodeficiency virus (FIV)-coinfected symptomatic cats. *J Vet Intern Med*, 2004; 18(4):477-82.

Hartmann, A., Wilheulum, N., Balzarini, J., Hartmann, K. Clinical efficacy of the acyclic nucleoside phosphonate 9-(2-phosphonylmethoxypropyl)-2,6-diaminopurina (PMPDAP) in the treatment of feline inmunodeficiency virus-infected cats. *Jour Fel Med Surg*, 2014; 2:107-112.

Hartmann, K. Feline immunodeficiency virus infection: an overview. *Vet J*, 1998; 155:123-137.

Hartmann, K., Donath, A., Kraft, W. AZT in the treatment of feline immunodeficiency virus infection. Part 2. *Fel Pract*, 1995; 6:13-20.

Hartmann, K., Stengel, S., Klein, D., Egberink, H., Balzarini, J. Efficacy of the chemokine receptor inhibitor 1,1'-bis-1,4,8,11-tetraazazacyclotetradekan against feline immunodeficiency virus infection. Abstract, 6th International Feline Retrovirus Research Symposium. Amelia Island, USA, 2002; 26.

Hohdatsu, T., Pu, R., Torres, B.A., Trujillo, S., Gardner, M.B., Yamamoto, J.K. Passive antibody protection of cats against feline immunodeficiency virus infection. *J Virol*, 1993; 67(4):2344-8.

Horzinek, M., Addie, D., Lutz, H., Lloret, A., et al. Update of the 2009 guidelines. *J Fel Med Surg*, 2013; 15:530-532.

Hosie, M., Addie, D., Belak, S., et al. Feline Inmunodeficiency: ABCD Guidelines on prevention and management. *Jour Fel Med Surg*, 2009; 11:575-584.

Levy, J., Crawford, C., Hartmann, K., Little, S. 2008 American Association of Feline Practitioners' feline retrovirus management guideline. *J Fel Med Surg*, 2008; 10:300-316.

MacDonald, K., Levy, J.K., Tucker, S.J., Crawford, P.C. Effects of passive transfer of immunity on results of diagnostic tests for antibodies against feline immunodeficiency virus in kittens born to vaccinated queens. *J Am Vet Med Assoc*, 2004; 225:1554-1557.

Most, K., Egberink, H.J., Addie, D., Frymus, T., Hartmann, K., et al. Prevention of infections diseases in cats helters. ABCD guidelines. *J Fel Med Surg*, 2013; 15:546-554.

Pedretti, E., Passeri, B., Amadori, M., Isola, P., Di Pede, P., Telera, A., Vescovini, R., Quintavalla, F., Pistello, M. Low-dose interferon-alpha treatment for feline immunodeficiency virus infection. *Vet Immunol Immunopathol*, 2006; 109(3-4):245-54.

Tafin, E., Paepe, D., Goris, N., Auwers, J., Debille, M., et al. Antiviral treatment of feline immunodeficiency virus-infected cat with (R)9-(2phosphonylmethoxypropyl)-2,6-diaminopurina. *Jour Fel Med and Surg*, 2014; 1-8.

CASE STUDIES

CASE STUDY 1: *Bree*

Review: non-neutered male adult cat of indeterminate age.

Reason for consultation: poor general appearance. Examination prior to addition to a cat colony.

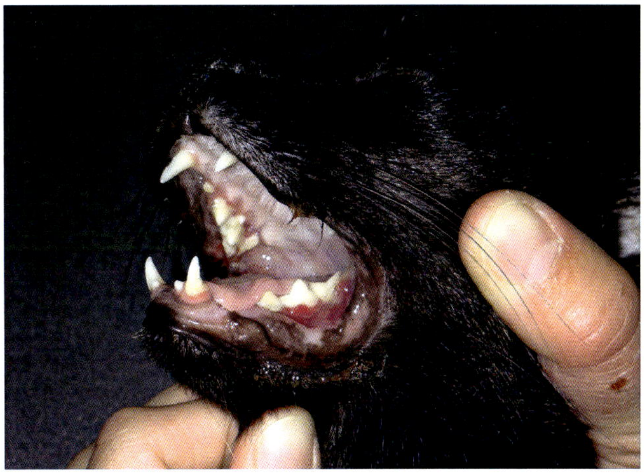

Figure 1. Oral mucosa of the patient.

Medical history

Bree has recently joined an apparently controlled colony of sterilised cats that are negative for feline leukaemia virus and feline immunodeficiency virus.

Physical examination and diagnostic tests

The cat is very thin, with a body mass index of 2/9, and has a dirty haircoat due to poor grooming behaviour. It presents with bilateral otitis externa, chronic gingivitis affecting the entire oral mucosa covering the teeth, and inflammation and necrosis of the caudal oral mucosa and the palatoglossal arch (Figs. 1 and 2). The retropharyngeal lymph nodes are enlarged.

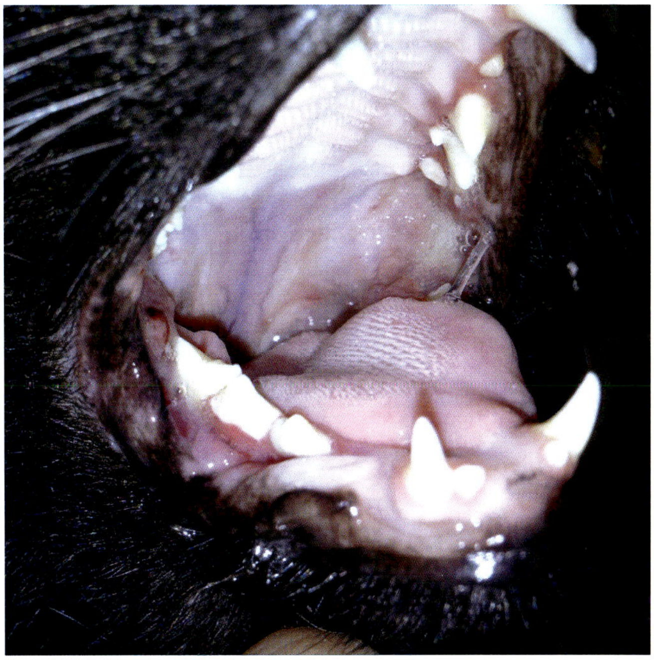

Figure 2. Oral examination of *Bree*, revealing chronic gingivitis.

Table 1. Results of blood tests.

Analysis		Result	Reference
Complete blood count	Erythrocytes	4.5×10^{12}/l	$5.0–10 \times 10^{12}$/l
	Platelets	123×10^{9}/l	$175–400 \times 10^{9}$/l
	Leukocytes	2.3×10^{9}/l	$5.5–19.5 \times 10^{9}$/l
	Neutrophils	1.3×10^{9}/l	$2.5–12.5 \times 10^{9}$/l
	Lymphocytes	0.8×10^{9}/l	$0.4–6.8 \times 10^{9}$/l
Biochemistry	ALT	175 IU/l	25-45 IU/l
	AST	145 IU/l	25–75 IU/l
	Alkaline phosphatase	455 IU/l	<145 IU/l
	Blood urea nitrogen (BUN)	0.5 mg/dl	7–32 mg/dl
	Creatinine	0.8 mg/dl	0.6–1.6 mg/dl
	Total protein	9.5 g/dl	5.5–7.5 g/dl
	Albumin	0.5 g/dl	2.1–4.0 g/dl

Table 2. Results of viral test.

Test	Result	Reference
FIV (Ab ELISA)	Positive	Negative
Calicivirus (PCR)	Positive	Negative

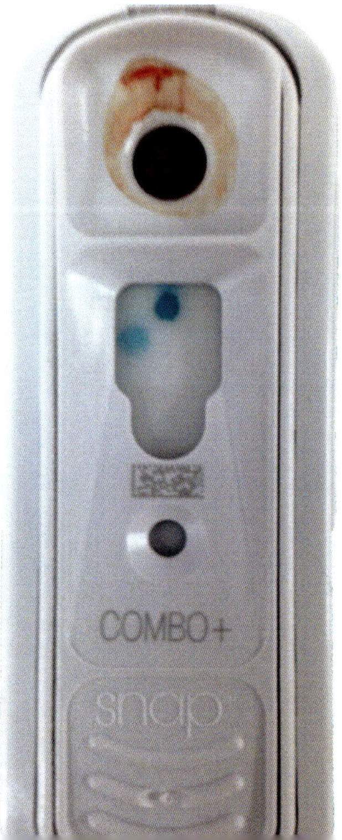

Figure 3. Rapid ELISA test positive for FIV.

A general blood test is performed, the results of which are shown in Table 1.

A rapid retrovirus test and a PCR test for calicivirus are performed (Table 2, Fig. 3).

Recommended treatment

The animal is hospitalised due to dehydration and its temperature monitored. Fluid therapy is applied (see appendix on fluid therapy).

Antibiotic treatment is administered (marbofloxacin, 2 mg/kg IV every 24 hours), as well as the analgesic buprenorphine (20 mg/kg IV every 8 hours).

Oral gavage is attempted, but the cat refuses food. After two days of hospitalisation, *Bree* is more active and eats of his own volition, albeit in insufficient quantities.

It is decided to perform a complete dental extraction to improve the chronic gingivitis (see appendix on feline oral disease) and to insert an oesophagostomy tube.

After three days of hospitalisation, *Bree* is moved to a shelter run by a cat protection association with instructions to feed at home and to continue oral marbofloxacin and buprenorphine treatment, as well as anti-inflammatory treatment with oral meloxicam (0.1 mg/kg on first day and 0.05 mg/kg per day thereafter).

Follow-up

Two weeks after the dental extraction, *Bree* is able to feed without an oesophagostomy tube.

Oral examination reveals a marked improvement of the oral mucosa surrounding the teeth, as well as the caudal oral mucosa and palatoglossal arch. Antibiotic treatment is withdrawn and the feeding tube is removed. Analgesic and anti-inflammatory (meloxicam) treatment are maintained.

Bree is lost to follow-up for 6 months due to constant changes from one foster home to another. At the next examination, *Bree* is extremely thin (BMI, 2/9), dehydrated, and has a wiry haircoat. The anamnesis indicates that Bree has visited the veterinary clinic numerous times and has received oral and intralesional interferon treatment as well as periodic treatment with slow release methylprednisolone. Despite initial improvements, none have been observed in recent visits.

A new blood test is performed, the results of which are shown in Table 3.

Bree is hospitalised again and an oesophagostomy tube inserted. After one week of analgesic, anti-inflammatory, and antibiotic treatment, *Bree* is sent home to be tube-fed and is prescribed zidovudine (AZT) at a dose of 5 mg/kg PO every 12 hours for 8 weeks.

On the next visit, the inflammation of the oral mucosa has almost fully abated. Oral zidovudine and meloxicam treatment is withdrawn.

From this point *Bree* undergoes regular evaluations. Zidovudine and meloxicam treatment is instituted each time the inflammation of the oral mucosa worsens, and is withdrawn as soon as haematocrit values approach 20 %.

Four years after the first consultation, *Bree* is diagnosed with hyperthyroidism, which is controlled with oral methimazole every 12 hours.

Table 3. Results of blood tests.

Analysis		Result	Reference
Complete blood count	Erythrocytes	3.2×10^{12}/l	5.0–10 × 10^{12}/l
	Platelets	274 × 10^9/l	175–400 × 10^9/l
	Leukocytes	10.5 × 10^9/l	5.5–19.5 × 10^9/l
	Neutrophils	7.3 × 10^9/l	2.5–12.5 × 10^9/l
	Lymphocytes	2.3 × 10^9/l	0.4–6.8 × 10^9/l
Biochemistry	ALT	225 IU/l	25–45 IU/l
	AST	195 IU/l	25–75 IU/l
	Alkaline phosphatase	350 IU/l	<145 IU/l
	Blood urea nitrogen (BUN)	0.9 mg/dl	7–32 mg/dl
	Creatinine	1.2 mg/dl	0.6–1.6 mg/dl
	Total protein	9.1 g/dl	5.5–7.5 g/dl
	Albumin	1.2 g/dl	2.1–4.0 g/dl

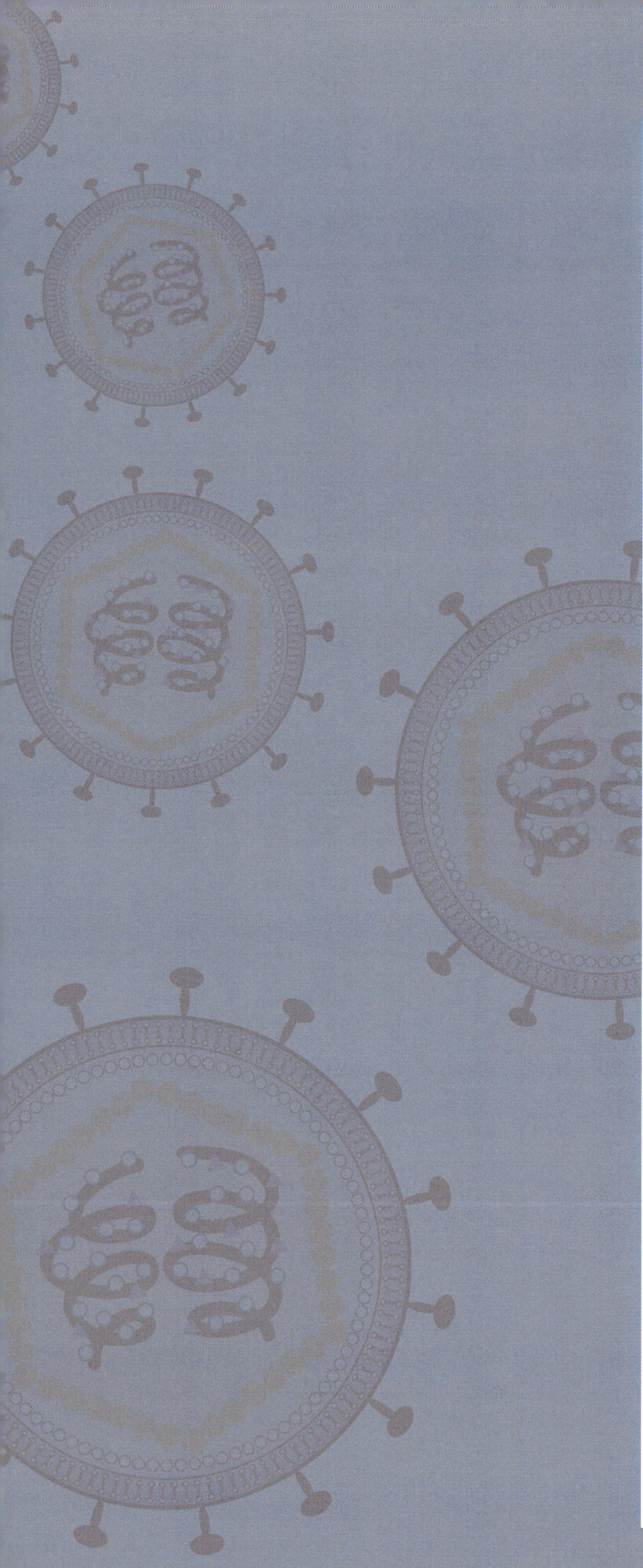

Feline leukaemia virus

Feline leukaemia virus

Feline leukaemia virus (FeLV) is a retrovirus of the genus *Gammaretrovirus*. It has a worldwide distribution and affects domestic cats as well as wild feline species including the bobcat, lynx, and panther (Horzinek et al., 2013; Levy et al., 2008; Lutz et al., 2009).

It consists of an enveloped ribonucleic acid (RNA) strand. The single strand makes contact with the host cell, and is integrated into its genome and transcribed into its DNA to form a **provirus** (Hofmann-Lehmann et al., 2001).

FeLV has three associated genes: *gag*, *pol*, and *env*. These genes encode proteins that account for the virus's special features, including its oncogenic capacity:

- The *gag* gene encodes structural proteins, which are found in all subtypes.
- The *pol* gene encodes polymerase, which is responsible for viral replication mediated by protease, integrase, and reverse transcriptase enzymes.
- The *env* gene encodes the envelope protein, which facilitates penetration and integration of the virus into the host genome. The most important proteins are gp70 and p15e. Anti-gp70 antibodies are specific to each subgroup. These neutralise the virus and confer immunity to reinfection. The p15e protein promotes viral persistence.

The presence of an envelope makes this virus extremely labile in the environment, where it is rapidly inactivated, and highly sensitive to any disinfectant.

All cats harbour endogenous virus, the result of the adaptation of ancestral forms via multiple mutations over many generations. These endogenous viruses are not pathogenic, but can exchange genetic information with exogenous retroviruses to produce other highly pathogenic retroviruses. The most important of these are the endogenous feline leukaemia virus (enFeLV) and the RD114 virus. Exogenous retroviruses are transmitted directly. The most important are FeLV, which causes chronic leukaemia, and feline sarcoma virus (FeSV), which causes acute leukaemia.

Four subtypes of FeLV are described; A, B, C and T, which differ in terms of cell tropism and pathogenesis:

- **Subtype A:** involved in all infections and found in all viraemic cats. This subtype produces tumours when combined with subtypes B or C.
- **Subtype B:** this is the result of recombination between subtype A and enFeLV. It is not transmitted. It is associated with the development of lymphomas.
- **Subtype C:** this is the result of a mutation in the *env* gene. This rare subtype causes alterations of red blood cells including anaemia and erythroid leukaemia.
- **Subtype T:** variant of subtype A. Shows tropism for T lymphocytes, causing immunosuppression of variable severity.

Subtypes B and C require subtype A to cause infection (Horzinek et al., 2013; Levy et al., 2008; Lutz et al., 2009).

Epidemiology

FeLV has a worldwide distribution. Its prevalence, which is influenced by the density of cats living in a given territory, has changed in recent years. FeLV also exhibits geographical variability. In some European countries, as well as the United States and Canada, its prevalence is very low (less than 1 %), while in other countries or specific regions its prevalence can reach 20 %. Its prevalence has declined in recent years thanks to a better understanding of its pathogenesis, increased availability of diagnostic tests, and the introduction of highly effective vaccines (Lutz et al., 2009).

Infection is transmitted by viraemic cats. Transmission occurs via saliva, nasal secretions, faeces, and milk. Risk factors for transmission include high population density, young age, and poor hygiene.

Viraemic pregnant females may experience abortions or stillbirths, or kittens may be born viraemic and very weak. Rapid perinatal death is frequent. Females in the latent phase of infection generally do not transmit FeLV when pregnant, although some kittens may become viraemic after birth as a result of transmission via the mammary glands (milk). The virus can remain dormant in the mammary gland, meaning that the animal tests negative for FeLV, but can be reactivated during lactation and can be contagious for kittens.

Kittens are especially vulnerable to FeLV infection, and become more resistant with age, although infection is always possible and depends on many factors (Levy et al., 2008).

Pathogenesis

When the virus first makes contact with the cat initial viral replication occurs in the cells (lymphocytes and macrophages) of the oropharyngeal cavity (Horzinek et al., 2013; Levy et al., 2008; Lutz et al., 2009). Viral RNA is intergrated into the host cell and is transcribed into DNA (provirus).

Next, depending on the capacity of the immune system, replication can occur in lymphocytes and blood monocytes, the thymus, spleen, lymph nodes, and salivary glands. This viraemic phase generally lasts between 3 and 16 weeks, but can be prolonged to up to one year.

The outcome of this phase varies depending on the immune response of the cat, as described below.

Immunocompetent cat

The immune response is effective, limiting the process to preinfection of the oropharynx with no systemic dissemination. This occurs in between 2 % and 30 % of cases. The cat will be serologically negative for p27 protein and in most cases it will never be evident that the cat contracted FeLV, unless PCR analysis of oropharyngeal samples is performed. These cats have high titres of neutralising antibodies (Ab) and are resistant to subsequent exposure. This is known as **abortive viraemia**.

Immuncompromised cat

Infection results in an insufficient, non-neutralising immune response, leading to primary viraemia in the oropharynx and subsequent systemic dissemination of the virus. The infection produces mild clinical signs including fever, malaise, and lymphadenopathy. This can give rise to several possible scenarios:

1. **Transient regressive viraemia:** between 30 % and 40 % of immunocompromised cats experience transient regressive viraemia lasting 3 to 4 weeks, during which they are contagious and serologically positive for p27 protein. After this period they can overcome the infection. They become serologically negative for p27 protein, but DNA-PCR, which is a highly sensitive technique (Gomes-Keller et al., 2006; Tandom et al., 2005), can detect the presence of the provirus in blood lymphocytes and monocytes. While cats do not completely eliminate the virus, they are not infectious and viral replication does not occur.
2. **Progressive or persistent viraemia:** between 30 % and 40 % of immunocompromised cats develop progressive or persistent viraemia. Viraemia lasts more than three weeks, and the immune system

fails to produce neutralising antibodies to eliminate the virus. The virus invades the cells of the bone marrow, after which the immune system is unable to eliminate the virus. The cat becomes persistently serologically positive for p27 protein and enters an asymptomatic latency phase, which lasts from 3 months to 3 years. This is ultimately followed by death from some pathogenic manifestation of the disease. The probability of this outcome depends on the cat's age and immune status at the time of infection, the duration of exposure, and the viral load.

3. **Latent infection:** some cats mount a delayed immune response that eliminates the viraemia but does not completely eliminate the infection. These cats remain with a persistent latent viral infection of the bone marrow. They are serologically negative for p27 protein, but test positive in DNA-PCR analyses of bone marrow samples. These animals show no clinical signs and are not infectious to other cats. Stressful situations can result in reactivation of the disease. The probability of reactivation is greater during the first year after infection, and subsequently decreases.
4. **Discordant cats:** less than 5 % of cats develop atypical infections. These animals are serologically positive for p27 protein but are negative in RNA-PCR analyses. Tests for the detection of p27 reveal incomplete portions of the virus from different FeLV-infected tissues in which the virus may be harboured, including the bladder, eye, and glandular system. The virus does not replicate in either blood or bone marrow, and thus is not infectious.

In these animals the virus triggers a CD8+ T-lymphocyte-mediated **cellular immune response** 1 to 2 weeks after infection. This response eliminates FeLV-infected cells and precedes the development of antibodies.

The subsequent **humoural immune response** is characterised by the generation of antibodies against p27 and the envelope glycoprotein gp70, and the formation of circulating antigen-antibody (Ag-Ab) immune complexes. Deposition of these immune complexes on organ surfaces will trigger immune-mediated disease in the affected organs.

Clinical signs

FeLV infection can cause a wide range of clinical signs, which affect most persistently infected animals. These include immunosuppression, anaemia, and tumoural diseases associated with the presence of FeLV (Hornisek et al., 2013; Levy et al., 2008; Lutz et al., 2009).

Immunodepression

This is a rather complex situation that results in atrophy of the thymus as well as lymphopaenia, neutropaenia, abnormal neutrophil function, and the loss of CD4+ and CD8+ T lymphocytes.

It can result in the development of concurrent infections such as salmonellosis, cryptococcosis, toxoplasmosis, mycoplasmosis, and other viral infections, the consequences of which are exacerbated. Immunodepression can also result in the complication of chronic rhinitis, subcutaneous abscesses, and chronic gingivostomatitis (see appendix on feline oral disease).

Anaemia

FeLV-infected animals can develop different types of anaemia. The most common form is non-regenerative anaemia, but regenerative anaemia associated with haemolysis secondary to opportunistic infections such as mycoplasma or immune-mediated haemolysis can also occur.

Non-regenerative anaemia occurs in cats infected with FeLV subtype C, which interferes with the heme binding protein, or as a result of chronic inflammatory mechanisms, myelodestruction, myelosuppression, or myeloproliferative disease.

Other cytopaenias that may be observed include thrombocytopaenia and neutropaenia, caused by immune-mediated mechanisms triggered by the action of the virus and by myelosuppression.

Cancer

Several types of cancer have been associated with FeLV infection. These include lymphoma (Weis et al., 2010) and leukaemia, as well as other malignant non-hematopoietic tumours such as fibrosarcoma (observed in young viraemic animals), which is associated with FeSV or recombination of FeLV subtype A with cellular oncogenes.

FeLV induces the development of lymphomas as a consequence of myeloproliferative alterations. Lymphomas can develop in different locations, and include thymic or cranial mediastinal lymphoma, alimentary lymphoma, which can affect various digestive organs (stomach, intestine, colon, liver, pancreas) (Figs. 1–7), multicentric lymphoma, and atypical or extranodal lymphoma, an isolated form that can affect organs such as the kidney, the central nervous system, or the skin.

Injection-site sarcomas have not been associated with either FeLV or FeSV (Lutz *et al.,* 2009).

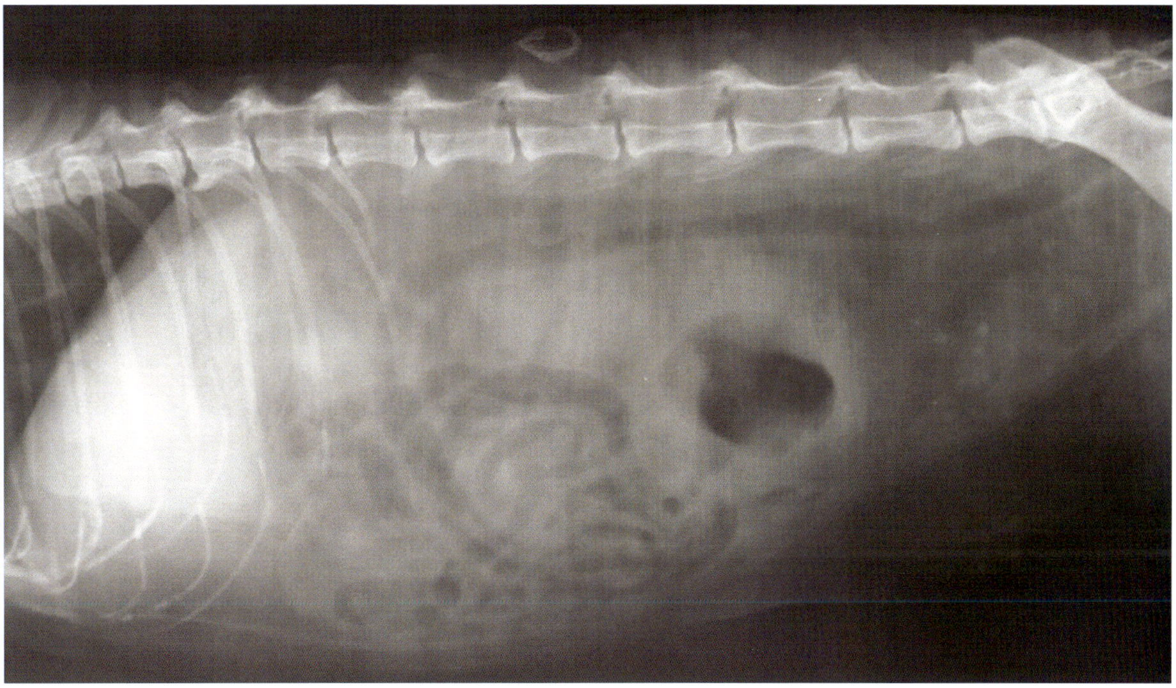

Figure 1. Laterolateral abdominal radiograph of a cat that had lost weight in the preceding weeks, but had retained its appetite and experienced no vomiting. An air-containing structure, the exact location of which cannot be determined, is observed in the mid-abdomen.

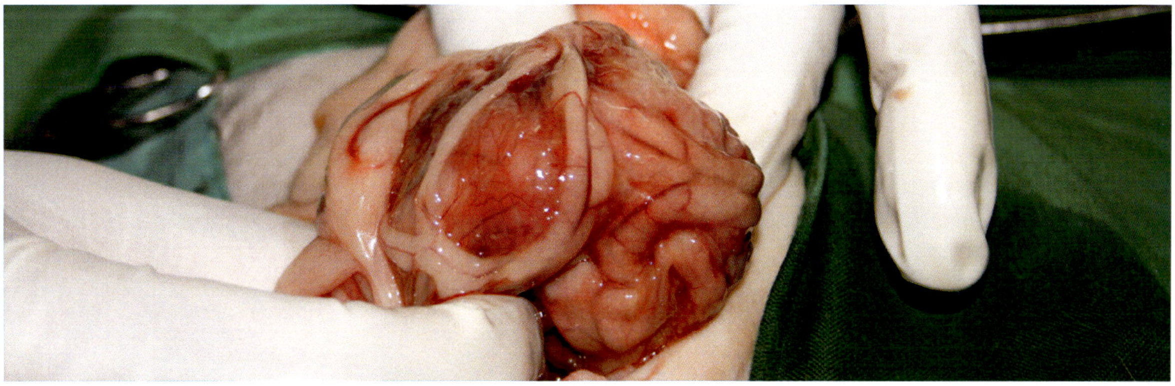

Figure 2. Exploratory laparotomy of cat from previous image, revealing a large mass almost completely covered in omentum.

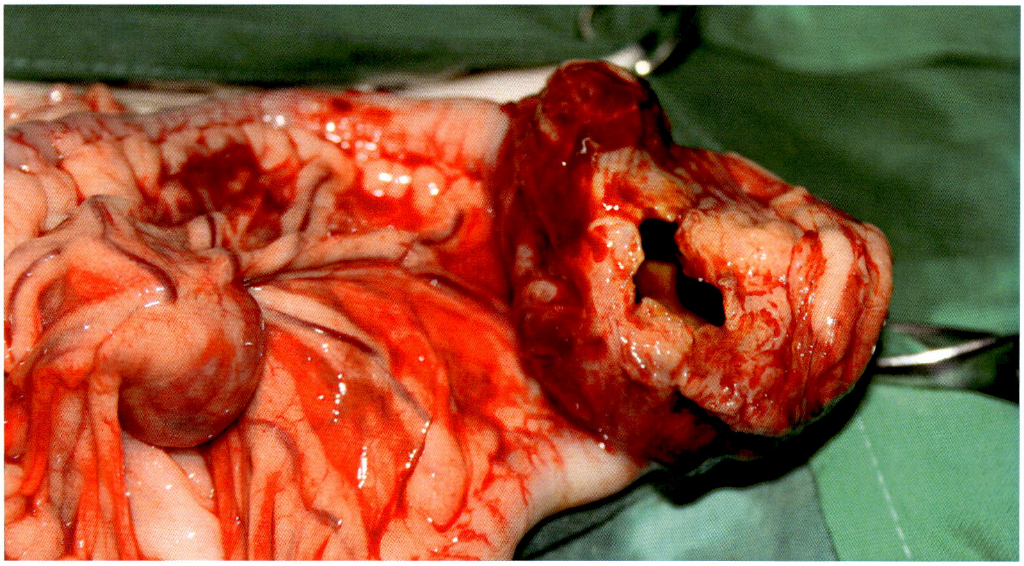

Figure 3. Cat from preceding images: removal of the omentum reveals a perforated, cavitated mass corresponding to a segment of jejunum. A diagnosis of high-grade intestinal lymphoma is established. Analyses reveal that the cat is positive for FeLV.

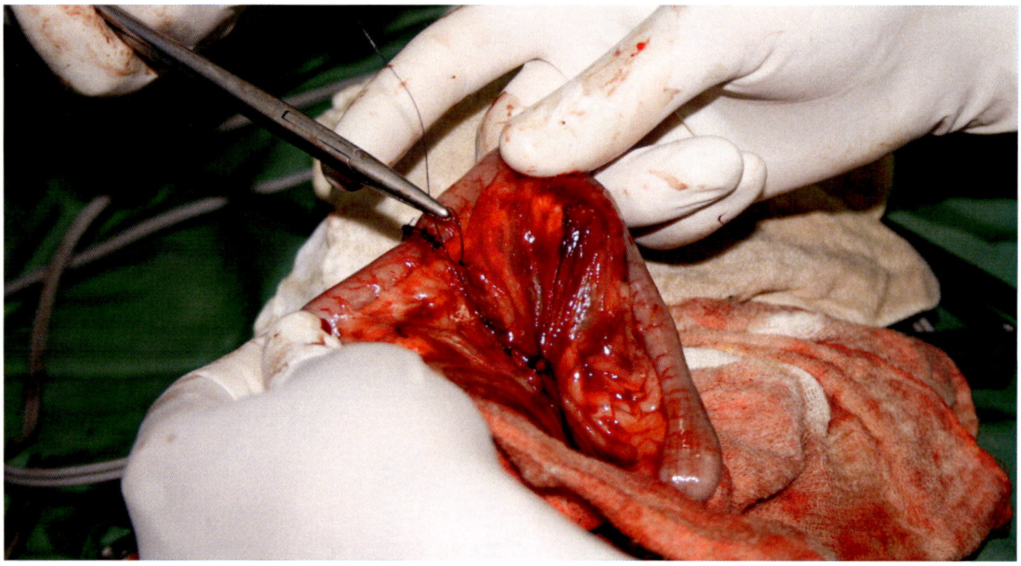

Figure 4. Wide intestinal resection, with margins, and subsequent termino-terminal anastomosis.

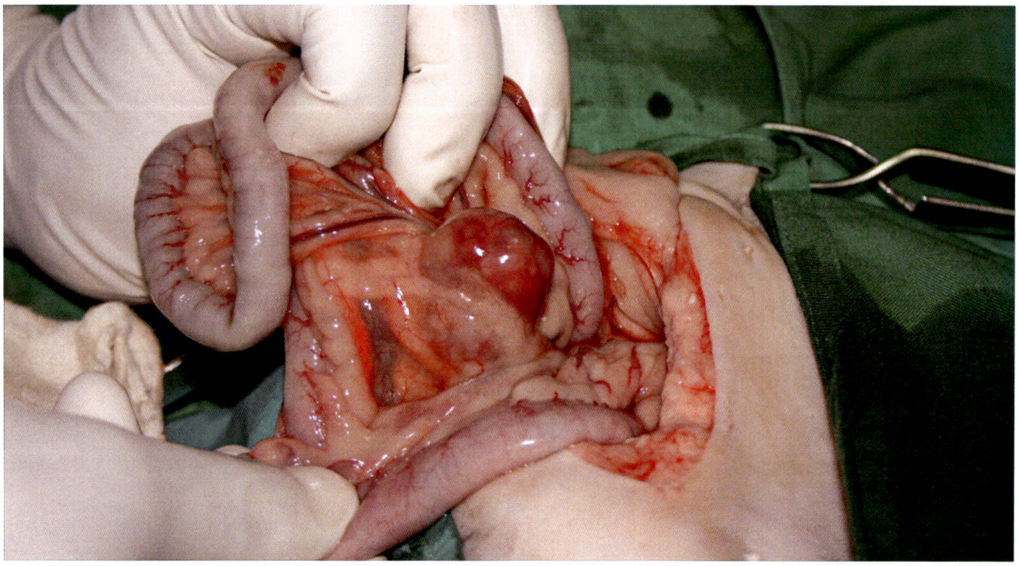

Figure 5. Caudal mesenteric lymph node of an FeLV-positive cat with an infiltrative lymphocytic process compatible with lymphoma.

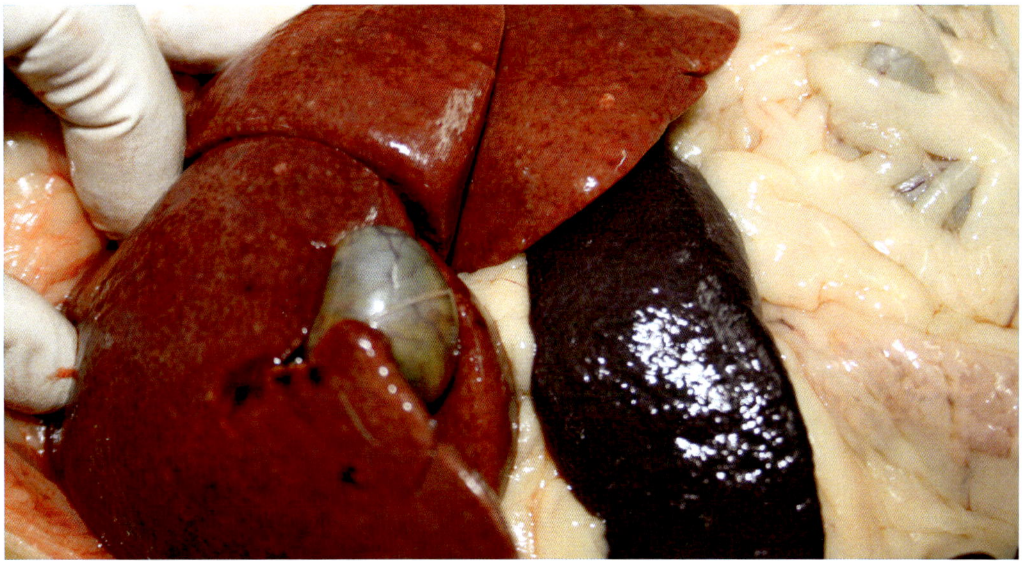

Figure 6. Liver of an FeLV-positive cat with an infiltrative lymphocytic process compatible with lymphoma.

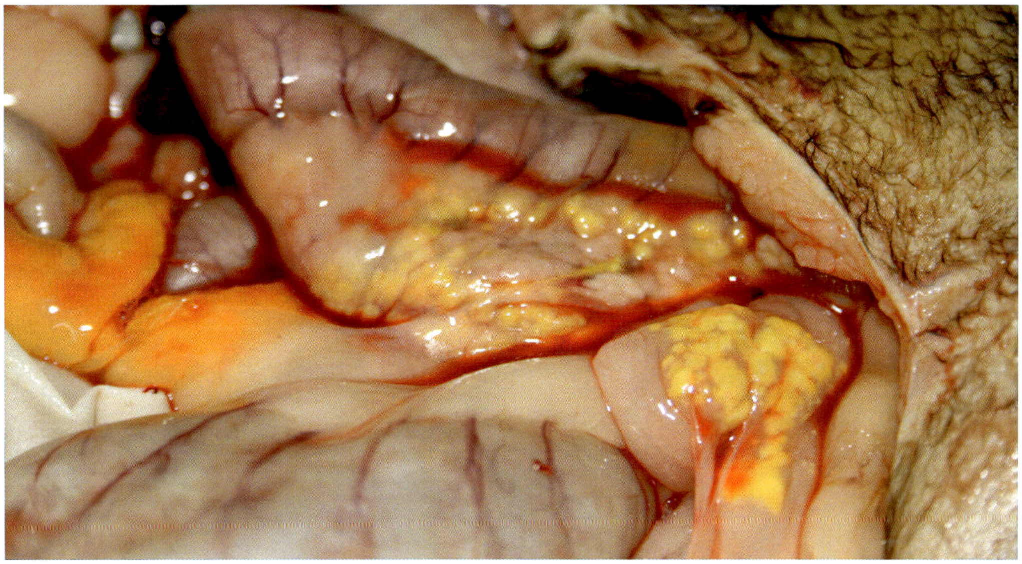

Figure 7. Pancreas of a FeLV-positive cat with an infiltrative lymphocytic process compatible with lymphoma.

Other diseases associated with FeLV infection include glomerulonephritis (Figs. 8 and 9) and polyarthritis, consequences of Ag-Ab immune complex deposition or the loss of regulatory T-cell activity. Chronic enteritis with degeneration and necrosis of the intestinal crypts caused by the presence of FeLV has also been described. Other problems associated with the presence of FeLV include reproductive disorders and the birth of weak kittens that die soon after birth.

FeLV can also cause other neurological manifestations that are not the result of neurological lymphomas or opportunistic infections. These include peripheral neuropathies such as anisocoria, mydriasis, Horner syndrome (Fig. 10), urinary incontinence, abnormal vocalisation, hyperaesthesia, paresis, and paralysis, all of which are direct consequences of the action of the virus.

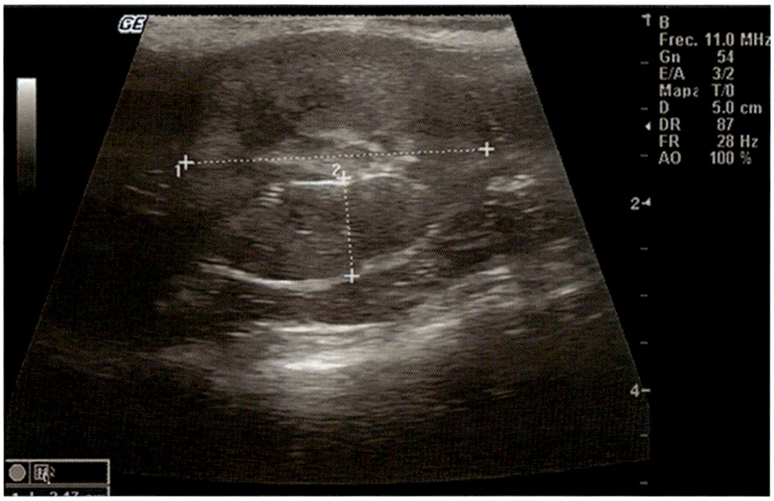

Figure 8. Renal ultrasound of a FeLV-positive cat that has developed glomerulonephritis, which ultimately proved fatal.

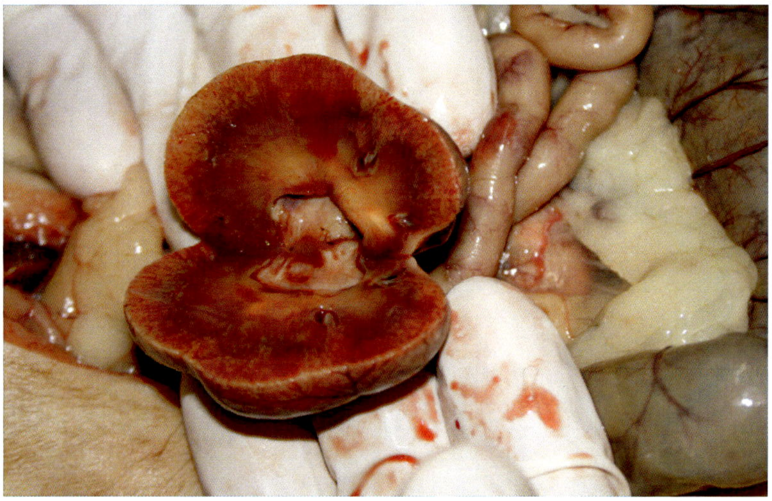

Figure 9. Kidney as seen during necropsy of cat from previous image.

Diagnosis

Virus isolation

Virus isolation in cell culture is the definitive test for the presence of FeLV. In the early stages of the disease, virus isolation is the most sensitive approach, but is generally not the first method of choice (Horzinek et al., 2013).

ELISA (p27)

Enzyme-linked immunoassay demonstrates the presence of FeLV antigen by detecting p27 protein (positive antigenaemia) in whole blood, plasma, or serum (Fig. 11), using a single monoclonal antibody. The advantage of ELISA is that it is a highly sensitive and specific test, depending on the gold standard selected. One study (Hofmann-Lehmann et al., 2001), in which the method of choice was proviral DNA-PCR, reported ELISA sensitivity and specificity of 90 % and almost 100 %, respectively. If virus isolation is the method of choice, ELISA has a sensitivity and specificity of 90 % and 98 %, respectively (Hartmann et al., 2001).

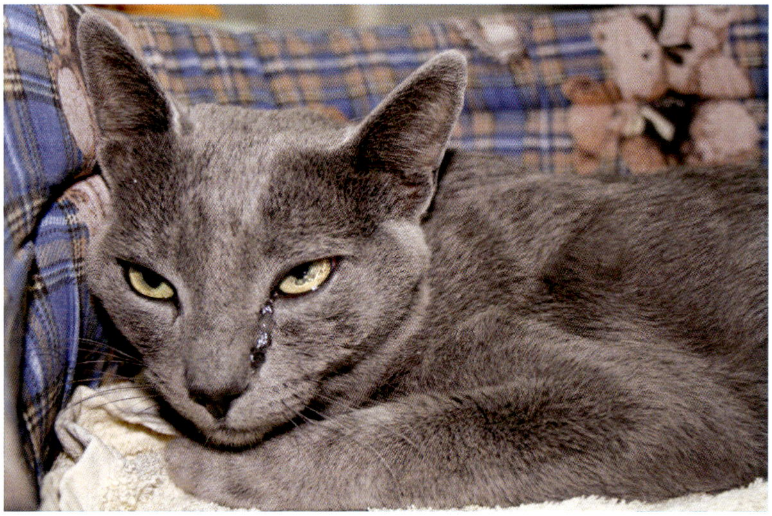

Figure 10. FeLV-positive cat with neurological signs including anisocoria and Horner syndrome.

FeLV-infected cats will test positive in analyses performed 28 days or more post-infection.

Immunochromatography

This method is similar to ELISA, and detects p27 with comparable sensitivity and specificity (Hartmann et al., 2007; EBM grade 1).

Immunofluorescent antibody test

The immunofluorescent antibody (IFA) test was the first method used for the detection of FeLV in field conditions (Gomes-Keller et al., 2006). It detects viral p27 antigen within infected cells, particularly platelets and neutrophils. The sensitivity of this test, with virus isolation as the method of choice, is almost 100 %. Cats with positive IFA results are persistently infected. This test was used until the development of PCR and its subsequent universal standardisation as the method of choice for confirming the presence of FeLV infection. IFA detects persistent infection, rather than the mere presence of the disease, and thus does not detect infection in early stages.

False negatives can be obtained in animals with cytopaenia, neutropaenia, and thrombocytopaenia.

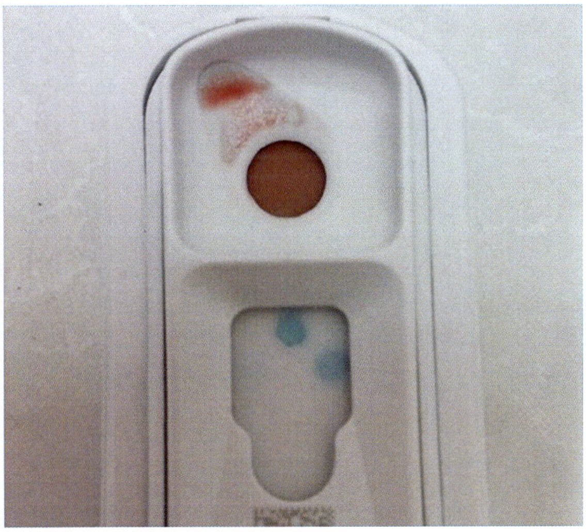

Figure 11. Positive result in a rapid ELISA test for FeLV.

PCR for detection of provirus (DNA-PCR)

Since the development of real-time PCR, this technique has enabled the identification and quantification of provirus DNA (Hofmann-Lehmann et al., 2001; Pinches et al., 2007; Tandom et al., 2005). It offers high sensitivity and specificity, depending on the clinical condition of the cat.

Some cats that have been exposed to the virus and have recovered from viraemia retain viral genetic material in their genome, and thus may test positive despite a lack of clinical significance.

PCR is useful in the following cases:

- When ELISA and IFA results are contradictory.
- In cats to be used as donors; despite the absence of infection, the presence of viral genetic material in the cat's genome can give rise to infection.
- If there is a suspicion of latent infection, which can be confirmed by detection of the presence of the virus in bone marrow.

Using RT-PCR, a study of discordant animals with positive ELISA and negative virus isolation results found that 85 % of these animals were positive for FeLV (Pinches et al., 2007).

Another study (Weis et al., 2010) found that at least 80 % of T-cell lymphomas and 60 % of B-cell lymphomas contain FeLV proviral DNA, which can be detected by RT-PCR. Analysis of these same cases using ELISA (p27) would have produced negative results.

PCR for detection of viral RNA (RNA-PCR)

With this technique FeLV genetic material (RNA) is directly detected in whole blood, plasma, serum, saliva, or faeces. It allows the detection, identification, and quantification of FeLV in the absence of cells into which it has been integrated. RNA-PCR and DNA-PCR do not provide the same information. Many animals that have overcome viraemia still harbour provirus, and thus will test positive in DNA-PCR tests but negative in RNA-PCR tests. Therefore, RNA-PCR is used to detect viraemic animals (Gomes-Keller et al., 2006; Tandon et al., 2005).

Serology

This is no longer a commonly used technique, owing to the presence of endogenous FeLV antibodies and the availability nowadays of vaccines against FeLV.

Interpretation of test results

The fastest means of determining whether an animal is positive for FeLV is virus isolation, followed by PCR, ELISA, and finally IFA assay (Lutz et al., 2009). The most commonly used tests are ELISA and immunochromatography for the detection of p27 antigen.

The predictive value of each test depends on multiple factors. Currently, owing to the reduced incidence of the disease, more false positives are obtained. A positive result in a p27 antigen detection test is less likely in a healthy population than in a population of animals showing signs of disease.

FeLV-positive cats can overcome viraemia within a few (8–12) weeks, although this period may be prolonged, and these animals should be reanalysed to determine their FeLV status.

Cats that eliminate the virus from plasma are negative in virus isolation tests, ELISA, immunochromatography, IFA, and RNA-PCR, but remain positive in the DNA-PCR test and are considered latent carriers (Gomes-Keller et al., 2006; EBM grade 1).

Between 2 % and 3 % of cats remain positive in ELISA or immunochromatography assays, but lack detectable virus in plasma samples. These animals (discordant cats), which are potential sources of infection, have a focus of infection in a tissue outside of the bone marrow that releases p27 into the circulation.

Therefore, p27 antigen detection by ELISA or immunochromatography should be the first test conducted. If any inconsistencies are observed in the results, additional tests should be performed to determine the animal's FeLV status (preferably DNA-PCR of bone marrow samples).

Management of infection

Animals infected with FeLV should be confined indoors, both to avoid infection of other cats and to protect them against other infectious process that could complicate the clinical picture (Hartmann, 2005; Horzinek et al., 2013; Hosie et al., 2013).

In the case of asymptomatic FeLV-infected animals, a health assessment should be performed and disease prevention measures applied every six months, without waiting for the appearance of clinical signs of disease. This should include blood tests with a complete blood count and biochemical analyses, as well as urinalysis.

Deworming and vaccination measures should also be strictly applied, although the latter remains a topic of debate. Inactivated vaccines are recommended since modified live vaccines can produce clinical signs in immunocompromised animals.

FeLV-infected animals should be sterilised to minimise stress and to avoid exposure of other animals to the virus.

A rapid and effective means of establishing diagnosis is required to ensure that treatment can be instituted as soon as possible in order to avoid rapid deterioration. As a result of immunodepression, some infected animals can develop infectious diseases that require antibiotic treatment. In these cases, the use of corticosteroids and immunosuppressive drugs should be avoided as much as possible, except in situations in which they are recommended for specific conditions associated with FeLV (e.g. cancer and immune-mediated diseases).

Animals should be provided with the best care possible depending on their clinical status. They may require fluid therapy, antibiotic treatment, management of conditions such as chronic gingivostomatitis, blood transfusions in cases of severe anaemia, interventions such as abdominal or thoracic puncture/drainage (see corresponding appendices), or chemotherapy in the case of lymphomas associated with the presence of FeLV.

Immunomodulators

There is little scientific evidence supporting the use of these drugs to stimulate the immune system and improve the quality of life or life expectancy of FeLV-infected animals (Hartmann et al., 2006).

Antiviral drugs

There are few studies of the efficacy of specific antiviral drugs, some of which have many adverse effects (Hartmann, 2005 and 2006).

Feline interferon ω

This inhibits viral recombination *in vitro* and can alleviate clinical signs in persistently viraemic animals (De Mari et al., 2004; EBM grade 1) at doses of 10^6 IU/kg SC, administered daily for 5 consecutive days, and repeated up to 3 times at intervals of several weeks.

Zidovudine (AZT)

AZT (3-azido-2',3'-dideoxythymidine) is a nucleoside derivative that blocks the action of reverse transcriptase in retroviruses. It inhibits replication of FeLV both *in vitro* and *in vivo* in experimentally infected animals, reducing viral load and improving both immune system function and clinical status. It is administered in doses of 5–10 mg/kg every 12 hours, PO or SC. High doses may cause adverse effects such as regenerative anaemia (Hartmann, 2005; EBM grade 1).

However, a study by Stuetzer and coworkers (2012) reported no improvements compared with controls in animals treated with AZT or human interferon α, either alone or in combination.

Raltegravir

This antiretroviral drug is used to treat HIV AIDS in human medicine, and inhibits the action of integrase during FeLV replication (Cattori et al., 2011; Horzinek et al., 2013). In experimental conditions treatment for 15 weeks significantly improves the clinical status of infected animals, markedly decreasing viral load, albeit without completely eliminating viraemia. At the time of writing, no studies have replicated these effects observed in experimental conditions in naturally infected animals. However, in our experience using raltegravir for 2.5 years, results observed in FeLV-infected cats are very encouraging. Raltegravir is administered at 40 mg/kg per day, divided into two doses.

Prevention

FeLV is not one of the viruses covered by the essential vaccine program (core vaccines) (Brunner et al., 2006, Hofmann-Lehmann et al., 2006 and 2007).

Significant research effort has been devoted to the production of vaccines against FeLV, resulting in the development of inactivated adjuvanted vaccines and recombinant (non-adjuvanted) vaccines. A new vaccine has been recently released in Europe, and is licensed for revaccination of animals up to every three years. All provide a high degree of protection against disease, but not against infection, and therefore prevent animals from developing the fatal form of the disease.

Many vaccines produce immunity to FeLV for at least 12 months, which is the interval after which most manufacturers recommend revaccination. However, in the opinion of expert panels (Horzinek et al., 2013; Levy et al., 2008; Lutz et al., 2009), such vaccine pressure is unnecessary, and animals can be revaccinated every 2 or 3 years depending on their risk of FeLV infection. Primary vaccination is recommended, especially in kittens, with a first dose administered at 8 to 9 weeks of age, followed by a second dose at 12 to 13 weeks and revaccination one year later.

Disease control in specific situations

» **Homes with multiple cats**
If an animal is diagnosed with FeLV, all animals should be retested.
Those who test positive should be moved. It is important to identify FeLV-positive cats to prevent infection of other animals, even though they may be vaccinated (Horzinek et al., 2013; Hosie et al., 2013).

» **Cat shelters**
The prevalence of FeLV is typically much higher in cat shelters. Expert panels continue to recommend euthanasia of infected animals to prevent infection of other animals, and given their low life expectancy and minimal chances of adoption. However, nowadays this practice is much less common thanks to social awareness and the creation of protective associations that identify these animals and treat them with new therapies, offering them a chance of survival that was not previously possible.

In these rescue centres periodical testing for FeLV every 2 to 3 years is recommended, and all new cats should be tested before entering.

References

BRUNNER, C., KANELLOS, T., MELI, M.L., SUTTON, D.J., GISLER, R., GOMES-KELLER, M.A., HOFMANN-LEHMANN, R., LUTZ, H. Antibody induction after combined application of an adjuvanted recombinant FeLV vaccine and a multivalent modified live virus vaccine with a chlamydial component. *Vaccine*, 2006; 24(11):1838-46.

CATTORI, V., WEIBEL, B., LUTZ, H. Inhibition of feline Leukaemia virus replication by the integrasa inhibitor Raltegravir. *Veterinary Microbiology*, 2011; 152: 165-168.

DE MARI, K., MAYNARD, L., SANQUER, A., LEBREUX, B., EUN, H.M. Therapeutic effects of recombinant feline interferon-omega on feline leukemia virus (FeLV)-infected and feline immunodeficiency virus (FIV)-coinfected symptomatic cats. *J Vet Intern Med*, 2004; 18(4):477-82.

GOMES-KELLER, M.A., GONCZI, E., TANDON, R., RIONDATO, F., HOFMANN-LEHMANN, R., MELI, M.L., LUTZ, H. Detection of feline leukemia virus RNA in saliva from naturally infected cats and correlation of PCR results with those of current diagnostic methods. *J Clin Microbiol*, 2006; 44(3):916-22.

HARTMANN, K., GRIESSMAYR, P., SCHULZ, B., GREENE, C.E., VIDYASHANKAR, A.N., JARRETT, O., EGBERINK, H.F. Quality of different in-clinic test systems for feline immunodeficiency virus and feline leukaemia virus infection. *J Feline Med Surg*, 2007; 9(6):439-45.

HARTMANN, K., WERNER, R.M., EGBERINK, H., JARRETT, O. Comparison of six inhouse tests for the rapid diagnosis of feline immunodeficiency and feline leukaemia virus infections. *Vet Rec*, 2001; 149(11):317-20.

HARTMANN, K. Antiviral and inmunomodulatory chemotherapy. En: Green, C.E. (Ed.). *Infectious Diseases of the Dog and Cat*. 3rd edition. Elsevier Saunders, St Louis, USA, 2006; pp. 10-25.

HARTMANN, K. FeLV treatment strategies and prognosis. *Suppl Compend Contin Educ Pract Vet*, 2005; 27:14-26.

HOFMANN-LEHMANN, R., CATTORI, V., TANDON, R., BORETTI, F.S., MELI, M.L., RIOND, B., PEPIN, A.C., WILLI, B., OSSENT, P., LUTZ, H. Vaccination against the feline leukaemia virus: Outcome and response categories and long-term follow-up. *Vaccine*, 2007; 25(30):5531-5539.

HOFMANN-LEHMANN, R., HUDER, J.B., GRUBER, S., BORETTI, F., SIGRIST, B., LUTZ, H. Feline leukaemia provirus load during the course of experimental infection and in naturally infected cats. *J Gen Virol*, 2001; 82(Pt 7):1589-96.

HOFMANN-LEHMANN, R., TANDON, R., BORETTI, F.S., MELI, M.L., WILLI, B., CATTORI, V., GOMES-KELLER, M.A., OSSENT, P., GOLDER, M.C., FLYNN, J.N., et al. Reassessment of feline leukaemia virus (FeLV) vaccines with novel sensitive molecular assays. *Vaccine*, 2006; 24(8):1087-94.

HORZINEK, M., ADDIE, D., HARTMAN, K., et al. Update of the 2009 guidelines on prevention and management of feline infections diseases. *J Fel Med Surg*, 2013; 15:520-539.

HOSIE, M., ADDIE, D., BELAK, S., et al. ABCD recomendations for indoor/outdoor cats, rescue shelter cats and breeding catteries. *J Fel Med Surg*, 2013; 15:540-544.

LEVY, J., CRAWFORD, C., HARTMAN, K., HOFMANN-LEHMANN, R., LITLLE, S., SUNDHAL, E., THAYER, V. American Association of Feline Practitioners feline retrovirus management guideline. *J Fel Med Surg*, 2008; 10:300-316.

LUTZ, H., ADDIE, D., BELAK, S., et al. Feline Leukaemia: ABCD Guideline on prevention and management. *J Fel Med Surg*, 2009; 11:565-574.

PINCHES, M.D., DIESEL, G., HELPS, C.R., EGAN, K., GRUFFYDD-JONES, T.J. Diagnostic of feline leukaemia virus infection by semi-quantitative real time polymerase chain reaction. *Journal of Feline Medicine and Surgery*, 2007; 9:8-13.

STUETZER, B., BRUNNER, K., LUTZ, H., HARTMAN, K. A trial with 3′-azido-2′3′-dideoxythimidina and human interferon alfa in cats naturally infected with feline leukaemia virus. *J Fel Med Surg*, 2013; 15(8):667-671.

TANDON, R., CATTORI, V., GOMES-KELLER, M.A., MELI, M.L., GOLDER, M.C., LUTZ, H., HOFMANN-LEHMANN, R. Quantitation of feline leukaemia virus viral and proviral loads by TaqMan real-time polymerase chain reaction. *J Virol Methods*, 2005; 130(1-2):124-32.

WEIS, A., KLOPFLEISH, R., GRUBER, A. Prevalence of feline leukaemia provirus DNA in feline lymphomas. *J Fel Med Surg*, 2010; 12:929-935.

CASE STUDIES

CASE STUDY 1: *Lucas*

Summary: neutered male cat of indeterminate age.

Reason for consultation: poor overall appearance.
Comes from a colony of cats positive for feline leukaemia virus.

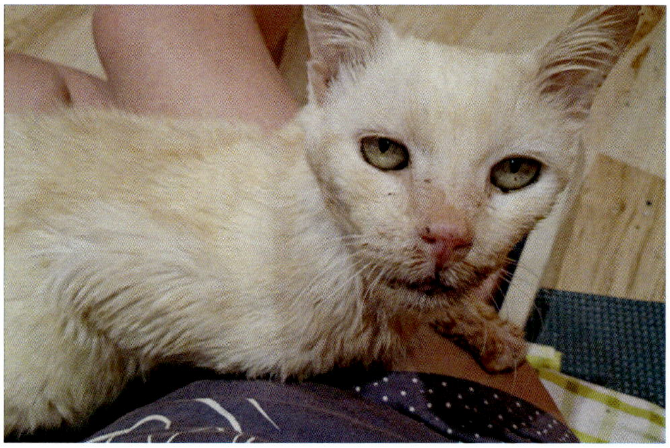

Figure 1. Image of *Lucas* in which emaciation and poor haircoat appearance are evident.

Medical history

The patient is a neutered male cat of indeterminate age that comes from a colony of FeLV-positive cats. He is currently housed in a foster home for FeLV- and FIV-positive cats, after long-term hospitalisation in a veterinary centre where he was diagnosed with FeLV and FIV by rapid immunochromatographic assay.

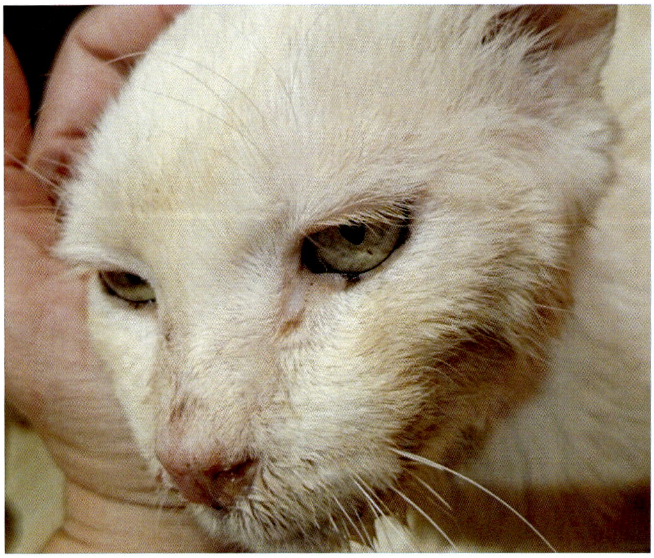

Figure 2. Mucoid haemorrhagic nasal discharge.

Physical examination and diagnostic tests

The animal is very thin, with a body mass index of 3/9 (Fig. 1).

The haircoat is very dirty due to poor grooming and the cat has various injuries in different parts of the body that are dirty and infected. The retropharyngeal lymph nodes are enlarged.

The cat had undergone a complete dental extraction in the previous veterinary centre due to chronic gingivitis and other unspecified oral and dental alterations.

The cat presents with respiratory stridor with mucoid haemorrhagic nasal discharge (Fig. 2). It has been treated with various antibiotics and other unspecified drugs.

Oral examination reveals marked inflammation of the gums in the areas surrounding the teeth and of the oral mucosa and palatoglossal arch. The inflammation is moderate to severe, with ulceration and necrosis.

A general blood test is performed (Table 1) as well as a rapid ELISA for the detection of retroviruses and a PCR test for calicivirus (Table 2).

Table 1. Results of blood tests.

Analysis		Result	Reference
Complete blood count	Erythrocytes	4.0 × 10^{12}/l	5.0–10 × 10^{12}/l
	Platelets	123 × 10^9/l	175–400 × 10^9/l
	Leukocytes	22.3 × 10^9/l	5.5–19.5 × 10^9/l
	Neutrophils	17.3 × 10^9/l	2.5–12.5 × 10^9/l
	Lymphocytes	3.3 × 10^9/l	0.4–6.8 × 10^9/l
Biochemistry	ALT	475 IU/l	25–45 IU/l
	AST	245 IU/l	25–75 IU/l
	Alkaline phosphatase	455 IU/l	<145 IU/l
	Blood urea nitrogen (BUN)	0.5 mg/dl	7–32 mg/dl
	Creatinine	1.3 mg/dl	0.6–1.6 mg/dl
	Total protein	11.3 g/dl	5.5–7.5 g/dl
	Albumin	2.2 g/dl	2.1–4.0 g/dl

Table 2. Results of virus test.

Test	Result	Reference
FIV (Ab ELISA)	Positive	Negative
FeLV (Ag ELISA)	Positive	Negative
Calicivirus (PCR)	Positive	Negative

The following diagnostic imaging tests are performed: radiographs of the oral cavity and skull, abdomen, and vertebral column, and abdominal ultrasound.

Radiographs of oral cavity and skull reveal an abnormal nasal turbinate, with differences between one side and the other. Collection of fluid from the pharynx following its instillation into the nasal cavity is difficult on one side, and impossible on the side on which the radiograph revealed an abnormality of the nasal turbinate. Accumulation of material is observed in the nasal and frontal sinuses, in which air content is reduced, and the walls of the tympanic bullae display bilateral thickening and irregularities (Fig. 3).

An abdominal radiograph indicates dilation of the stomach and the rest of the intestine and colon, with high gas content as a result of respiratory distress.

Areas of diskospondylosis-diskospondylitis are evident in the coccygeal vertebrae, as evidenced by swelling and inflammation of soft tissue, as well as considerable pain and immobility of the tail (Fig. 4).

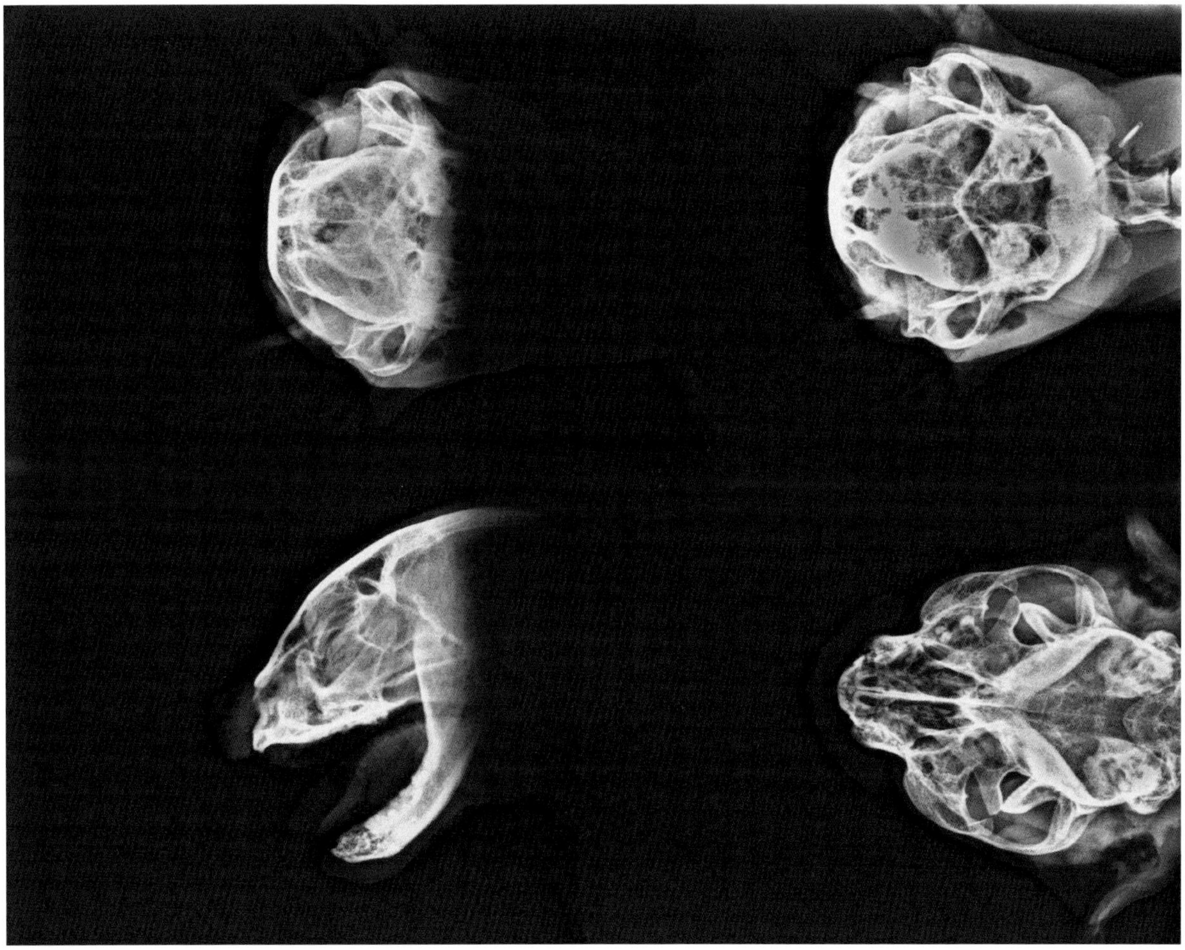

Figure 3.
Radiographs of the skull, nasal and frontal sinuses, nasal cavity, and tympanic bullae of *Lucas*.

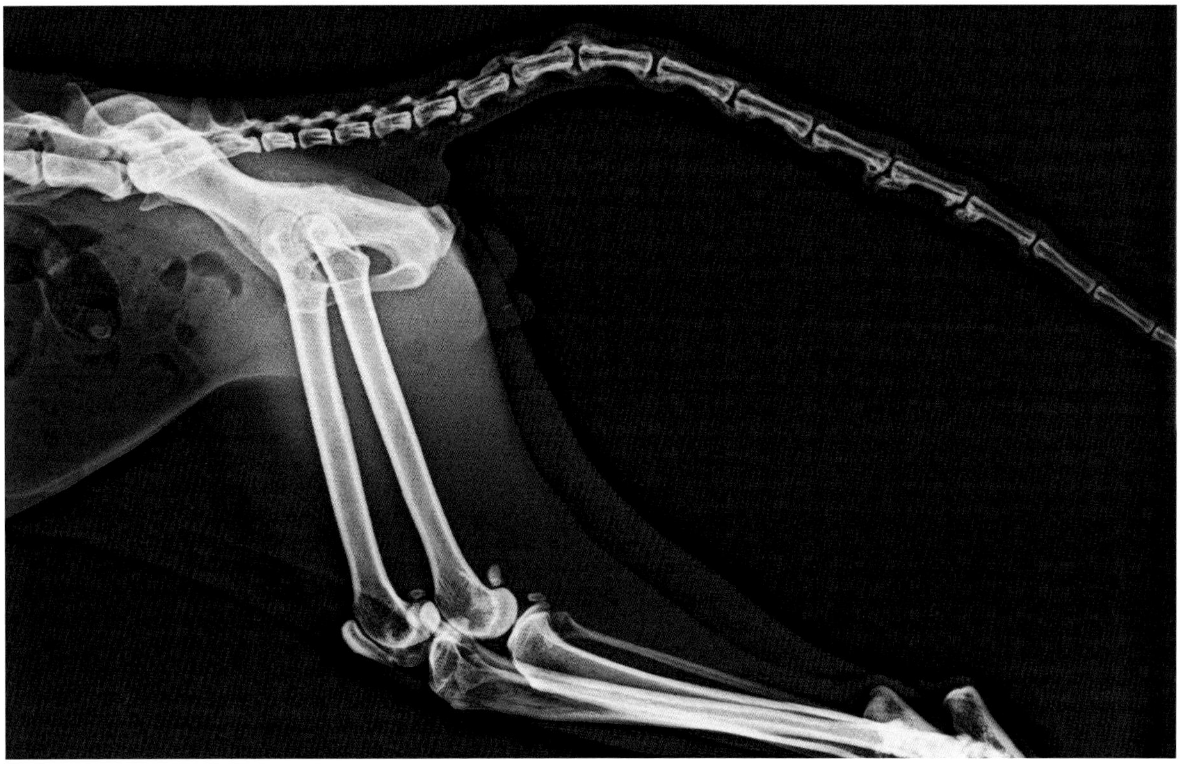

Figure 4.
Radiograph of the vertebral column (lumbosacral and coccygeal vertebrae).

Enlargement of the liver is observed in the abdominal ultrasound, with heterogeneous echogenicity and marked dilation of the gallbladder (Fig. 5).

Recommended treatment

Lucas is hospitalised due to dehydration, and his temperature monitored. Fluid therapy is applied (see appendix on fluid therapy).

After two days in hospital, *Lucas* is returned to the shelter to follow the following treatment regimen:

- Oral meloxicam (anti-inflammatory): 0.1 mg/kg for one day, subsequently decreasing to 0.05 mg/kg per day.
- Oral transmucosal buprenorphine (analgesic): 20 µg/kg every 12 hours.
- Oral pradofloxacin (antibiotic): 5 mg/kg every 24 hours.
- Oral zidovudine (antiretroviral): 5 mg/kg every 12 hours.

Follow-up

After two weeks of treatment, oral examination reveals a significant improvement in the mucosa surrounding the teeth, and a greater improvement in the oral mucosa and palatoglossal arch. *Lucas* has less difficulty breathing and no nasal discharge is observed. He eats normally and has gained 500 g. No changes in the treatment regimen are proposed.

At a subsequent examination three months later, *Lucas* is extremely thin (BMI 2/9) and dehydrated, and his haircoat is in poor condition. The oral mucosa is very pale, with no inflammation, and the capillary refill time is 3 seconds. His pulse is rapid and weak. Bloating and hepatomegaly are evident upon palpation, and ultrasound indicates widespread thickening of the abdominal wall and the presence of free abdominal fluid. The abdominal ganglia are very enlarged.

A blood test is performed, the results of which are shown in Table 3.

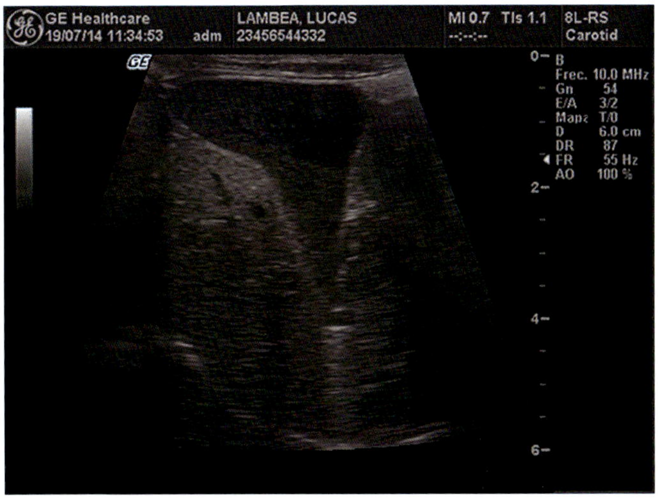

Figure 5. Liver ultrasound.

This reveals marked anaemia, as well as advanced impaired liver function. Zidovudine treatment, the adverse effects of which include marked anaemia, is withdrawn. Antibiotic, anti-inflammatory, and analgesic treatment had been withdrawn at some point without veterinary consultation.

After three weeks without medication the presence of free abdominal fluid is no longer detected. However, the anaemia becomes severe and is accompanied by a heart murmur. A decision is made to perform a blood transfusion. Abundant nasal discharge and dyspnoea are observed once again.

Treatment with raltegravir is instituted at 50 mg every 12 hours, as well as oral doxycycline at 10 mg/kg per day.

After three weeks of treatment the nasal discharge, abdominal distension, and hepatomegaly have resolved and laboratory tests reveal a marked improvement in the red blood cell count, with a significant increase in the regeneration rate (Table 4).

After another three months of raltegravir treatment, the results of laboratory analyses are within the normal range (Table 5). Lucas continues with the same antiretroviral regimen, without antibiotic treatment, and has a body mass index of 5/9, a good condition haircoat, and no oral alterations. Upper airway respiratory sounds are still detected, but nasal discharge is absent.

Table 3. Results of follow-up blood tests.

Analysis		Result	Reference
Complete blood count	Erythrocytes	2.9×10^{12}/l	$5.0–10 \times 10^{12}$/l
	Platelets	274×10^{9}/l	$175–400 \times 10^{9}$/l
	Leukocytes	10.5×10^{9}/l	$5.5–19.5 \times 10^{9}$/l
	Neutrophils	7.3×10^{9}/l	$2.5–12.5 \times 10^{9}$/l
	Lymphocytes	2.3×10^{9}/l	$0.4–6.8 \times 10^{9}$/l
Biochemistry	ALT	555 IU/l	25–45 IU/l
	AST	195 IU/l	25–75 IU/l
	Alkaline phosphatase	475 IU/l	<145 IU/l
	Blood urea nitrogen (BUN)	5.7 mg/dl	7–32 mg/dl
	Creatinine	1.5 mg/dl	0.6–1.6 mg/dl
	Total protein	12 g/dl	5.5–7.5 g/dl
	Albumin	1.3 g/dl	2.1–4.0 g/dl

Table 4. Results of blood tests after three weeks of raltegravir treatment.

Analysis		Result	Reference
Complete blood count	Erythrocytes	3.9×10^{12}/l	$5.0–10 \times 10^{12}$/l
	Haematocrit	23 %	30–45 %
	Haemoglobin	6.8 g/dl	9.0–15.0 g/dl
	Reticulocytes (%)	4 %	-
	Reticulocytes	0.07×10^{12}/l	$0.05–0.1 \times 10^{12}$/l
Biochemistry	ALT	65 IU/l	25–45 IU/l
	AST	34 IU/l	25–75 IU/l
	Alkaline phosphatase	67 IU/l	<145 IU/l
	Blood urea nitrogen (BUN)	12 mg/dl	7–32 mg/dl
	Creatinine	1.5 mg/dl	0.6–1.6 mg/dl
	Total protein	9 g/dl	5.5–7.5 g/dl
	Albumin	2.9 g/dl	2.1–4.0 g/dl

Table 5. Results of follow-up blood tests.

Analysis		Result	Reference
Complete blood count	Erythrocytes	6.7×10^{12}/l	$5.0–10 \times 10^{12}$/l
	Haematocrit	29.5 %	30–45 %
	Haemoglobin	11 g/dl	9.0–15.0 g/dl
	Reticulocytes (%)	4 %	-
	Reticulocytes	0.023×10^{12}/l	$0.05–0.1 \times 10^{12}$/l
Biochemistry	ALT	35 IU/l	25–45 IU/l
	AST	27 IU/l	25–75 IU/l
	Alkaline phosphatase	98 IU/l	<145 IU/l
	Blood urea nitrogen (BUN)	15 mg/dl	7–32 mg/dl
	Creatinine	1.6 mg/dl	0.6–1.6 mg/dl
	Total protein	8.5 g/dl	5.5–7.5 g/dl
	Albumin	3.8 g/dl	2.1–4.0 g/dl

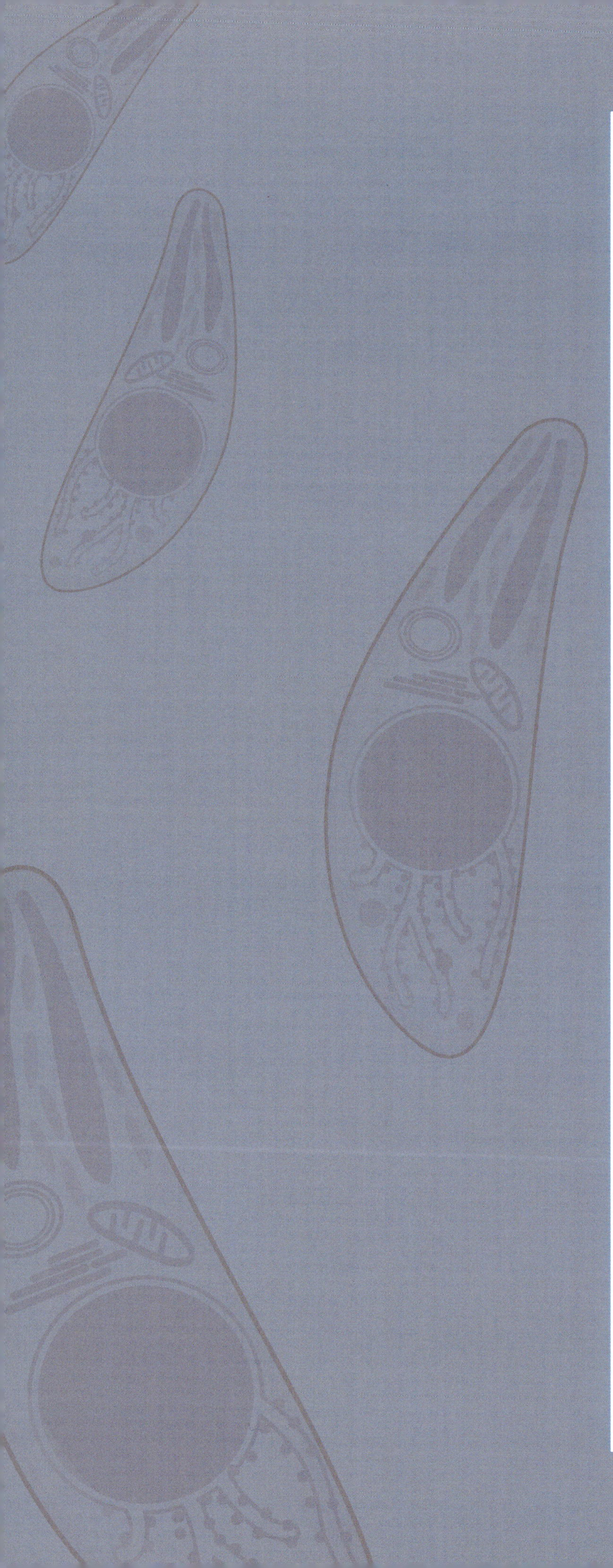

Intestinal protozoa of cats

Intestinal protozoa of cats

The gastrointestinal tract is affected by many protozoan species with a wide geographical distribution. Here we will focus on those with the highest prevalence, those which produce the most important clinical signs, and those which should be considered in the differential diagnosis of diarrhoeic processes in cats. These are *Giardia* spp., *Cryptosporidium* spp., *Cystoisospora* spp., *Toxoplasma gondii*, and *Tritrichomonas foetus* (Table 1).

Young cats often show clinical signs, especially in cases of coinfection with viruses or bacteria.

The clinical management of enteric infections caused by protozoa poses several challenges:

- Diagnosis: in some cases several serial samples are required for stool analysis. A negative result does not rule out infection, and specific PCR laboratory tests are required for definitive diagnosis.
- Available treatments are not very effective, are not registered for use in cats, or have toxic effects that should be considered before prescribing.
- *Cryptosporidium* spp. and *Toxoplasma* spp. are agents with zoonotic potential.

Table 1. Main gastrointestinal protozoa of cats.

Gastrointestinal protozoa		Type of diarrhoea
Flagellates	*Giardia* spp.	Small intestine
	Tritrichomonas foetus	Colon
Coccidia	*Toxoplasma gondii*	Not associated with diarrhoea
	Cryptosporidium spp.	Subclinical / small intestine
	Cystoisospora spp.	Colon

Giardia

Parasites of the genus *Giardia* are flagellate protozoa capable of infecting many mammalian species, including humans.

Seven subtypes (A–G) have been described. Cats are infected by subtype F and humans by subtypes A and B. As transmission of *Giardia* from cats to humans has not been described to date, **it should not be considered a zoonotic disease.**

Giardia spp. has a direct biological cycle, with active and mobile forms called trophozoites that adhere to epithelial cells of the small intestine, where they evolve into cysts that are eliminated intermittently in the faeces.

It is transmitted between cats via the faecal-oral route. Trophozoites that are shed in the faeces survive for short periods in the environment, whereas cysts can remain infective for years. Indirect transmission through contaminated material is thus a common route of infection.

Prevalence rates vary from study to study, ranging from 1 % to 20 % depending mainly on the diagnostic method used, the age of the cat, and its origin, with no differences observed between cats with or without diarrhoea (Bouzid et al., 2015).

Clinical signs

Cats of less than one year of age are more susceptible to infection and associated intestinal diseases.

Giardia spp. produces lesions on epithelial cells of the small intestine (Fig. 1), inducing an inflammatory response in the small intestine, inhibition of the enzymatic function of enterocytes, and changes in the intestinal flora, resulting in diarrhoea, malabsorption syndrome, and hypersecretion.

The diarrhoea has the typical characteristics of small intestine diarrhoea, and can be intermittent or persistent, with steatorrhea, anorexia, vomiting, weight loss, and apathy.

Diagnosis

Several different diagnostic methods can be used:

- Direct examination of faeces.
- Faecal flotation method.
- Faecal antigen ELISA.
- Direct immunofluorescence of faecal samples.
- PCR.

Direct examination is achieved by mixing a small amount of fresh faeces with a drop of saline. Motile trophozoites, which exhibit a movement pattern similar to that of a falling leaf, can be observed by microscope at 100× or 400×. Motile forms will not be observed if the sample is not fresh or has been refrigerated.

For stool analyses samples taken on three different days should be tested, given that *Giardia* spp. is shed intermittently. Flotation should be performed using zinc sulfate, which also allows detection of other intestinal parasites that may be implicated in the clinical picture.

ELISA offers high sensitivity and specificity, and results obtained using this technique correlate well with those obtained by direct immunofluorescence. ELISA combined with faecal flotation offers a specificity of 97.8 %, and this combination is recommended in cases of suspected *Giardia* enteritis (Mekaru et al., 2007).

Even if faecal analysis is negative, it is appropriate to initiate treatment and observe the clinical response.

Treatment

The first goal of treatment is to control diarrhoea. Metronidazole (15–25 mg/kg PO every 12 or 24 hours for 5–7 days) is an effective treatment for *Giardia* spp. and for *Clostridium* spp. overgrowth, and also helps control the associated inflammatory process. Metronidazole can cause neurotoxicity at high doses or due to dose accumulation when administered for prolonged periods (Scorza and Lappin, 2004).

Another alternative is fenbendazole treatment (50 mg/kg PO every 24 hours for 3–5 days). It can be used alone or in combination with metronidazole (Table 2).

In cases of suspected infection with cestodes or nematodes fenbendazole can be combined with pyrantel and praziquantel.

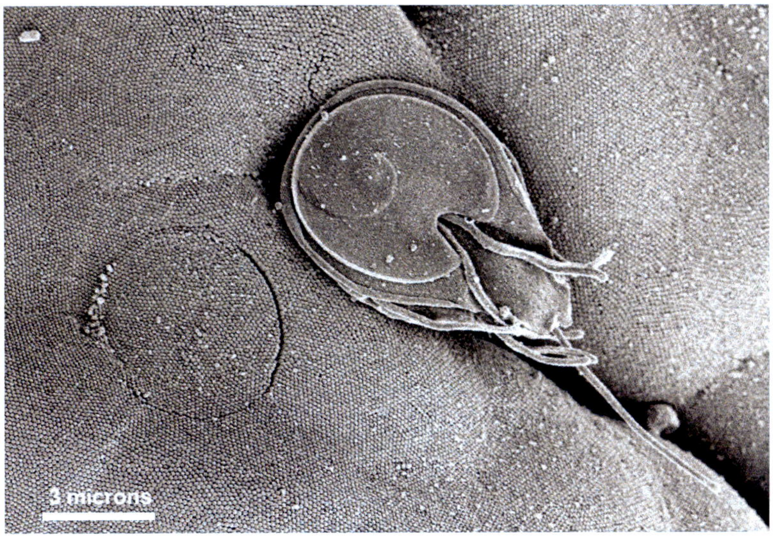

Figure 1. Electron microscopy image showing a circular lesion on the epithelial surface of the intestine caused by firm adhesion of a protozoan of the genus *Giardia* (Image courtesy of Dr. Stan Erlandsen, Centers for Disease Control and Prevention).

If clinical signs persist or a partial treatment response is observed, other processes such as intestinal inflammatory disease, pancreatic exocrine insufficiency, reinfection, or coinfections with other pathogens should be considered.

Table 2. Recommended treatment for gastrointestinal protozoa of cats.

Protozoa	Drug	Dose
Giardia	Fenbendazole	50 mg/kg PO every 24 hours for 3–5 days.
	Metronidazole	15–25 mg/kg PO every 12–24 hours for 5–7 days.
Tritrichomonas foetus	Ronidazole	20–30 mg/kg PO every 24 hours for 14 days.
Toxoplasma gondii	Clindamycin	10 mg/kg PO every 12 hours for 4 weeks.
	Sulfamethoxazole + trimethoprim	15 mg/kg PO every 12 hours for 4 weeks.
	Azithromycin	10 mg/kg PO every 24 hours for 4 weeks.
***Cystoisospora* spp.**	Toltrazuril	9–20 mg/kg PO, single dose.
	Diclazuril	2.5–5 mg/kg PO, single dose.
***Cryptosporidium* spp.**	Azithromycin	10 mg/kg PO every 24 hours until resolution of clinical signs.
	Paromomycin	150 mg/kg PO every 12–24 hours for 5 days.
	Tylosin	11 mg/kg PO every 8–12 hours for 21 days.

Tritrichomonas foetus

Tritrichomonas foetus is a highly mobile flagellate protozoan that targets the mucosa of the large intestine of cats and can cause diarrhoea, especially in animals of less than one year of age that live indoors in groups.

The life cycle is direct, with the formation of trophozoites in the large intestine without a cyst stage.

Transmission occurs via the faecal-oral route and trophozoite survival in the external environment is very limited.

T. foetus infection is more common in groups of cats of less than one year of age that live in closed environments, such as catteries and shelters, where prevalence can be high in cats with or without diarrhoea.

Clinical signs

The infection can be subclinical or can manifest as chronic large intestine diarrhoea that does not respond to antibiotic treatment or worsens when treatment is withdrawn. Affected cats tend to have good body condition.

Pathogenicity is associated with the cytotoxic effects of *T. foetus* on the intestinal mucosa, which produces an inflammatory response, although not all infected cats develop diarrhoea.

Faeces are liquid or semi-liquid, with tenesmus and the presence of mucus and occasionally blood. Some cats may become faecally incontinent.

The prognosis in the short and medium term is usually good and 88 % of cats achieve spontaneous resolution within two years of the onset of clinical signs. However, 54 % of cats may have intermittent diarrhoea related to reinfection, stress, or changes in the intestinal flora.

Diagnosis

Diagnosis of *T. foetus* can be established by examining fresh faeces under a microscope (200× or 400×) for the presence of trophozoites, which exhibit erratic movements distinct to those of *Giardia* spp. However, the sensitivity of this technique is low. Trophozoites of *T. foetus* should also be differentiated from commensal *Pentatrichomonas hominis*, which can be isolated from cats and dogs.

Unlike other protozoans, *T. foetus* can be grown in commercial media in which neither *P. hominis* nor *Giardia* spp. grow.

Direct detection by PCR is another means by which the species can be identified.

Treatment

The treatment of choice is ronidazole (20–30 mg/kg PO every 24 hours for 14 days). This dose is lower than that initially recommended, in order to minimise the associated neurotoxic effects. Treatment can be effective following a single cycle, or may need to be repeated (Table 2).

Each cat should be managed individually, as many patients show improvements in diarrhoea in response to high-fibre diets and antibiotics such as metronidazole or doxycycline.

Prevention

Kittens living in closed communities are the most vulnerable to infection with *T. foetus*. Care should be taken to clean the litter boxes, food bowls, and surfaces in the area in which the kitten lives.

T. foetus can survive at room temperature for seven days. It is thus easy to control infection by applying routine cleaning measures.

Toxoplasma gondii

Toxoplasma gondii is an obligate intracellular coccidia parasite, which can infect all warm-blooded species, including humans. Cats are the definitive hosts, while all other species serve as intermediate hosts (Dubey et al., 2006).

Three infectious stages are described:

- **Sporozoites:** oocysts that are eliminated in the faeces.
- **Tachyzoites:** stage of active multiplication.
- **Bradyzoites:** stage of slow multiplication, encysted in tissues (Fig. 2).

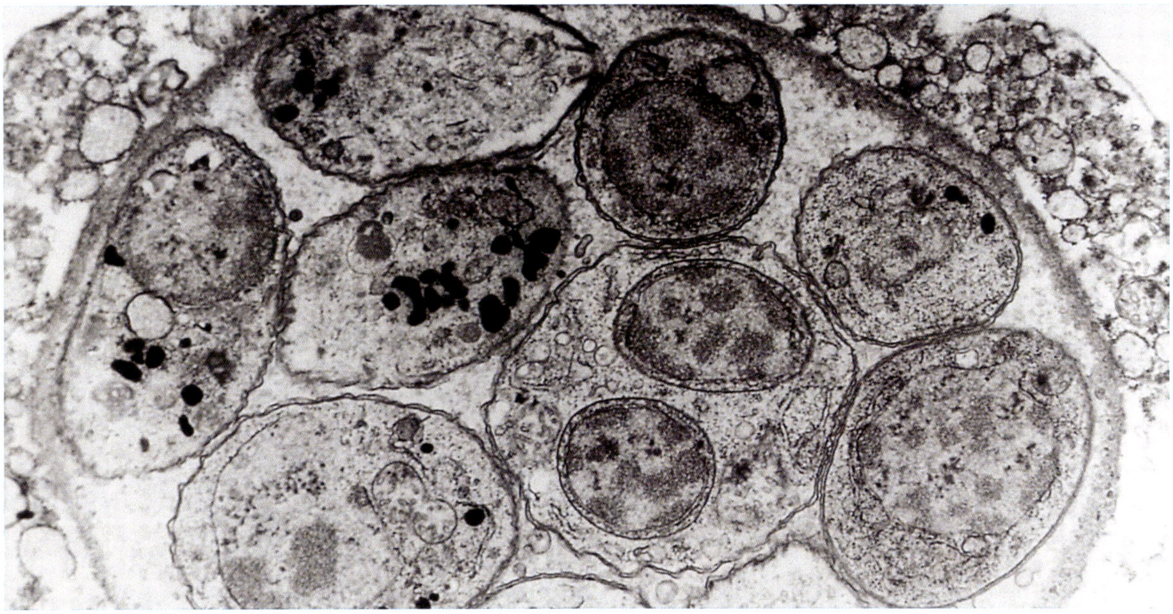

Figure 2. Electron microscopy image showing some ultrastructural details of a *Toxoplasma gondii* tissue cyst containing developing bradyzoites. (Image courtesy of Centers for Disease Control and Prevention).

Prevalence data vary depending on the lifestyle of the cat. Higher prevalence is likely in those with access to the outdoors and with the potential to engage in hunting. A study of 12,628 cats found that 31.6 % harboured antibodies to *T. gondii* (Vollaire et al., 2005). Although prevalence is high, the period of oocyst shedding is less than 21 days. Accordingly, the rate of detection of oocysts in faeces is low (<1 %).

Cats can become infected by eating mice or birds containing bradyzoites in their tissues or by ingesting sporulated oocysts, although the latter route is less common. Oocysts excreted in the faeces are not immediately infectious; sporulation in the external environment in the appropriate conditions of humidity and temperature takes at least 24 hours (usually 2–5 days). Oocysts can contaminate water, moist soil, or food, all of which serve as sources of contamination of intermediate hosts.

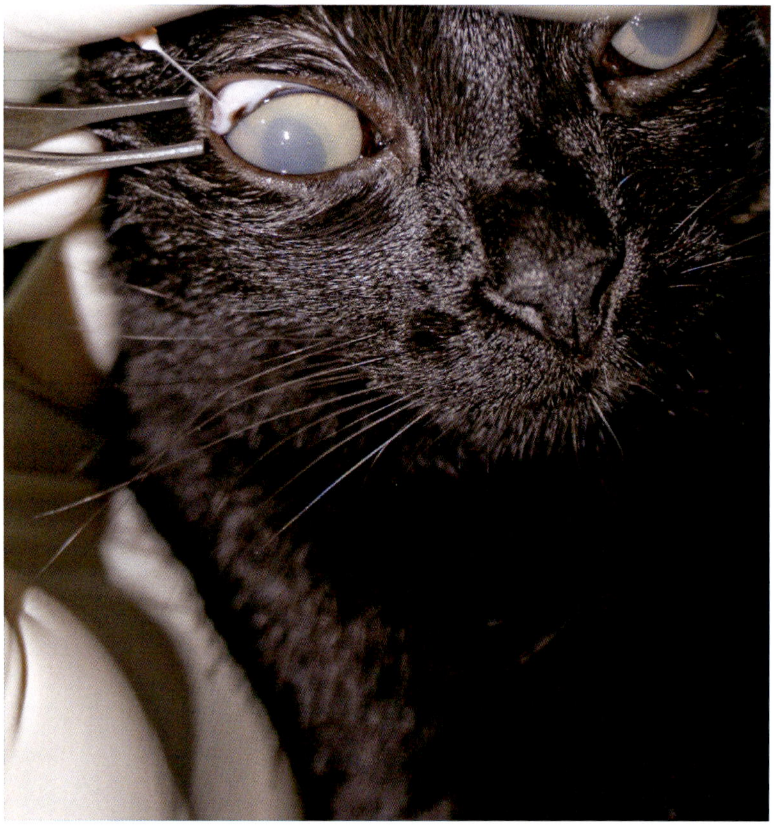

Figure 3. Uveitis caused by infection with *T. gondii*. Diagnosis was established by PCR of a sample of aqueous humour.

Clinical signs

Acute clinical signs are rare, but may be observed in animals that are immunosuppressed due to infection with feline leukaemia virus (FeLV), feline immunodeficiency virus (FIV), or due to treatment with immunosuppressive drugs such as cyclosporine.

Infection with *T. gondii* can cause fever, anorexia, abdominal pain, dyspnoea, uveitis, and neurological disorders (Fig. 3). Intestinal signs are rare.

T. gondii should be included in the differential diagnosis of cats with the following clinical signs:

- Non-regenerative chronic anaemia.
- Neutrophilic leukocytosis.
- Lymphocytosis.
- Monocytosis.
- Eosinophilia.
- Neutropaenia.
- Proteinuria.
- Bilirubinuria.
- Hyperproteinaemia.
- Bilirubinaemia.
- Increased liver enzyme levels.

Pulmonary toxoplasmosis is characterised by a diffuse interstitial pattern or an alveolar pattern (Fig. 4).

Diagnosis

Diagnosis can be established by combining the following:

1. Serological evidence of the presence of *T. gondii* antibodies.
2. IgM titres >1/64 or large increases in IgG, suggesting active infection.
3. Clinical signs associated with infection with *T. gondii*.
4. Exclusion of other diseases.
5. Treatment response.

Diagnosis is best established by antibody detection or based on positive *T. gondii* results in PCR analyses of aqueous humour samples from cats with uveitis or cerebrospinal fluid samples from cats with neurological signs.

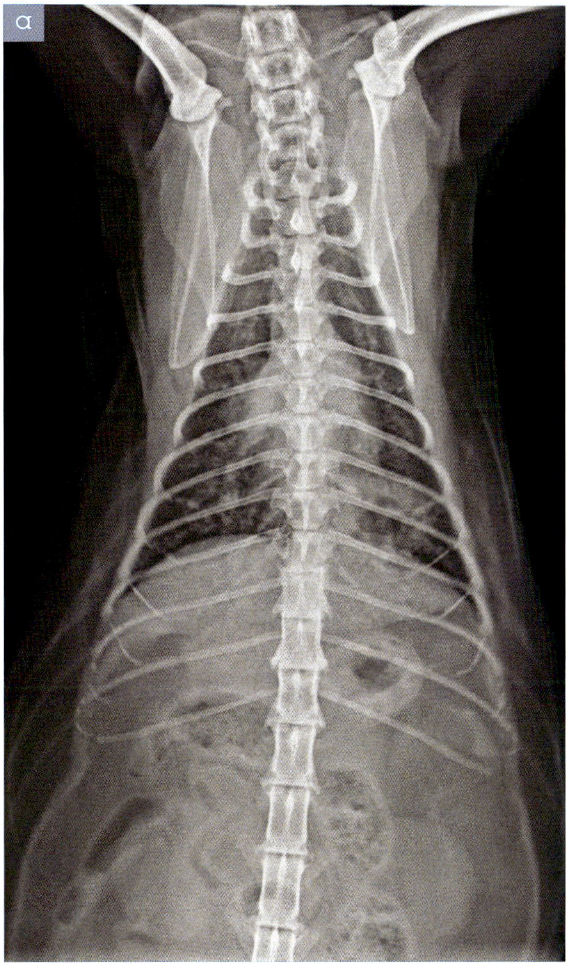

Treatment

The treatment of choice is clindamycin (10 mg/kg PO every 12 hours). During the first week of treatment an improvement in clinical signs may be observed. However, the treatment duration should not be less than 4 weeks as relapses can occur. If no improvement is observed, treatment with sulfamethoxazole + trimethoprim and azithromycin may be required (Table 2). There is no evidence that treatment results in the complete elimination of *T. gondii* from tissue, and recurrences are common.

The prognosis for cats with hepatic or pulmonary toxoplasmosis, uveitis, or neurologic signs is reserved, and is poorer still in cats with diseases that cause immunosuppression.

The best preventive measure is to avoid feeding cats raw or undercooked food.

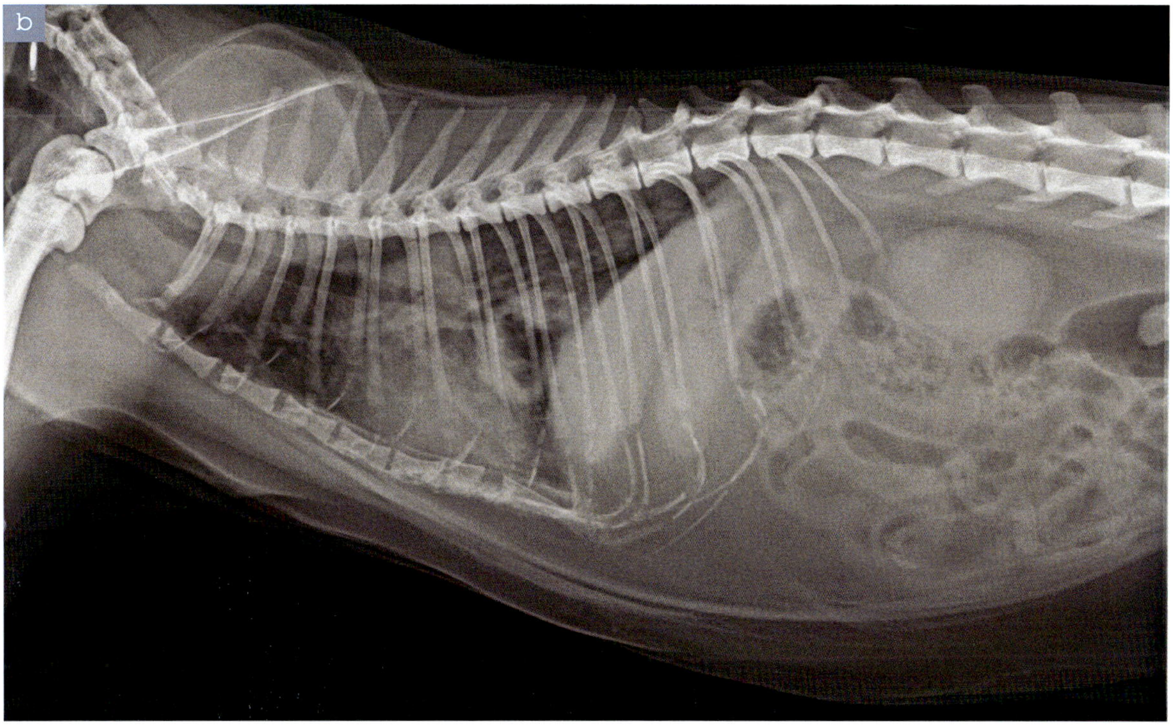

Figure 4. Chest radiographs of a cat with pulmonary toxoplasmosis: (a) dorsoventral and (b) lateral projection.

Cystoisospora

Cystoisospora felis and *Cystoisospora rivolta* are coccidia that can infect cats and cause enteric processes.

Cats are infected via the faecal-oral route, by ingestion of sporulated oocysts. Multiplication of intestinal phases occurs within the epithelial cells of the small and large intestine.

Cystoisospora species are ubiquitous and oocysts can be found in the faeces of both ill and clinically healthy animals.

Primary infections usually occur during the lactation period, between 3 and 8 weeks of age. Thus, most clinical cases are diagnosed in puppies and kittens of less than 4 months of age.

Oocysts remain infective for several months in the environment and can accumulate in catteries and shelters with very high animal densities.

Clinical signs

Cystoisospora species are associated with enteritis in kittens and can cause diarrhoea, vomiting, abdominal pain, and bloody stools.

Diagnosis

Diagnosis is established using faecal flotation techniques (Fig. 5).

The presence of *Cystoisospora* spp. may not be the main cause of the enteric problem. If the kitten presents with lack of energy, dehydration, or blood test abnormalities, other infectious diseases such as feline panleukopaenia virus (FPV) should be included in the differential diagnosis.

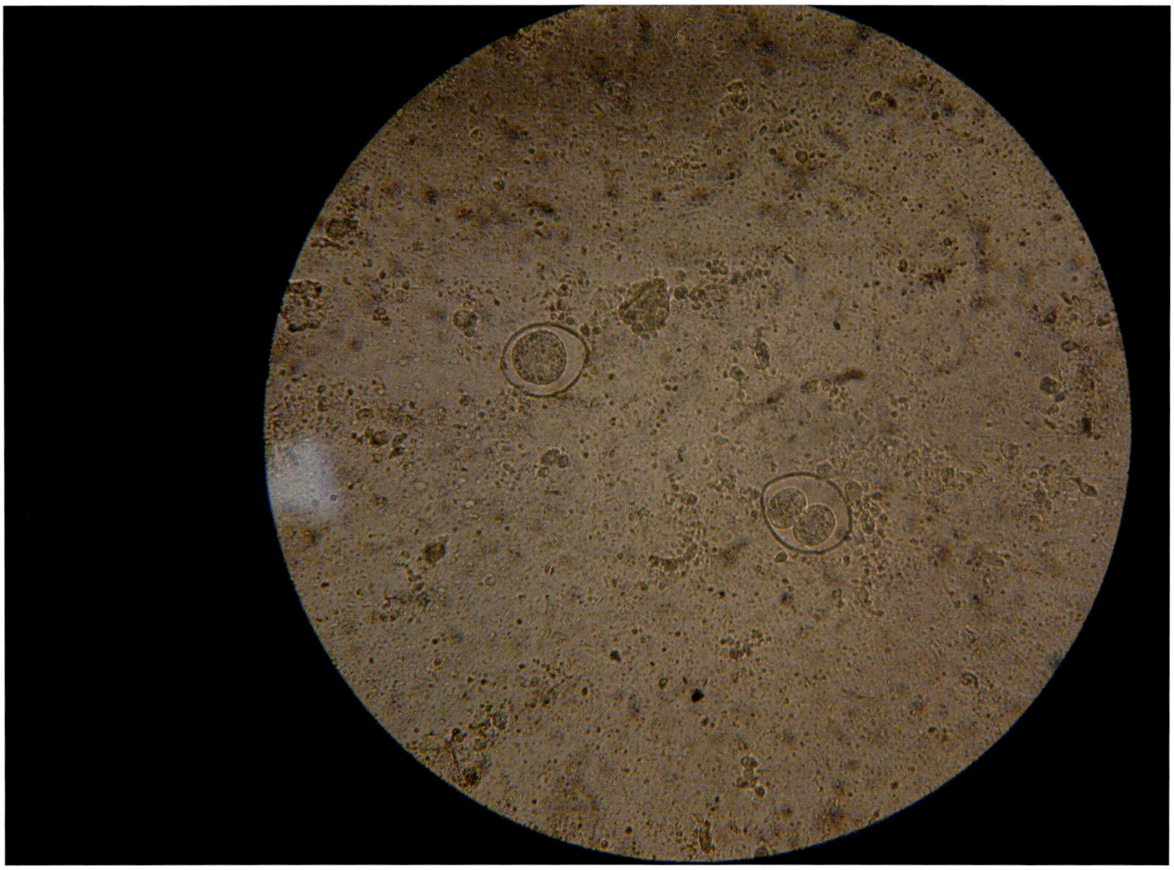

Figure 5. *Cystoisospora* spp. oocyst observed under a microscope at 400x. Photo courtesy of Joana Valente.

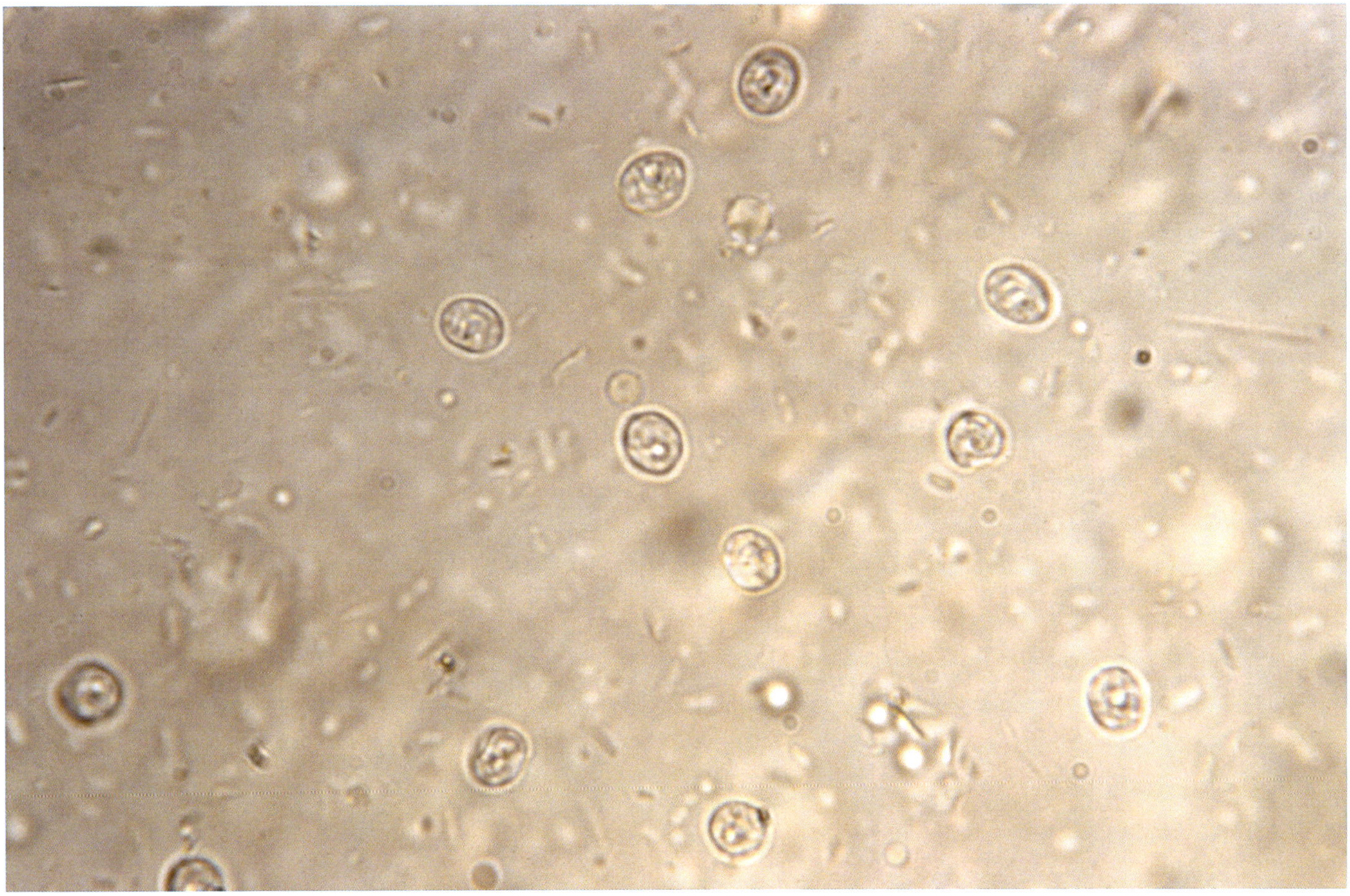

Figure 6. Faecal smears in which the presence of *Cryptosporidium parvum* is observed. Image courtesy of Dr. Peter Drotman, Centers for Disease Control and Prevention.

Treatment

Coccidiosis in kittens is usually a self-limiting disease and often resolves without specific treatment. However, drug administration may accelerate the resolution of clinical signs and prevent environmental contamination.

Daily administration of sulfonamides for 5 to 7 days is effective in controlling diarrhoea, but does not affect the excretion of oocysts. Diclazuril and toltrazuril and are the drugs of choice for the treatment of feline cystoisosporiasis (off-label use). The recommended doses are 9–20 mg/kg PO for toltrazuril and 2.5–5 mg/kg PO for diclazuril (both administered as a single dose). These drugs significantly reduce the presence of oocysts in animals and administration during the prepatent period successfully prevents the excretion of parasites and alleviates diarrhoea in infected animals (Table 2).

Cryptosporidium felis

Cryptosporidium felis is a coccidia that infects the small intestine of ruminants and other mammals, including humans, dogs, and cats (Fig. 6).

Given that molecular characterisation is necessary to distinguish between species, the exact prevalence in cats is unknown, although it is estimated at about 5 %.

C. felis infection begins with the ingestion of oocysts in the environment and invasion of the small intestinal epithelium by sporozoites, which then undergo intracellular multiplication. Endogenous replication ends with the production of sexual forms that give rise to oocysts, which undergo sporulation (producing infective forms) and are excreted in the faeces.

Some oocysts with thinner walls may be produced during the biological cycle. These forms are less resistant, and release their sporozoites within the intestine itself before reaching the exterior. This results in auto-infection in the patient, and the release of large numbers of oocysts in a short time.

Clinical signs

The main clinical signs associated with *C. felis* are small intestine diarrhoea, vomiting, and weight loss.

Most cats that show clinical signs are kittens that are coinfected with other infectious agents or other intestinal diseases such as inflammatory bowel disease, intestinal lymphoma, or immunosuppressive diseases.

Diagnosis

The presence of oocysts in faeces can be observed using the faecal flotation technique, but this test has low sensitivity given the small size of *C. felis* and the intermittent pattern of oocyst excretion.

While diagnosis can be achieved using PCR techniques, a positive result is not necessarily proof that the parasite is the cause of the intestinal process. It is advisable to use this technique only when the results of other diagnostic tests are negative and diarrhoea is chronic and persistent.

Treatment

The main objective is to control small intestine diarrhoea by prescribing a highly digestible diet specially formulated for cats. Supportive fluid therapy may be required in cases of dehydration (see appendix on fluid therapy).

Treatment protocols for *C. felis* published to date are based on isolated clinical cases. Azithromycin can be safely administered, but at least 10 days of treatment is necessary before improvements are observed, and resolution of infection can take several weeks.

Tylosin is an antibiotic with anti-inflammatory effects, but is poorly tolerated by cats due to its unpleasant taste and must be administered in capsules. Treatment generally results in improvement of clinical signs within one week, but should be continued for several more weeks.

Paromomycin should not be administered in cats that have bloody diarrhoea given the possibility of systemic distribution and the risk of renal toxicity and ototoxicity. Treatment should be continued for one week after the resolution of clinical signs (Table 2).

In immunocompetent animals resolution of *C. felis* infection can occur with or without treatment. However, in immunosuppressed cats these infections can be difficult to treat.

C. felis oocysts are extremely resistant in the environment. Although *C. felis* is a species-specific protozoan, it has been isolated in immunosuppressed people living with infected cats (Lucio-Forster et al., 2010).

It is recommended to maintain good sanitation and to wash hands regularly. Immunocompromised individuals should avoid keeping cats of less than 6 months of age.

References

Bouzid, M., Kapil, H., Danielle, J., et al. The prevalence of Giardia infection in dogs and cats, a systematic review and meta-analysis of prevalence studies from stool samples. *Veterinary Parasitology*, 2015; 207:181-202.

Dubey, J.P., Lindsay, D.S., Lappin, M.R. Toxoplasmosis and other intestinal coccidial infections in cats and dogs. *Vet Clin North Am Small Anim Pract*, 2009; 39:1009-1034.

Lucio-Forster, A., Griffiths, J.K., Cama, V.A., et al. Minimal zoonotic risk of cryptosporidiosis from pet dogs and cats. *Trends Parasitol*, 2010; 26:174-179.

Mekaru, S.R., Marks, S.L., Felley, A.J., et al. Comparison of direct immunofluorescence, immunoassays, and fecal flotation for detection of Cryptosporidium spp. and Giardia spp. in naturally exposed cats in 4 Northern California animal shelters. *J Vet Intern Med*, 2007; 21:959-965.

Scorza, A.V., Lappin, M.R. Metronidazole for the treatment of feline giardiasis. *J Feline Med Surg*, 2004; 6:157-160.

Vollaire, M.R., Radecki, S.V., Lappin, M.R. Seroprevalence of Toxoplasma gondii antibodies in clinically ill cats in the United States. *Am J Vet Res*, 2005; 66:874-877.

Recommended reading

- Control de protozoos intestinales de perros y gatos. Guía nº 6 de ESCCAP. www.esccap.org
- Guía de ABCD sobre *Giardia* spp. www.abcd-vets.org
- Guía de ABCD sobre Toxoplasmosis. www.abcd-vets.org
- Guía de ABCD sobre *Tritrichomonas* spp. www.abcd-vets.org
- Posicionamiento GEMFE sobre toxoplasmosis y embarazo. www.avepa.org

Appendices

Appendix 1

Fluid therapy

The administration of sera and solutions is a common practice in the therapeutic management of many feline diseases. For example, in feline infectious panleukopaenia, hypovolaemia and dehydration can become rapidly established as a result of anorexia, vomiting, diarrhoea, and fever.

Hypovolaemia and dehydration are distinct processes with different clinical signs, but can sometimes occur simultaneously, and it is important to identify and manage all situations concurrently.

Hypovolaemia occurs as a result of a decrease in intravascular volume (e.g. haemorrhage).

Dehydration initially occurs as a result of a reduction in the volume of interstitial fluid, but can be exacerbated by decreases in the volume of other compartments (e.g. **vomiting, diarrhoea**).

Hypovolaemia causes tachycardia, although eventually the patient can display normal frequencies or even develop bradycardia with hypotension, with an increase in capillary refill time. Dehydration causes skin tenting and dryness of mucous membranes, but does not alter heart rate or pulse quality.

Furthermore, electrolyte and acid-base balance disturbances often occur as a consequence of infection, with hypokalaemia caused by anorexia and by vomiting and diarrhoea, metabolic acidosis with bicarbonate deficit, and compensatory increases in CO_2 that result in various alterations as a result of overhydration.

Clinical evaluation, including physical examination and the collection of detailed data on the amount of vomiting or diarrhoea and the time passed without eating or drinking, are essential to determine the degree of dehydration (Table 1) and the severity of the situation, to establish emergency therapy, and to accurately calculate fluid therapy requirements.

Table 1. Physical examination to determine level of dehydration.

Level of dehydration	Examination findings
<5 %	Not detectable.
5–8 %	• Slight loss of skin elasticity. • Slightly dry and pale mucous membranes.
8–10 %	• Clear loss of skin elasticity (takes some time to return to its initial state after pinching). • Dry and sticky mucosa. • Slightly sunken eyes.
10–12 %	• Skin does not return to its initial position after pinching. • Dry and sticky mucosa. • Sunken eyes. • Increased CRT.
>12 %	• Skin does not return to its initial position after pinching. • Dry and sticky mucosa. • Sunken eyes. • Signs of shock (tachycardia/bradycardia, etc.). • Hypothermia, hypotension, poor pulse quality, increased CRT, weakness, syncope.

Physical examination

The percentage of dehydration should be calculated exhaustively. Vital parameters measured should include mental status, weight, heart rate, respiratory rate, pulse quality, capillary refill time (CRT), rectal temperature, and arterial blood pressure (ABP). Laboratory analyses include the measurement of haematocrit, total protein, and urine specific gravity.

All these data provide information on the animal's status and will enable subsequent evaluation of the effectiveness of fluid therapy.

Hypotension is characterised by ABP <90 mmHg, tachycardia or bradycardia, poor quality peripheral pulse, CRT >2 seconds, altered mental status, weakness, and hypothermia.

Treatment

The aim of fluid therapy is to reverse all signs of dehydration until the following values are obtained:

- ABP <100 mmHg.
- Heart rate: 120–180 bpm (beats per minute).
- CRT <2 seconds.
- Temperature: 38–39 °C.
- Urine output >1 ml/kg/hour.

Treatment begins with gentle, active auxiliary heating of the animal if hypothermia is observed, as this situation entails a weakened vascular response. This can be achieved using sleeping bags (snuggle bags), intravenous or intraperitoneal administration of warm sera, intensive care, etc.

Fluid

Fluid requirements change over time and with resolution of dehydration. Therefore, it is necessary to constantly monitor clinical signs.

Cats are very sensitive to volume overload and hypernatraemia. Liquids should be infused slowly and progressively. Fixed volumes should not be administered given that needs change with the progressive resolution of dehydration. The necessary steps are shown at the bottom of the page.

Fluid replacement can be administered empirically using the formula below, or alternatively based on the response to fluid therapy, adjusting the treatment according to clinical signs, vital signs, body weight, urine output, and laboratory data such as haematocrit, total protein, electrolyte levels, and urine specific gravity.

Large volumes or rapid infusion can result in excess hydration. This can cause serous nasal discharge, chemosis, tachycardia, crepitation upon cardiac auscultation, cough, tachypnoea, hypertension, and pleural/ascitic effusion.

The best route of administration, especially in emergency situations, is intravenous (IV), ideally using infusion pumps or automated infusion devices (Fig. 1), as these ensure an accurate rate of fluid administration. Other potential routes of administration include

1. Calculation of deficit	2. Maintenance needs	3. Ongoing losses
Liquid deficit (ml) = [Body weight (kg) × % dehydration/100] × 1000	2 ml/kg/hour 50 ml/kg/24 hours	Volume of fluids lost (in ml): • Vomiting • Diarrhoea • Urine

Vomiting or diarrhoea are estimated to account for losses of 4 ml/kg per episode. **Total requirements = 1 + 2 + 3.**

intraosseous and peritoneal. The subcutaneous route is not an option when animals are dehydrated.

Solutions

Saline dextrose is not recommended because dextrose is rapidly metabolised leaving a hypotonic solution that can cause further electrolyte disturbances.

Isotonic crystalloid solutions are the most widely used (e.g. 0.9 % saline or Ringer's lactate solution). These solutions initially accumulate in the intravascular space and are subsequently distributed rapidly into the interstitial space. They are low in potassium. Therefore, in severe cases involving vomiting and diarrhoea, which may result in metabolic acidosis with **excessive potassium loss, potassium should be supplemented.**

The effect of potassium administration should be considered even in animals with normal electrolyte levels.

Potassium supplementation depends on the animal's serum levels of potassium (Table 2). If the potassium level is less than 3.4 mmol/l, it should be supplemented intravenously with no more than 30 mmol/l to avoid irritation of the veins and tissues.

Shock management

In situations of low oncotic pressure, in animals with hypoalbuminaemia, or as a treatment for hypotension, colloidal solutions or even blood products such as plasma or whole blood are required.

When total protein levels are below 3.5 g/dl or albumin levels are less than 1.5 g/dl, approximately 40–60 ml/kg are required.

Treatment should begin with a quarter of that volume (10–20 ml/kg) of crystalloid solution for 15 minutes, after which the response should be evaluated. If satisfactory results are not obtained, the bolus should be readministered.

Table 2. Potassium supplementation.

Serum potassium (mmol/l)	Potassium (mmol/l) in 500 ml of 0.9 % saline
<2	40
2–2.5	30
2.5–3	20
3–3.5	14
3.5–5	10 (maintenance supplementation)

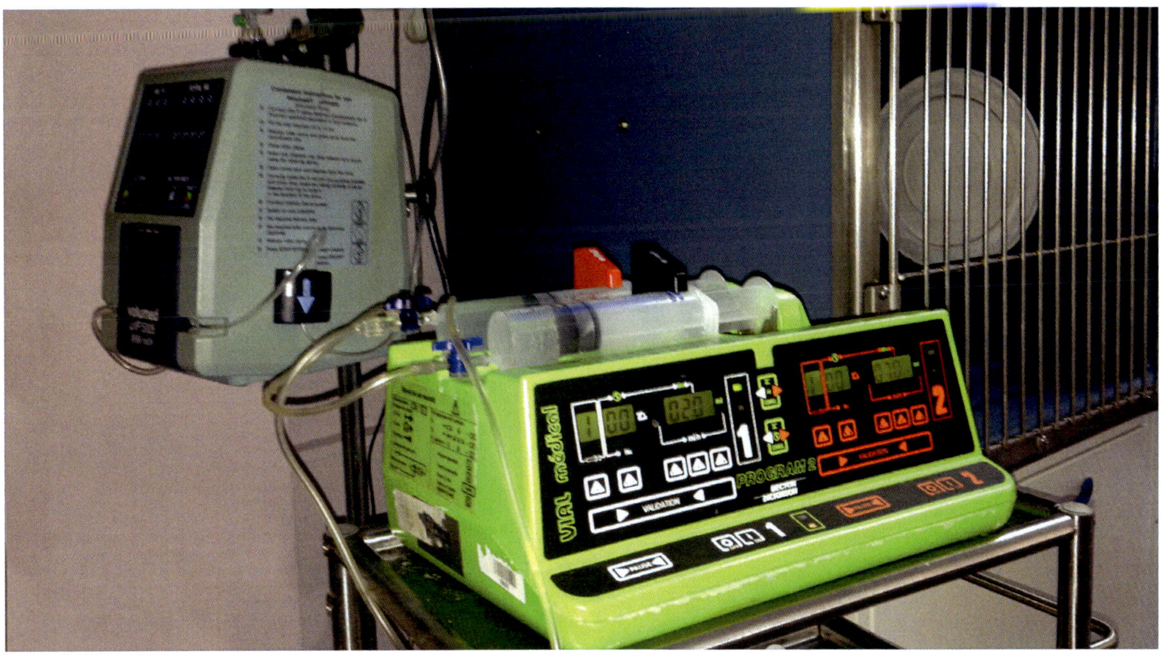

Figure 1. Infusion pumps for precise administration of fluid therapy.

Appendix 2

Vascular access routes

Central venous catheters

A central venous catheter (CVC) is defined as a catheter whose tip is located in the cranial or caudal vena cava. CVCs are inserted via the jugular vein (Figs. 1–4).

A CVC can be used for the following:

- Monitoring of central venous pressure (CVP): in this case, the tip should be located in the thoracic or abdominal vena cava in cats.
- Infusion of irritant or hyperosmolar solutions: e.g. total parenteral nutrition (TPN).
- Collection of blood samples for diagnosis without the need for repeated and uncomfortable venous puncture.

Catheter types:

- Single lumen.
- Multiple lumen (usually with 2 or 3 access ports and lumens): these catheters allow the infusion of incompatible solutions or the administration of liquid while simultaneously monitoring CVP.

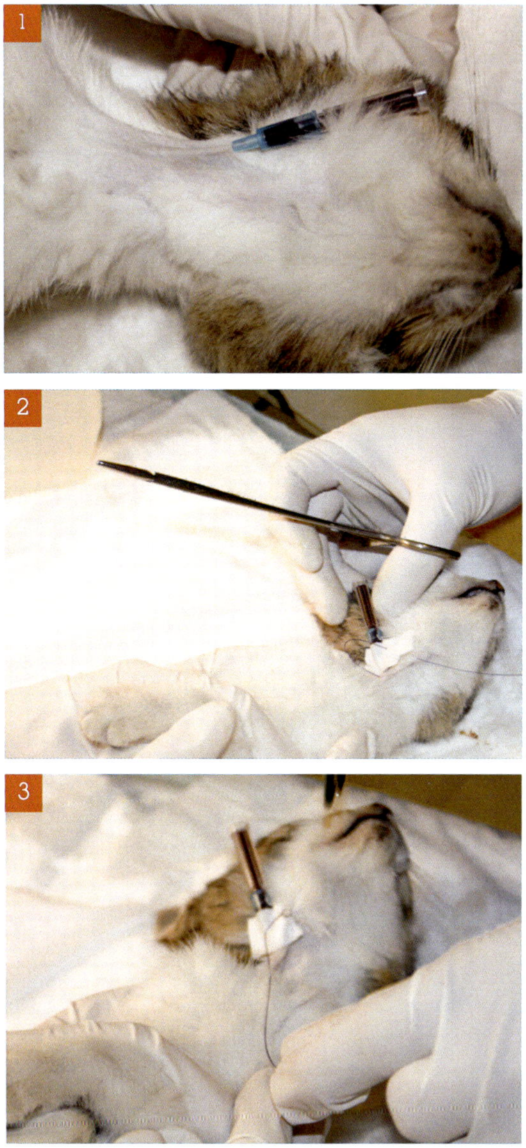

Figures 1–3. Placing a peripheral catheter into the jugular vein of a kitten in an emergency situation.

Contraindications for catheter placement

Thrombocytopaenia.

Coagulopathy.

Bleeding disorders.

Placement via the jugular vein is contraindicated in animals that have or are suspected to have high intracranial pressure; the pressure exerted upon the jugular vein during the procedure decreases venous return, which may further exacerbate intracranial pressure.

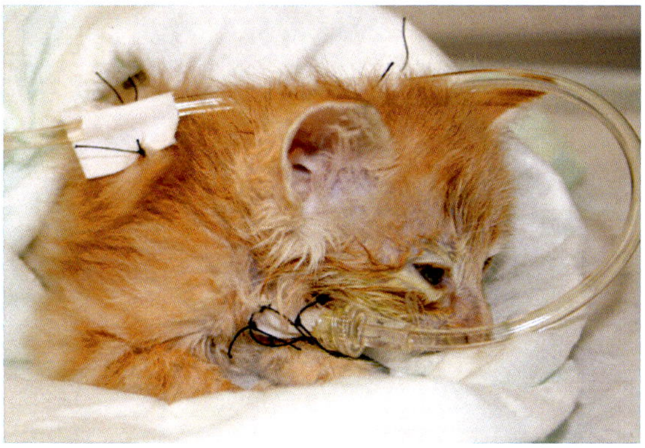

Figure 4. Placement of a central venous catheter in a patient in an emergency situation.

The following equipment is required for **placement** of a CVC:

- Clippers.
- Solutions for sterilisation of the area: **chlorhexidine**, povidone-iodine, saline, alcohol.
- A sterile drape (impermeable): self-adhesive drapes are useful, especially in conscious patients who may move during the procedure.
- Towel or bag containing liquid to be **placed under** the animal's neck.
- A catheter kit (some are sold as a complete package containing everything required for catheter placement) (Fig. 5).
- Sterile gloves (gown and mask optional).
- Scalpel blade.
- Sterile gauze.
- Topical local anaesthetics (0.5 ml lidocaine in a sterile syringe with a 25-G needle).
- Several syringes of heparinised saline.
- Suture thread.
- Needle holder.
- Suture scissors.
- Bandages.

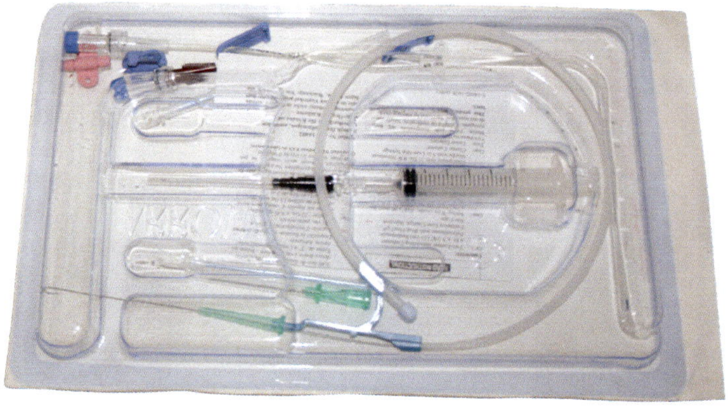

Figure 5. Central venous catheter kit.

Selecting a catheter

Several **models** of catheter are available:

- Over-the-needle catheters: usually rigid and easier to bend.
- Through-the-needle catheters: these have a single lumen and can result in bleeding and haematoma, since the hole created in the vein is larger than the catheter itself. This type is the most difficult to safely maintain in place.
- Catheters for implantation using the Seldinger technique: these are the most versatile and the easiest to secure in place for prolonged use. There are many commercially available catheters suitable for veterinary patients.

These models are available with a single or multiple lumen. Single-lumen catheters are preferable for cats.

The **length** of the catheter should be selected so that the tip lies in the cranial vena cava. This can be calculated by measuring from the point of placement (insertion) to approximately the second intercostal space (ICS). It is important to ensure that the length is appropriate to avoid causing arrhythmia.

The **diameter** selected should be as large as possible in order to minimise flow resistance: 22 G.

General catheter care

If a catheter is not being used, it should be rinsed every 2 to 4 hours with heparinised saline to prevent clotting of blood in the lumen.

Dressings should be removed daily to check for signs of infection (redness, swelling, or discharge) at the point of entry.

All injection ports should be cleaned with alcohol before administering injections, and a sterile procedure should be followed each time intravenous fluid infusion equipment is changed.

How long can a catheter be left in place?

With proper care, it can be left in place for up to 14 days. Peripheral catheters are usually removed when no longer needed (e.g. after anaesthesia), but can be left in place for several days. Intraosseous catheters can stay in place for up to 72 hours.

Placement of a central venous catheter using the Seldinger technique

» If the animal is conscious, it should be placed in right or left lateral recumbency on a comfortable surface to minimise movement.

» A wide area is clipped, with the mandible forming the cranial border, the sternum forming the caudal border, and the dorsal midline forming the dorsal border. Hair should also be clipped below the site of entry and as far across as the opposite jugular (Fig. 6).

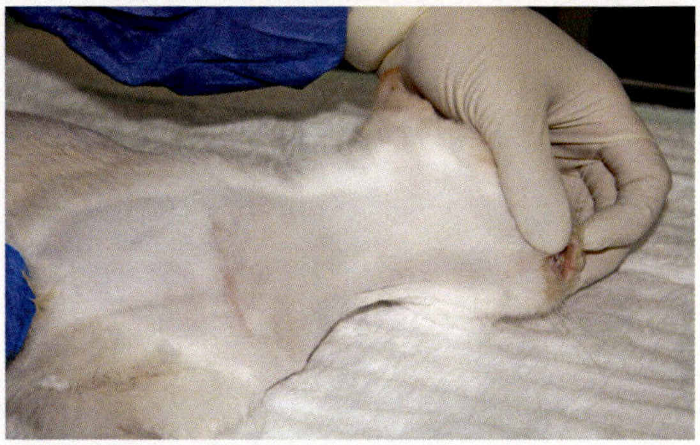

Figure 6. Localisation of the jugular.

» If a topical local anaesthetic cream is to be used, it should be applied at this point to ensure that it exerts its effect. Topical local anaesthetics increase the likelihood of effective placement in cats and have no side effects.

» The area is prepared as for surgery using the appropriate solution. Just before washing for the last time the site of catheter insertion can be numbed by infiltrating the dermis and subcutaneous tissues with a small volume of lidocaine (Fig. 7).

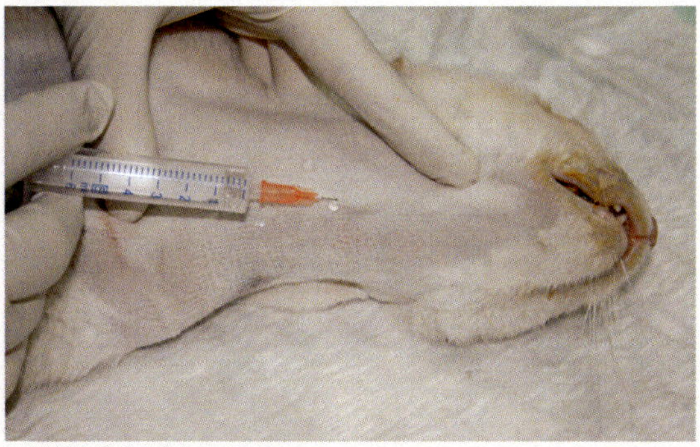

Figure 7. Infiltration of the skin with local anaesthesia.

» Place the rolled towel or bag of **IV** liquid under the neck to help stretch the skin and facilitate visualisation of the jugular vein.

» Place the surgical drape with a pre-existing hole (or create one using sterile scissors) over the point of entry into the jugular vein (approximately 1/3 of the distance between the caudal portion of the mandible and the thoracic inlet).

» Open the catheter kit or arrange the equipment on a sterile drape. Rinse the catheter with heparinised saline.

» Have an assistant apply pressure to the jugular vein, occluding it at the thoracic inlet (beneath the drape).

» Once the entry point has been identified, release the pressure on the jugular and use the tip of the scalpel to create a small cutaneous incision of 3–5 mm, orienting the blade away **from the vein** to avoid accidental laceration (Fig. 8).

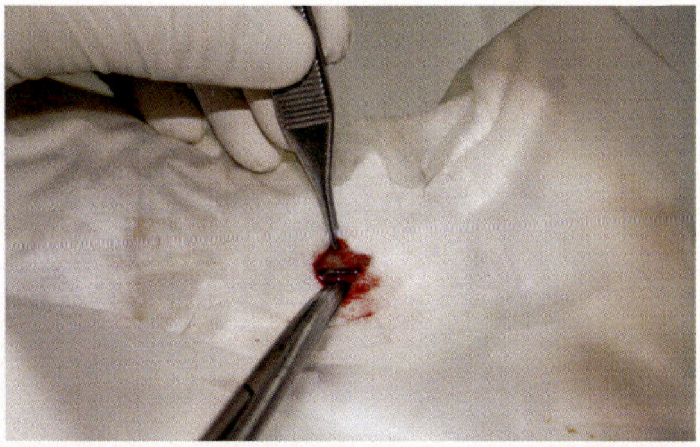

Figure 8. Dissection of the jugular vein.

» Occlude the vein once again and insert the introductory needle or needle and catheter into the jugular vein. Once in place (verified by the passage of blood through the needle or catheter), connect to a syringe with heparinised saline. This avoids the generation of an air embolism and allows confirmation of correct catheter placement by removing the plunger and observing the influx of blood (Fig. 9).

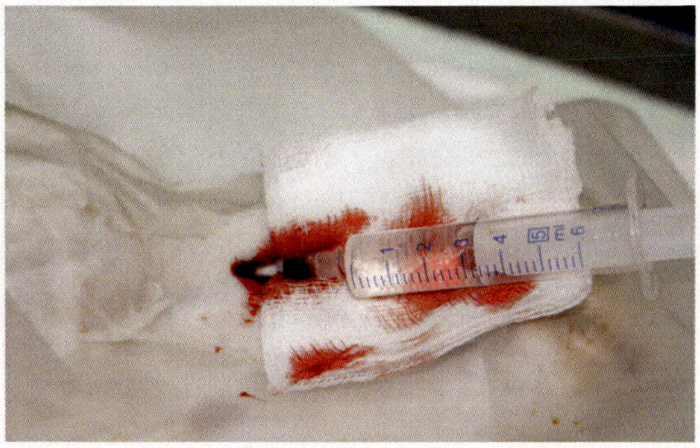

Figure 9. Canalisation of the vein.

Placement of a CVC using the Seldinger technique (*continued*)

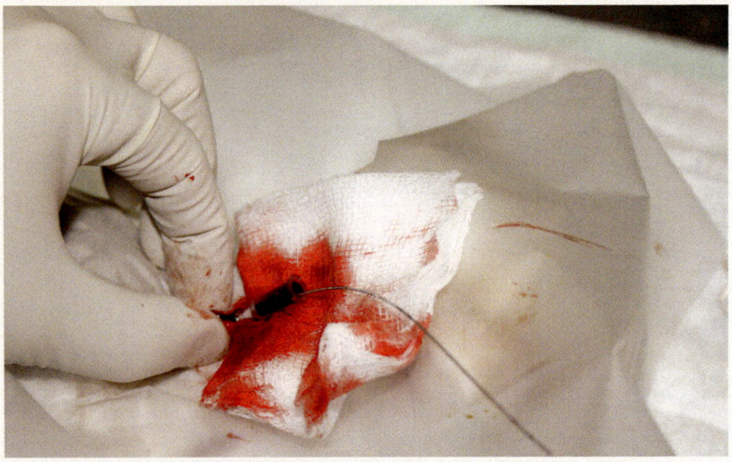

Figure 10. Insertion of the guidewire into the vein.

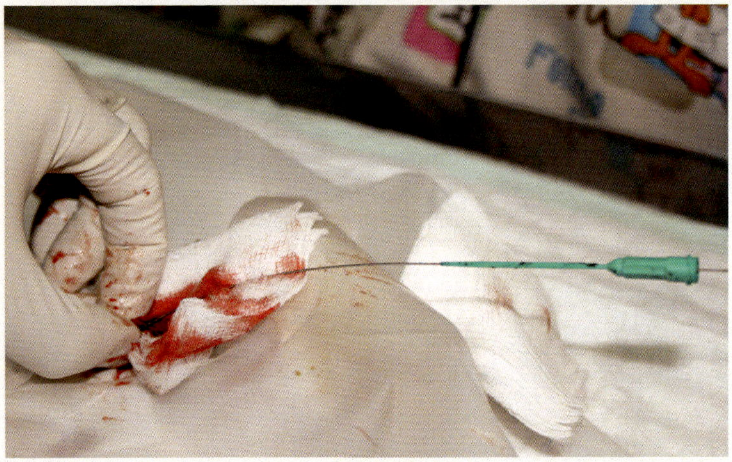

Figure 11. Threading of the vascular dilator onto the guidewire.

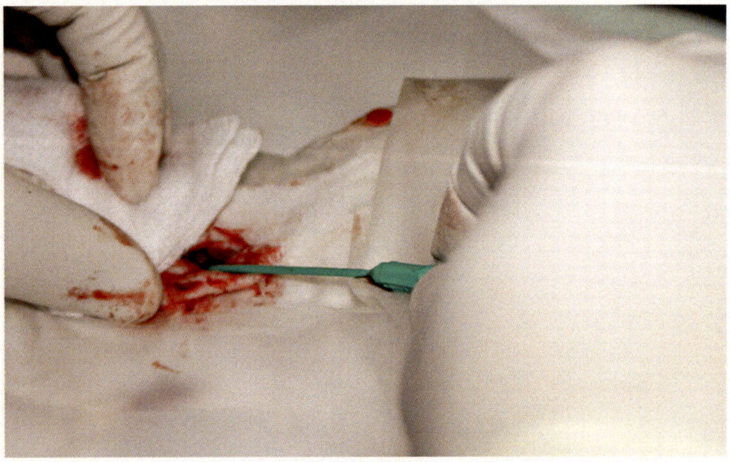

Figure 12. Dilation of the vein. Enlargement of the venipuncture hole to accommodate the diameter of the central venous catheter.

» Next, the guidewire (Fig. 10), which usually has a J-shaped tip, is inserted through the introductory needle or catheter as far as the second ICS.

» The introductory needle or catheter is pulled to separate it from the guidewire.

» Next, the vascular dilator (supplied with the catheter) is slid onto the guidewire and into the jugular vein (creating a tunnel through which the catheter slides easily) (Figs. 11 and 12).

» The dilator is removed, leaving only the guidewire in the jugular vein; at this point some bleeding may be observed, in which case gauze can be applied to the entry point to keep the field clean (apply some pressure to prevent the formation of a haematoma).

» The catheter is threaded over the guidewire and is advanced until the guidewire protrudes from the proximal end of the catheter.

» Maintaining a hold of the guidewire, the catheter is advanced into the jugular vein.

» The guidewire is removed, and the position of the catheter in the lumen of the vein is confirmed. At this point the catheter should be aspirating blood (Figs. 13 and 14).

» Attach an injection cap to each injection port.

» Suture the catheter at three points: the neck of the catheter and the two "wings" of the suture clip (Fig. 15).

» Clean and dry the area with sterile gauze, and place a sterile dressing over the insertion point and a light and comfortable elastic bandage around the neck. Although it may be tempting to use a large bandage to ensure that the catheter remains in place, experience has shown that the animal is less likely to interfere with a smaller, more comfortable bandage.

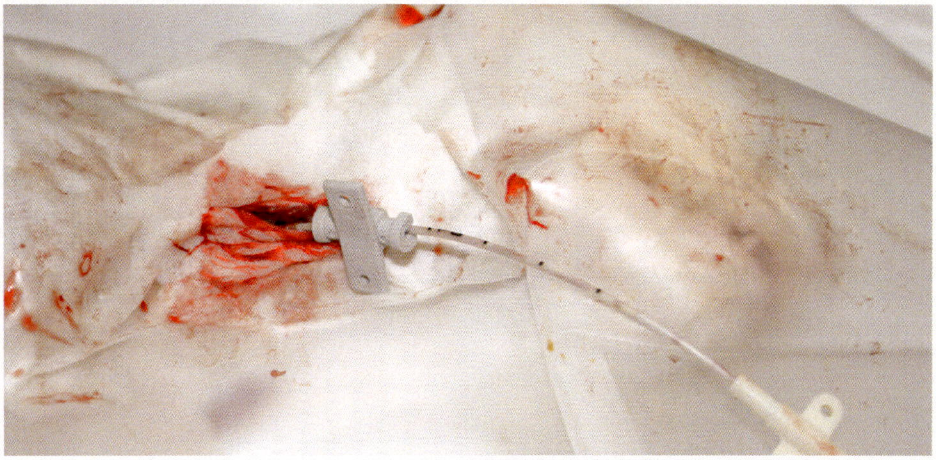

Figure 13. Introduction of the central venous catheter into the vein.

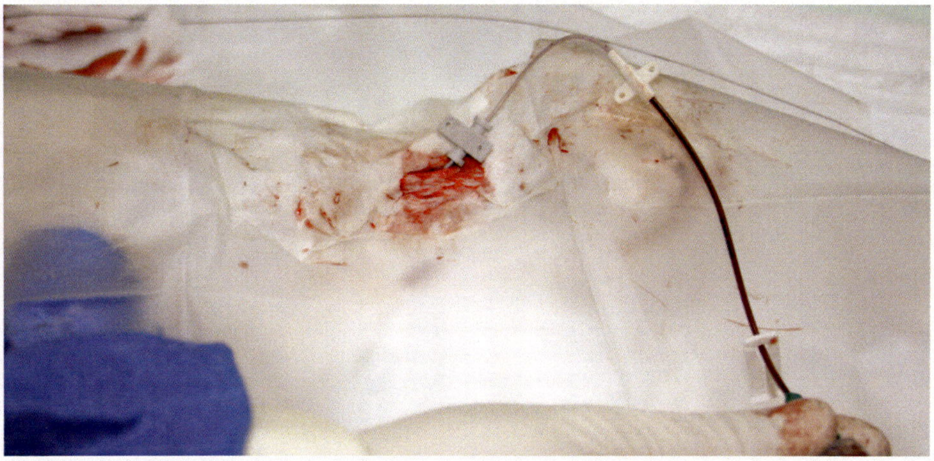

Figure 14. Verification of the location of the central venous catheter.

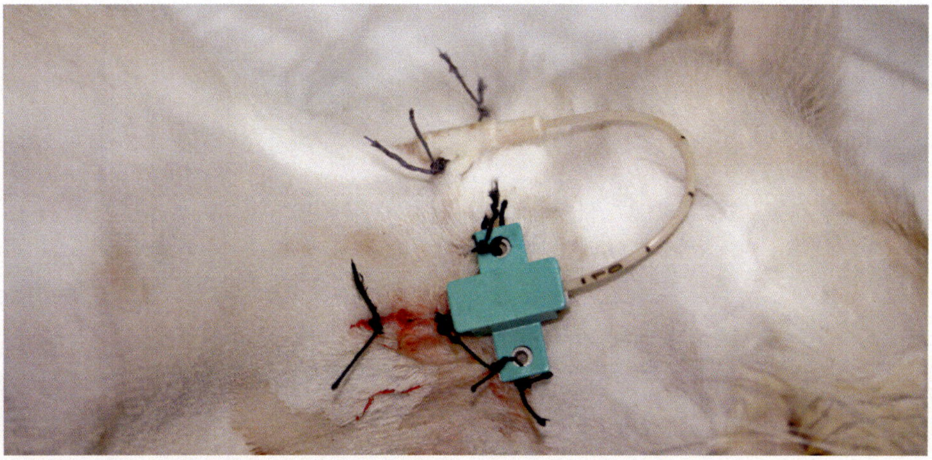

Figure 15. Suturing of the central venous catheter to the skin.

Catheter-related complications
Occlusion.
Removal of the catheter by the patient.
Contamination/infection.
Sepsis.
Thrombophlebitis.
Thrombosis.
Air embolism.
Infection rates of about 7 % have been reported.

Intraosseous access

Intraosseous access is another very important vascular access technique in emergency care when percutaneous access in not possible. It has the advantage of allowing very rapid access.

The rate of absorption of fluids, transfusions, or drugs administered via intraosseous access is practically equivalent to that of intravenous access, and possibly even higher than that obtained via the peripheral vein in cases of peripheral vasoconstriction.

An infusion pump or syringe is required to provide greater infusion pressure, although gravity alone can provide rates of 10–20 ml per minute.

This route can be used to administer hypertonic or hyperoncotic solutions and any blood product.

The most important access points are:

- Crest or wing of the ilium.
- Proximal femoral epiphysis in the trochanteric fossa.
- Proximal epiphysis of the humerus, located by palpating the proximal tuberosity or greater tubercle of the humerus.
- Proximal tibia on the medial side.

Material

In addition to general material required for aseptic preparation and anaesthesia of the area, the technique also requires a Rosenthal or Jamshidi needle for bone marrow puncture. The recommended size is 18–21 G depending on the size of the cat. In kittens, needles of 18–22 G may be sufficient given the softness of the cortical bone. It may be necessary to create a small incision in the skin to insert the needle.

Technique

Once the infusion area has been selected it is clipped and prepared aseptically, after which the skin, subcutaneous tissue, and periosteum are infiltrated with lidocaine or bupivacaine. A scalpel blade is used to make a minimal incision to facilitate insertion of the needle.

The needle is inserted until it reaches the periosteum. From this point the needle is advanced further using a firm twisting motion until it pierces the cortical bone, as indicated by a marked decrease in resistance to the needle (Fig. 16). To verify the location of the needle in the medullary canal, bone marrow, which is similar to blood, can be extracted. In situations of hypovolaemia it may be impossible to extract any material. In these cases physiological saline can be infused to determine whether this results in subcutaneous oedema.

The catheter is fixed to the skin with adhesive tape and silk sutures, and connected to the fluid infusion system (Figs. 17 and 18).

These catheters are difficult to maintain in animals with normal mobility, and thus should be replaced as soon as possible with a peripheral catheter.

Complications that may arise include bleeding, trauma, or infection of tissues adjacent to the bone or of the bone itself.

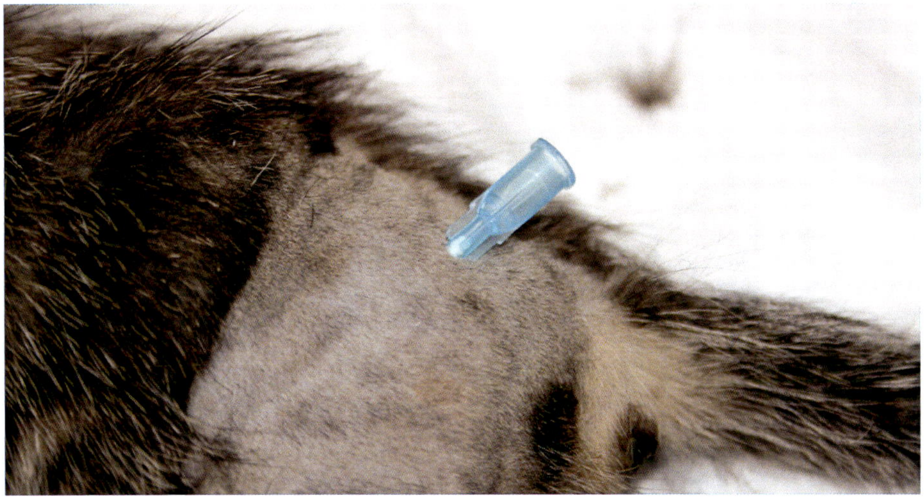

Figure 16. Placement of a needle into the trochanteric fossa of the femur.

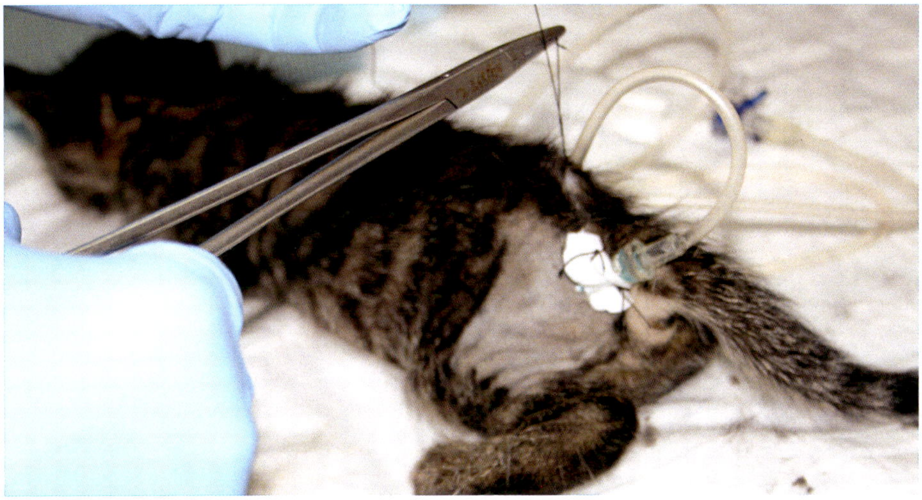

Figure 17. Connection of fluid therapy extension tubing and fixation to the skin with sutures.

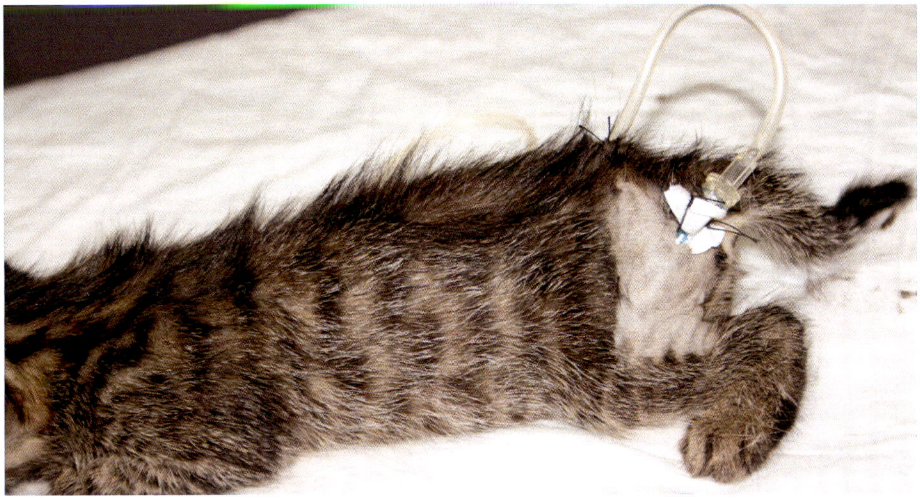

Figure 18. Completion of catheter fixation.

Appendix 3

Feeding in critical situations

Cats whose nutritional intake does not fulfil their requirements pose a challenge. Many diseases and traumatic processes result in inadequate feeding.

Cats have large protein and amino acid requirements. If insufficient calories are consumed, traumatised or sick animals catabolise body mass. Glycogen is consumed initially, but depletion of reserves results in rapid catabolism of fat and muscle.

This gives rise to metabolic alterations, including a decrease in circulating insulin levels and an increase in glucose, lactate, cortisol, glucagon, and norepinephrine levels.

In cases of inadequate intake, energy is derived from accelerated proteolysis. These animals may have some intact fat deposits, but lose a significant amount of muscle mass.

Healing and the immune system are impaired, with increased morbidity and mortality.

The objective of feeding in critical states is to provide nutrients and energy necessary to ensure the following:

- Successful recovery.
- Correct functioning of the internal organs.
- Correct healing.
- Limited loss of muscle mass associated with inflammation or hypermetabolic states.

The moment of intervention is key in situations of malnutrition. Generally, nutritional support is necessary in cases of loss of appetite, inability to eat, or persistent vomiting due to various disease processes.

Nutritional support should be provided to any sick animal that has had inadequate intake for three days. Emergency intervention is required for animals with insufficient intake for five days or more.

Nutritional support should not be instituted in animals that are haemodynamically unstable, dehydrated, or have electrolyte and acid-base imbalances, as this can result in serious metabolic disorders. First, the patient should be stabilised.

Parenteral nutrition

Significant advances have been made in the development of new formulations for parenteral nutrition. However, research has primarily focused on identifying patients that will benefit most.

The first study of total parenteral nutrition (TPN) in cats was conducted in 1977 (Lippert *et al.*). Seven normal cats were fed for 14 days according to their maintenance energy requirements (MER), which were calculated as 1.4 × RER (resting energy requirements). Cats that received excess calories developed vomiting, oral ulcers, and hyperglycaemia. All developed anaemia, thrombocytopaenia, hypertriglyceridaemia, atrophy of the intestinal villi, and hepatocellular alterations.

More recent studies have also investigated TPN in cats, primarily in those with pancreatitis and liver disease. Mechanical and septic complications arose in 18 % of patients, while 48 % developed hyperglycaemia.

Those studies found that calculation of the energy needs by multiplying by a correction factor corresponding to the disease resulted in an increased mortality rate.

Patient selection

In some patients TPN can increase the risk of complications and result in deterioration of the animal's health. It is therefore essential to properly select patients and provide them with the appropriate care.

Cats selected for TPN should be those in which this approach will be beneficial, although in reality the selection criteria in both human and veterinary medicine are unknown.

TPN is indicated in situations in which the patient neither eats voluntarily nor tolerates enteral nutrition, as occurs in the following situations:

- Vomiting.
- Regurgitation.
- Acute pancreatitis.
- Intestinal obstruction.
- Severe malabsorption.
- Paralytic ileus.
- Inability to maintain respiratory airway.

Before instituting TPN, it is necessary to correct fluid and electrolyte alterations and acid-base imbalances.

Nutrition can be administered via a central (TPN) or peripheral (PPN) venous catheter:

- TPN (total parenteral nutrition) covers all the animal's caloric and protein needs.
- PPN (partial parenteral nutrition) only covers a portion of those needs (calories, proteins, and other nutrients).

Indications for partial parenteral nutrition (PPN)
Maintenance of nutritional status, rather than recovery of the patient.
Animals with average nutritional needs.
When short-term nutrition is required (<5 days) in non-debilitated patients.
To supplement oral or enteral feeding.
In cases in which a central venous access catheter is not available.

When an animal requires parenteral nutrition TPN should ideally be administered, as this provides all the necessary nutrients, proteins, and calories in a more physiological manner. However, this approach has some drawbacks (e.g. requires a central venous catheter) and is associated with a greater risk of metabolic disorders.

Determination of parenteral nutrition needs

Caloric needs

RER is the number of calories the animal needs for maintenance at rest.

$$RER = 30 \times (BW \text{ in kg}) + 70$$

In cases of animals that are underweight, it is recommended to calculate RER using their actual weight.

The purpose of parenteral nutrition is not to gain weight; this will be achieved when the disease is under control and the patient can tolerate oral or enteral feeding. Overfeeding to increase weight increases the risk of metabolic complications.

Traditionally, the RER is multiplied by a disease factor of between 1.0 and 2.0 (IER, illness energy requirements). Current guidelines recommend more conservative calculations to prevent overfeeding and high rates of metabolic complications (e.g. hyperglycaemia).

In PPN, caloric needs are calculated as 50 % of the IER.

In patients with glycaemia, adjustments are made based on the patient's RER, and the subsequent response is evaluated.

The key to successful nutritional support is careful monitoring to ensure that the nutritional contribution corresponds to the needs of the animal.

Components of parenteral nutrition

The mixture administered in parenteral nutrition consists of amino acids, dextrose, and lipids, as well as vitamins and minerals.

Amino acids

These solutions constitute a source of nitrogen and essential amino acids. Commercial solutions are available with concentrations ranging from 3.5 % to 10 %. The most commonly used solutions range from 8.5 % to 10 %.

They may or may not contain electrolytes. If parenteral nutrition is administered without electrolytes and the animal has an electrolyte imbalance, this should be corrected with the appropriate fluid therapy.

The standard amount of protein in the formulation is **6 g/100 kcal in cats.**

This should be reduced in animals with protein intolerance, as occurs in cases of kidney disease and hepatic encephalopathy, or increased in the case of greater needs (e.g. in animals with large wounds or hypoalbuminaemia).

Currently, commercial solutions specifically designed to provide essential amino acids are available for humans, but not cats. These solutions are thus not entirely satisfactory when used in cats, but can be useful for short-term administration.

Dextrose

For PPN 5–10 % dextrose is used, whereas for TPN a 50 % solution is used.

A 50 % dextrose solution provides 1.7 kcal/ml

In TPN half of the non-protein calories are administered as dextrose, although this may vary depending on the animal's needs (e.g. higher percentage of lipids in animals with diabetes).

Dextrose should not be infused at rates of over 4 mg/kg/min, given the ability of cats to oxidise dextrose and the risk of hyperglycaemia.

Lipids

Lipid solutions, derived from soybeans and egg yolks, are used to provide energy and essential fatty acids.

A 20 % lipid solution provides 2 kcal/ml

High lipid doses may cause immunosuppression due to granulocyte dysfunction. Ideally lipid doses should be limited to 2 g/kg/day to avoid immunosuppression.

Minerals

Commercial solutions may or may not contain electrolytes. It is more flexible to use solutions that do not contain electrolytes and to provide them as required via specific fluid therapy.

Vitamins

A combination of vitamin B complex with parenteral solutions is usually beneficial in hospitalised animals. Patients with liver disease can be treated with vitamin K supplements.

Composition of mixtures used for parenteral nutrition

The use of a mixture of different nutrients contained within in a single bag is generally preferred. The total osmolarity is equal to the sum of the different osmolarities of the individual components.

Solutions for TPN have an osmolarity of over 1000 mOsm/l and should be administered via a central venous catheter.

Mixtures used for PPN have an osmolarity of less than 700 mOsm/l and can be administered via a peripheral line.

The proportions of the different nutrients for cats are as follows: 25 % dextrose (concentration, 5 %), 25 % amino acids (8.5 %), and 50 % lipid solution (20 %).

Calculation of total parenteral nutrition

1» Resting energy requirements (RER)

RER = 30 × BW (kg) + 70 = kcal/day

2» Protein needs

Usually: 6 g/100 kcal

$\frac{\text{RER}}{100}$ × g/100 kcal = g protein needed/day

3» Volumes of nutrient solutions required per day

a) 8.5 % amino acid solution = 0.085 g protein/ml

$\frac{\text{g protein/day}}{\text{0.085 g protein/ml}}$ = ml amino acids/day

b) Non-protein calories

- The calories provided by the amino acids equal 4 kcal/g

  g protein/day × 4 kcal/g = kcal provided by proteins

  RER - kcal provided by proteins = kcal non-protein/day

- Non-protein calories: 50 % lipids + 50 % dextrose

  20 % lipid solution = 0.2 kcal/ml

  $\frac{\text{kcal lipids required}}{\text{2 kcal/ml}}$ = ml lipids

  50 % dextrose solution = 1.7 kcal/ml

  $\frac{\text{kcal dextrose required}}{\text{1.7 kcal/ml}}$ = ml dextrose

4» Total requirements

ml 8.5 % amino acid solution

ml 20 % lipid solution

ml 50 % dextrose

The calories provided by each of these formulas should be adjusted to the rate of fluid administration based on the bodyweight of each animal. In cats an adjustment is always necessary because the energy calculations for TPN will result in a total volume that is greater than that which is considered normal in terms of the rate of maintenance fluid administration.

Calculation of partial parenteral nutrition

- 25 % dextrose (5 %)
- 25 % amino acid (8.5 %)
- 50 % lipids (20 %)

1» Resting energy requirements (RER)

RER = 30 × BW (kg) + 70 = kcal/day

2» Partial energy requirements (PER)

Covers 70 % of RER: PER = RER × 0.7 = kcal/day

3» Nutrient composition

For cats in general, and especially kittens, formulas provide an amount of fluid greater than the fluid maintenance needs. It is important to make sure that the cat can tolerate the volume of fluid calculated, or otherwise to correct the infusion volume.

RER × 0.25 = kcal/day dextrose

RER × 0.25 = kcal/day protein

RER × 0.50 = kcal/day lipids

4» Volumes of nutrient solutions required per day

a) 5 % dextrose solution = 0.17 kcal/ml

$$\frac{\text{kcal dextrose}}{0.17\ \text{kcal/ml}} = \text{ml dextrose/day}$$

b) 8.5 % amino acid solution = 0.085 kcal/ml

$$\frac{\text{kcal amino acids}}{0.085\ \text{kcal/ml}} = \text{ml amino acids/day}$$

c) 20 % lipid solution = 2 kcal/ml

$$\frac{\text{kcal lipids}}{2\ \text{kcal/ml}} = \text{ml lipids/day}$$

5» Total requirements

ml 5 % dextrose solution

ml 8.5 % amino acid solution

ml 20 % lipid solution

Fluid can be added directly to the PPN solution.

Administration

Appropriate catheters should be used depending on whether the patient requires TPN or PPN. In both cases aseptic preparation is required; contamination is the most common cause of catheter-related complications.

Catheters should be long, and should not contain silicone or polyurethane, which are associated with a risk of thrombophlebitis. The catheter selected should be used for parenteral nutrition only. Alternatively, catheters with multiple ports can be used.

Nutrient solutions should be prepared on the day of use, also under strict aseptic conditions. It is advisable to use bags in which the various components can be easily manually mixed. If commercial preparations designed for human medicine are used, it can be very difficult to adjust caloric needs to the appropriate administration volumes. These preparations are therefore not very useful, at least in the medium-to-long term.

The mixture should not remain at room temperature for more than 24 hours and ideally should be administered using an infusion pump. Aseptic conditions should be maintained at all times and the different infusion lines should not be disconnected. If the animal needs to be moved, it should be moved together with the entire infusion system.

TPN should be administered gradually over 48 to 72 hours, using the same approach applied to enteral nutrition. In general, the amount of dextrose administered the first day should be 50 % of the total calculated, and blood glucose levels should be strictly controlled. If no problems are detected after 48 to 72 hours, the total calculated quantity can be administered. The intravenous administration of other fluids should also be adjusted to avoid fluid overload.

Complications

These are usually classified into three groups: mechanical, metabolic, and septic.

Mechanical causes are those related to the catheter, and thus are controlled by constant monitoring.

Metabolic complications are the most frequent, in particular hyperglycaemia. To avoid this type of complication, it is advisable to be conservative when calculating the daily nutritional needs based on the RER and to begin feeding gradually. TPN can also give rise to refeeding syndrome.

Constant monitoring of metabolism and of the concentrations of different ions is essential throughout the feeding process. Body weight should also be monitored daily.

RER should be used as a starting point for calculations, which can be modified upward or downward depending on the animal's progress.

The following clinical aspects and parameters should be monitored:

- Cardiorespiratory frequency.
- Catheter/skin interface.
- Attitude.
- Body weight.
- Temperature.
- Glucose.
- Electrolytes.

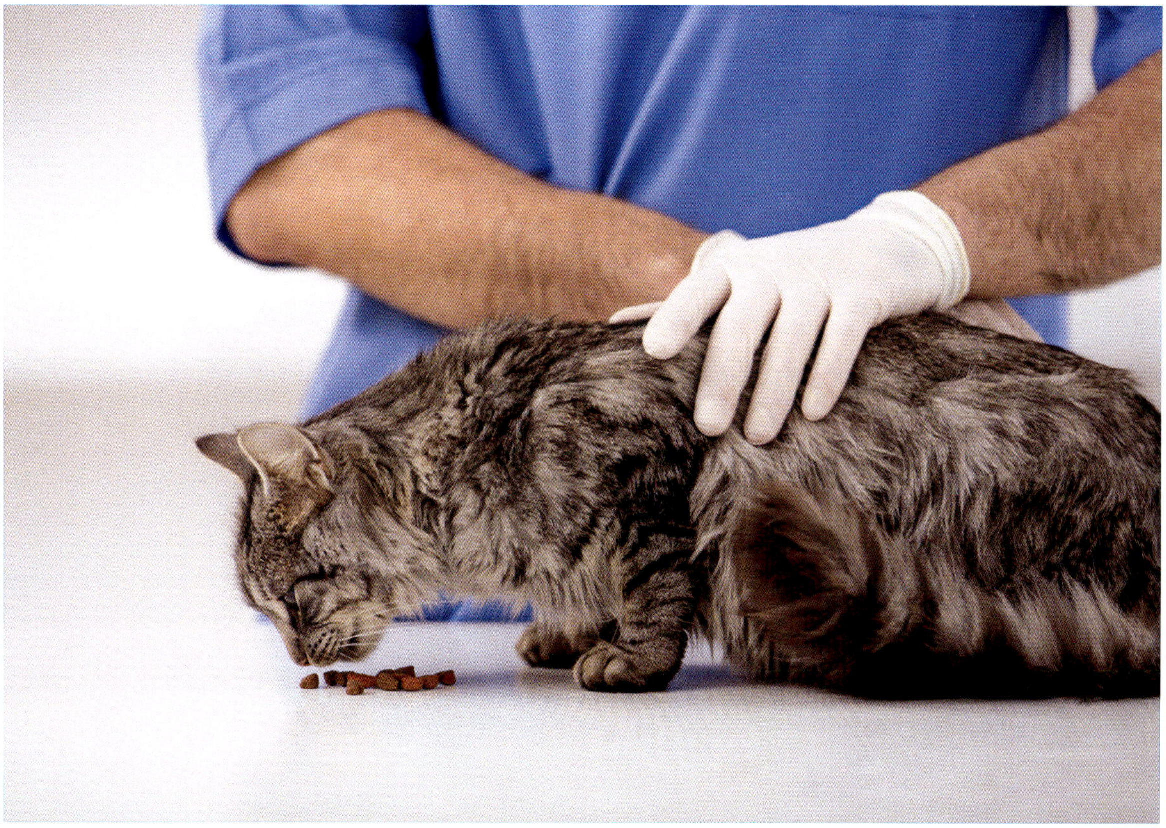

Figure 1. To the extent possible, the patient should be encouraged to eat (VGstockstudio, Shutterstock.com).

Interruption

The switch to oral ingestion or enteral feeding should be made as soon as possible to prevent atrophy of the intestine (Fig. 1). At least 50 % of RER should be provided via oral or enteral feeding before withdrawing parenteral nutrition. TPN should be removed gradually over 6 to 12 hours, always monitoring blood sugar levels, as this is a critical moment at which hypoglycaemia may occur.

Appendix 4

Blood transfusion

The objective of this supportive therapy is to correct deficiencies until the underlying cause can be treated. The risk/benefit ratio should be evaluated carefully before including blood transfusion in the patient's treatment plan.

Blood transfusion is indicated in the following cases:

- Hypoalbuminaemia.
- Severe anaemia.
- Haemorrhage.
- Lack of coagulation factors (e.g. poisoning).

Whole blood or components thereof can be transfused.

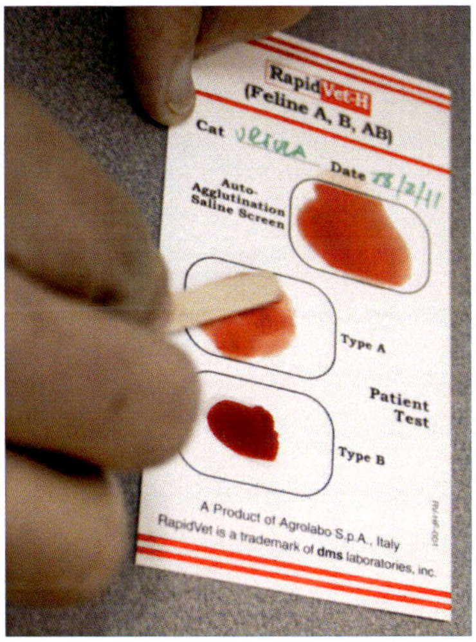

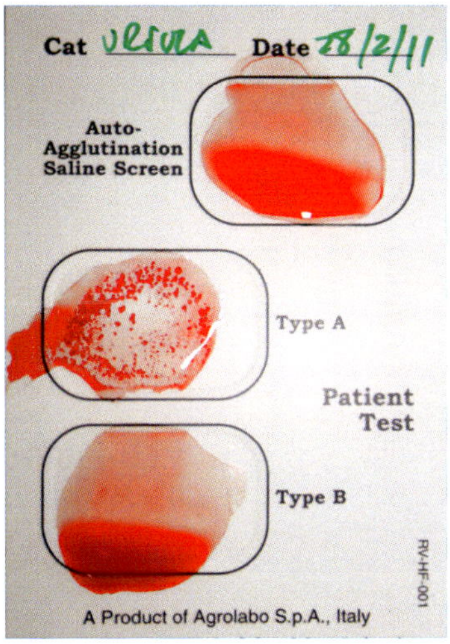

Figures 1 and 2. Agglutination test to determine blood group.

Table 1. Percentage of feline blood groups in Europe.

	A	B	AB
Common cats	87 %	8 %	5 %
Pure-bred cats	55 %	40 %	5 % (group B is more common in breeds such as shorthair, ragdoll, and rex)

Whole blood contains:

- Erythrocytes.
- Clotting factors.
- Proteins.
- Platelets.
- Leukocytes.

These last two components are inactivated following refrigeration.

Donor selection

Donors should be healthy and large (>4 kg), but not obese.

Blood type should be established before collecting blood (Figs. 1–3). In addition, the animal should undergo a general examination, including tests for blood-borne diseases such as feline immunodeficiency virus, feline leukaemia virus, feline infectious peritonitis, bartonellosis, and mycoplasmosis.

Ideally, the donor should have haematocrit levels of over 35 %. Cats have three blood groups; A, B, and AB. A new group, Mik, based on the expression of antigens on the surface of erythrocytes, has also been recently described.

The percentage of each group varies according to geographical regions and countries. The blood type distribution for Europe is shown in Table 1.

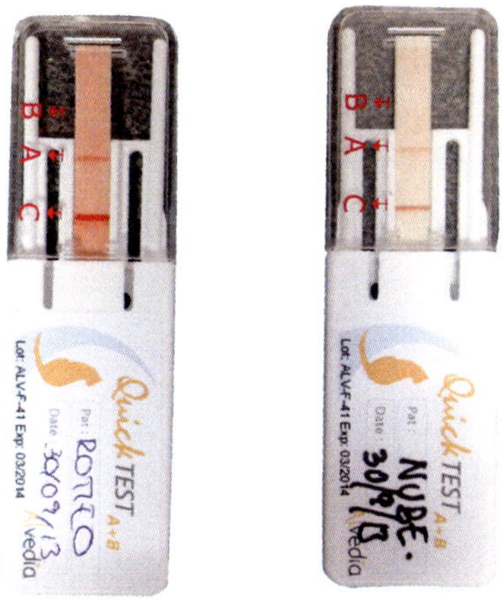

Figure 3. Rapid test for determining blood group.

These antigens are of clinical significance in transfusion medicine.

Adverse reactions associated with blood group

Blood transfusion haemolysis

Group A cats have few anti-B antibodies. Therefore adverse reactions to the transfusion of group B blood into group A animals are delayed and rarely severe. Extra- and intra-vascular haemolysis can occur.

Group B cats harbour large amounts of anti-A antibodies, and therefore can have very severe adverse reactions upon receipt of group B blood. These can occur within a few seconds, and are characterised by the following signs: apnoea, bradycardia, arrhythmias, hypotension, seizures, vocalisations, urination, defaecation, and depression.

Neonatal isoerythrolysis

This occurs when group B females give birth to kittens of groups A or AB. On the first day of life kittens receive maternal anti-A antibodies via the colostrum.

Manifestations can range from subclinical to very severe, with haemoglobinaemia, haemoglobinuria, anaemia, jaundice, growth problems, necrosis of the tail tip, or sudden death.

Tests can be performed to detect antibodies that can cross-react with the antigens present in erythrocytes. These tests are performed when the blood group is unknown and cannot be identified, or can be applied in combination with blood-typing tests.

If the cat has immune-mediated haemolytic anaemia, it will also have circulating antibodies to red blood cells and will test positive in the cross-matching blood test.

Collection of blood from donor

Generally sedation of the donor is necessary in order to manipulate the animal without causing hypotension or peripheral vasoconstriction.

Fluid therapy is administered to prevent hypovolaemia. In general the volume administered should be double the volume of blood to be extracted (Fig. 4).

Blood is extracted from the jugular vein using a butterfly needle or a catheter attached to an extension tube (Figs. 5 and 6). Blood is collected in a 50-ml syringe or in two 20-ml syringes containing 6 ml (or 3 + 3 ml) of anticoagulant extracted from a human blood transfusion bag (citrate).

Transfusion volume

In many cases the volume required cannot be extracted from a single donor.

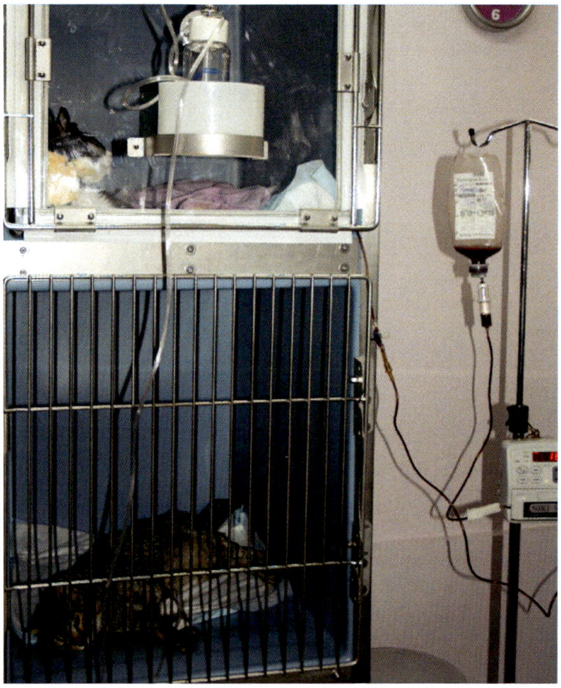

Figure 4. Infusion of blood into recipient animal. The volume of serum administered intravenously to the donor animal is twice the volume of the blood removed.

The volume of blood required for transfusion is calculated using the following formula:

$$\text{Volume of blood for transfusion} = 66 \times \text{patient BW} \times (\text{Ht desired} - \text{Ht patient})/\text{Ht donor}$$

In general the volume transfused is 10–22 ml/kg bodyweight.

Administration

Blood obtained is transferred into an empty serum bottle coupled to a drip chamber to ensure the absence of clots from the blood for transfusion (Fig. 7).

A three-way stopcock can be used to mix the blood with saline in order to avoid high blood density in the vein of the recipient. Alternatively, blood and saline can be mixed in the same bottle at a maximum ratio of 1:1, to avoid alterations (Fig. 8).

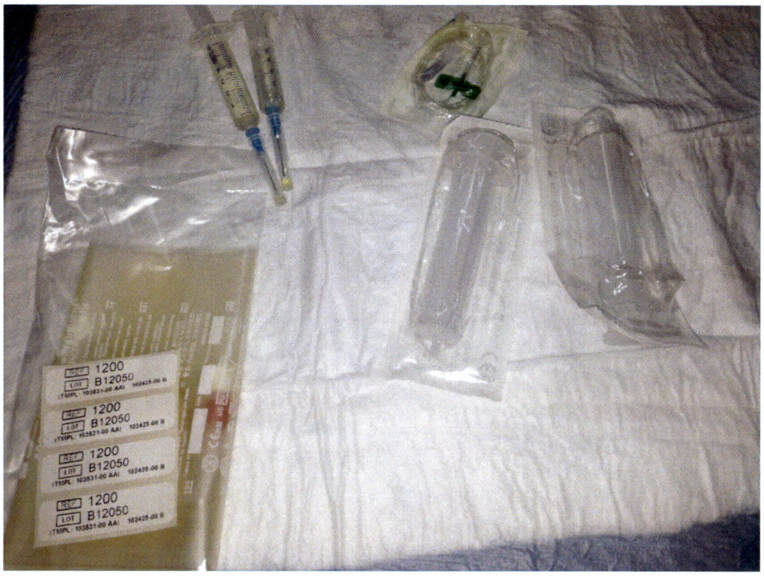

Figure 5. Material necessary for the extraction of blood from a donor.

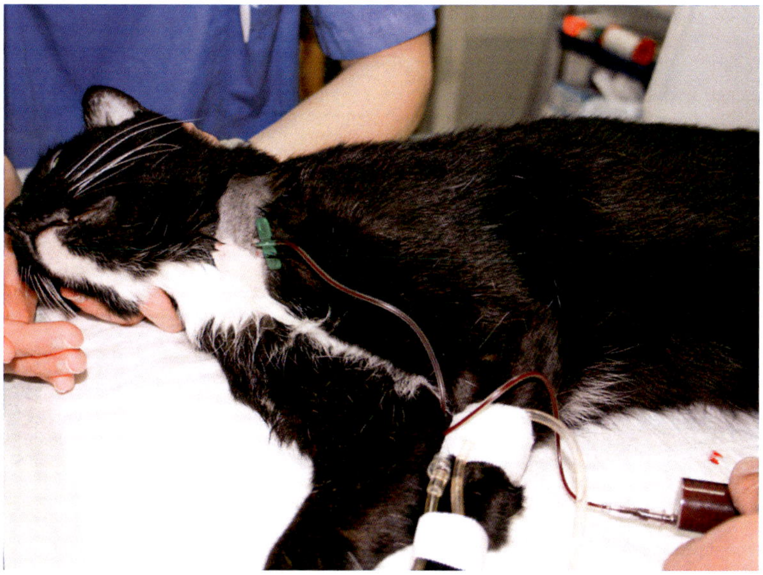

Figure 6. Animal under sedation for extraction of blood from the jugular vein.

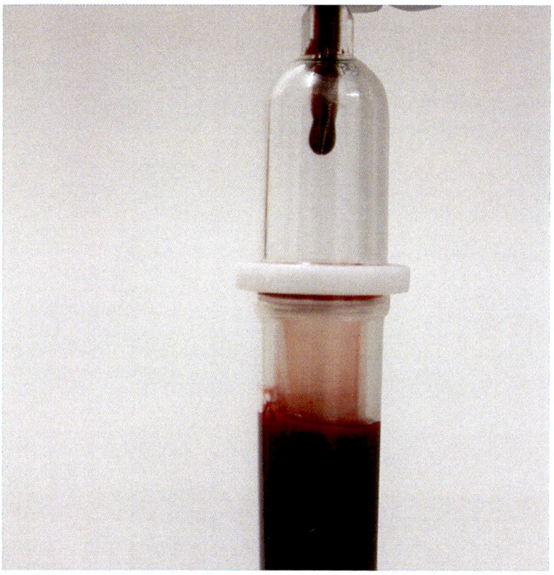

Figure 7. Transfusion system with anti-clotting filter.

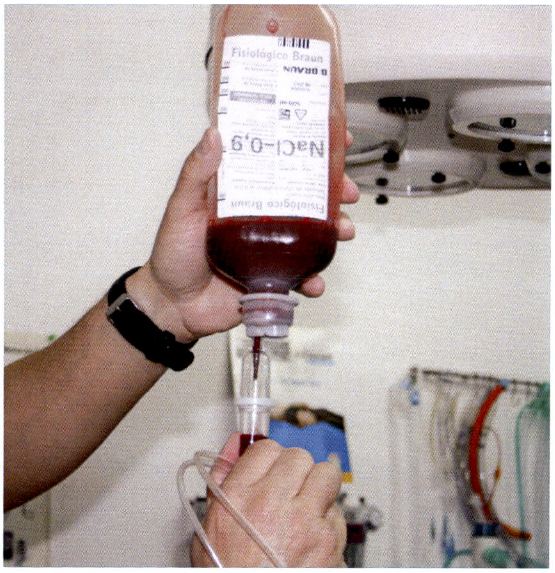

Figure 8. Mixture of extracted blood and warm 0.9 % saline.

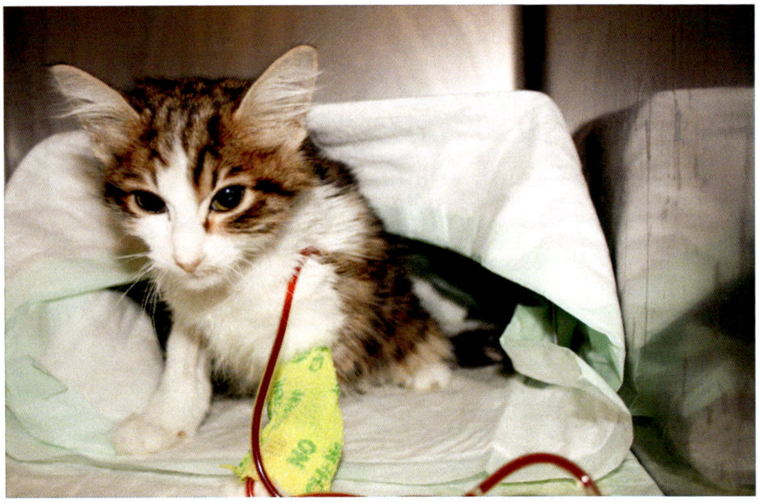

Figure 9. Cat receiving blood via the cephalic vein.

The route of administration is via the cephalic vein (Fig. 9). If this vein cannot be accessed (e.g. in very small animals), the transfusion can be administered via the intraosseous route or by central line.

The blood is gently heated to 27–30°C in a water bath to avoid haemolysis and clot formation.

Infusion begins slowly, at a rate of 0.5–1 ml/kg per hour for 10 to 15 minutes, during which the patient is monitored (Figs. 10 and 11). Subsequently, the rate of infusion is gradually increased to the normal rate.

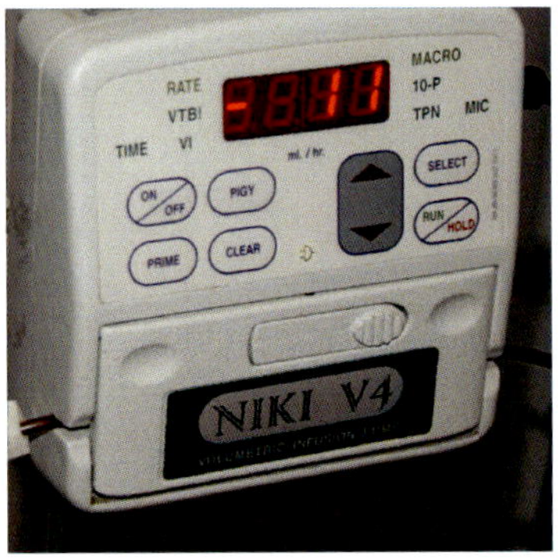

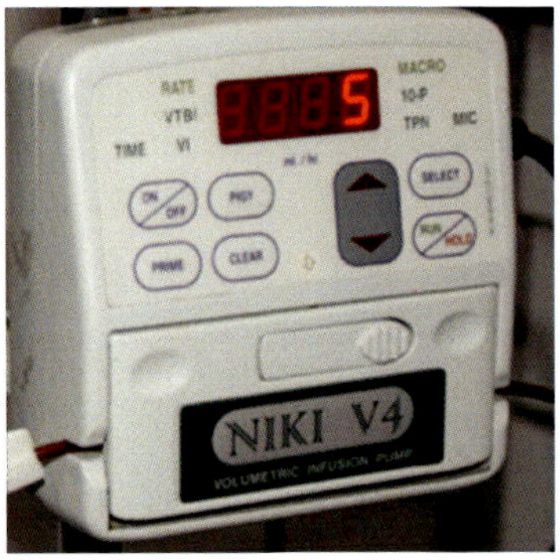

Figures 10 and 11. Infusion pumps set at slow initial transfusion rate.

Adverse transfusion reactions

In general, animals receiving transfusions should be constantly monitored, noting vital signs and the animal's behaviour. If haemoglobin appears in the urine, both blood and urine should be analysed.

The classification of adverse transfusion reactions is shown in Table 2.

Table 2. Classification of adverse reactions to blood transfusion.

Adverse reactions	Acute	Delayed
Immunological	• Haemolysis • Acute hypersensitivity • Platelet sensitivity • White blood cell sensitivity	• Haemolysis • Neonatal isoerythrolysis
Non-immunologic	• Circulatory overload • Bacterial contamination • Citrate toxicity • Hypothermia • Pulmonary embolism	• Transmission of infectious agents

Appendix 5

Punctures and drainage devices

Thoracentesis

Indications

The main indication is for the collection of pleural fluid for analysis when the presence of fluid is demonstrated by exploration and imaging tests (chest radiography and ultrasound).

When pleural fluid causes respiratory difficulties in cats, this procedure also facilitates removal of the fluid and improves respiratory function. Pleural fluid or gas can be removed using drainage devices either intermittently or continuously. This requires a needle and an intravenous catheter or a butterfly needle in the case of one-off or intermittent drainage. For continuous drainage a thoracostomy tube is required.

Complications

Potential complications include pneumothorax, haemothorax in the case of lesions of the intercostal arteries or lungs, and iatrogenic problems or infections.

Technique

The chest is shaved and the skin aseptically prepared with sterile drapes and gloves. Local anaesthesia of the insertion site is required.

The technique requires an intravenous catheter or butterfly needle (22 G) attached to an extension tube (so that the movements of the surgeon do not affect the patient). In turn, this tube is attached to a three-way stopcock and a collection system, which in this case should be a syringe of no more than 10 ml.

The patient is placed in lateral or sternal recumbency, whichever is most comfortable. This procedure must be performed rapidly, before any other diagnostic procedure.

It is advisable to prepare a large surgical field in order to be prepared for any eventuality (Fig. 1).

The puncture site should be between the 7th and 9th ICS at the cranial portion of the rib bone, since the neurovascular bundle runs along the caudal portion of the bone. The thorax should be virtually divided into three equal parts, and the puncture created in the ventral third to remove fluid, or the mid-dorsal third to remove gas.

Local anaesthesia is applied to the skin and subcutaneous tissue. It is important to be aware of the toxic

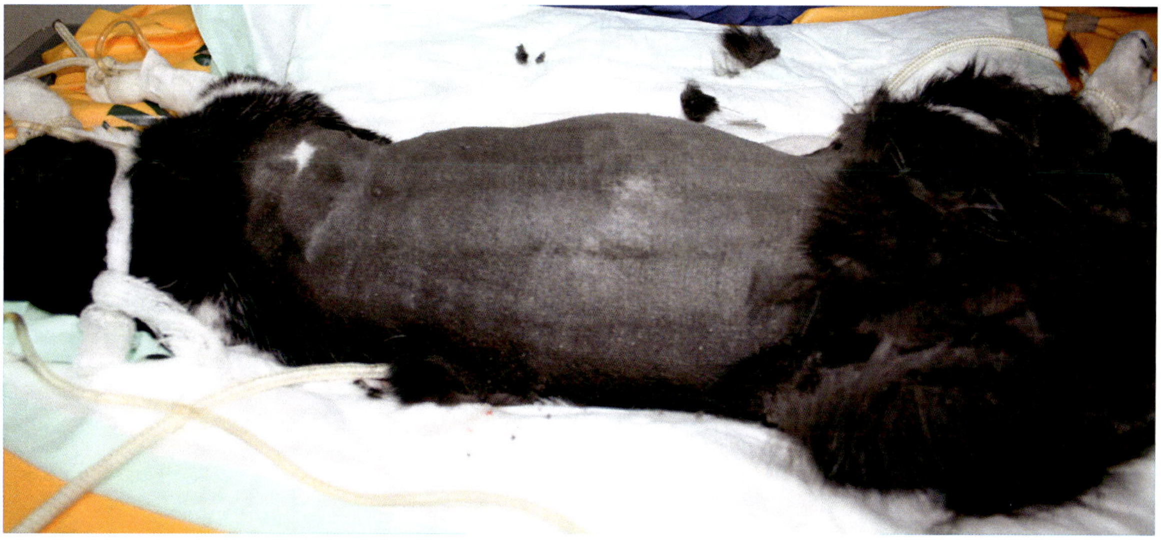

Figure 1. Clipping of both hemithoraces and even the abdomen in case additional interventions are required.

dose of the local anaesthetic used to avoid intoxication or other complications.

Since this is a one-off procedure, tunnelling of the catheter into the subcutaneous tissue to create a seal is not necessary.

The catheter or butterfly needle is inserted caudally with the bevel oriented towards the pleural cavity. After crossing the parietal pleura a change in resistance will be perceived. At this point the butterfly needle should be directed parallel to the chest wall to reduce the risk of pulmonary laceration. If using an intravenous catheter, the needle should be removed while introducing the catheter.

All connections must be well sealed to prevent contamination and the entry of air into the pleural cavity.

Open the stopcock and aspirate gently to avoid collapse of the butterfly needle or catheter. When the syringe is full, close the stopcock and open the collection bag. Repeat this process until the pleural space is empty.

When liquid is obtained, it should be collected (in EDTA tubes and in sterile tubes for culture) to perform the necessary analyses.

Once the procedure is complete, radiography is performed to verify that the drainage has been effective and that no complications have arisen. Subsequently, diagnosis can be established.

It may be necessary to perform this procedure on both hemithoraces.

Thoracic drainage

Objective

The objective is the same as that of thoracentesis:

- Restoration of intrapleural negative pressure.
- Improvement of respiratory function.

Indications

The indications for placement of a chest drain are:

- Persistence of clinical signs despite having undergone thoracentesis.
- Need for more than two thoracenteses procedures per day.
- Removal of more than 2 ml/kg of fluid per day.
- Processes lasting more than two days.
- Situations in which it is determined that the animal has a tension pneumothorax or pyothorax.
- In the postoperative period after thoracic surgery or in cases of penetrating chest wounds.

Complications

Potential complications associated with the technique include:

- Iatrogenic pneumothorax.
- Infections.
- Haemorrhage or haemothorax as a result of laceration of the vascular bundle that runs across the caudal portion of each rib or lesions of the pulmonary parenchyma.
- Drainage tube obstruction.
- Haemoperitoneum caused by abdominal lesions (spleen or liver).
- An undiagnosed diaphragmatic hernia could cause perforation of any organ in the thorax: stomach, spleen, liver, intestine, etc.

Preparing the patient

Some preliminary steps are advised to minimise the risks associated with this technique:

- Preoxygenation, shaving, and preparation of the surgical field, from the caudal edge of the scapula to the last rib. These steps should be performed while the animal is conscious, if possible. At this point an intercostal block is performed with local anaesthetic (lidocaine/bupivacaine) under mild sedation. The block is applied to the nerve of the ICS (7th–8th) into which the tube will be inserted as well as the adjacent cranial and caudal ICS. Local infiltration of the incision site is also necessary.

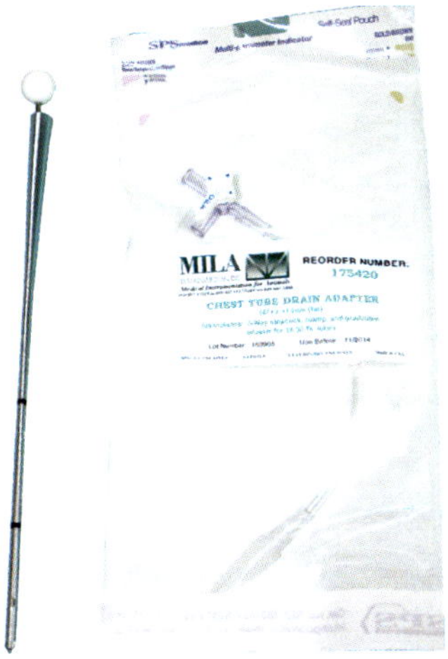

Figure 2. Material required for pleural drainage. Drainage tube with needle and extension with three-way stopcock.

Figure 3. Another type of drain with an external needle.

- Rapid induction of anaesthesia (IV) with patient in sternal recumbency so as not to compromise ventilatory function and insertion of chest drain.
- If the animal has serious respiratory difficulties, the procedure is as follows: stabilisation with oxygen first, followed by thoracentesis and rest until the situation improves.

Technique

The following equipment is required: a trocar for thoracic drainage, connectors for the chest drain, a three-way stopcock, two vent plugs, a fenestrated field, and a 10–20-ml syringe (Figs. 2 and 3). The size of the chest drain should be equivalent to the width of the main bronchus (7–10 Fr).

A small cutaneous incision is made at the level of the 10th ICS, in the top two thirds of the chest wall.

The procedure consists of the following steps:

- Insert the end of the chest drain beneath the skin and subcutaneous tissue and advance in a cranioventral direction, creating a tunnel up to about the 8th ICS (Figs. 5 and 6).
- Maintain the trocar/drain perpendicular to the 8th ICS (cranial to the rib) and carefully introduce it into the chest cavity, firmly grasping it by the base with the other hand to avoid uncontrolled or overly forceful insertion.
- Retract the trocar (a short distance) from the drain to protect the drain from the sharp tip.

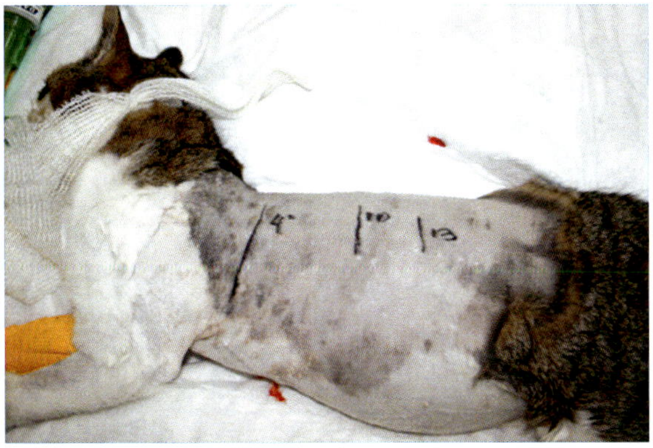

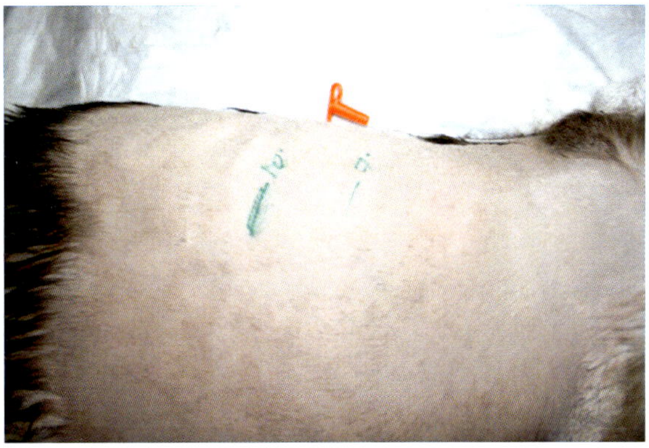

Figures 4 and 5. Anatomic location of rib number for placement of drain. If necessary this can be marked using a felt-tipped pen.

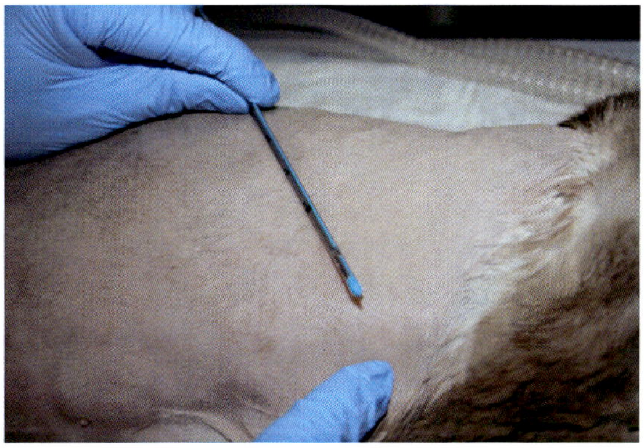

Figure 6. Assessment of tube to confirm direction of insertion and calculate necessary length.

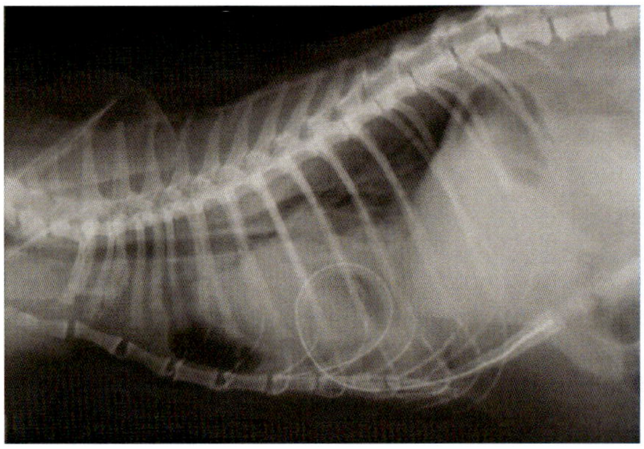

Figure 7. Radiographic verification of tube placement.

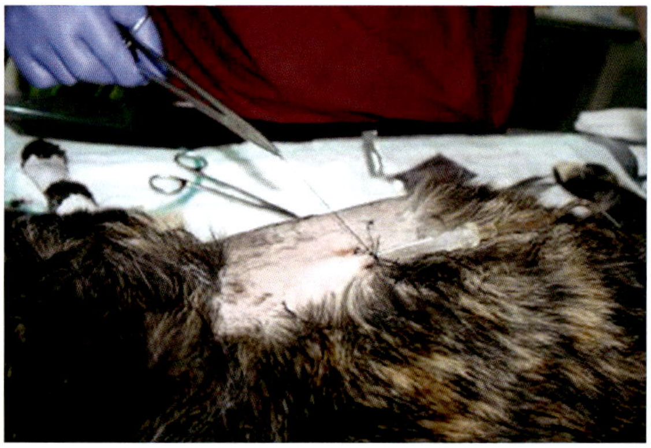

Figure 8. Attachment of tube to the chest wall using Chinese finger-trap sutures.

- Advance the trocar and drain in tandem, parallel to the chest wall, approximately as far as the 2nd rib ventrally.
- Retract the trocar while firmly maintaining the drain in position.
- It is not necessary to occlude the drain with compression forceps to prevent a tension pneumothorax while connecting the three-way stopcock. It is sufficient to simply ventilate manually so that the lungs do not collapse and respiratory function restarts while the drainage system is prepared and the tube is fixed to the chest wall (Figs. 7 and 8).
- Draining the pleural cavity using a syringe (Fig. 9). A syringe can be left connected to the system to facilitate periodic drainage depending on the amount of material to be removed. A drainage valve, specially designed for cats, that does not create an excessive vacuum (no more than -5 to -20 cmH_2O) can be used for continuous drainage.
- After drainage, the three-way stopcock is closed, the two vent plugs are put in place, and the chest drain secured using a "Chinese finger-trap" or "Roman sandal" suture.

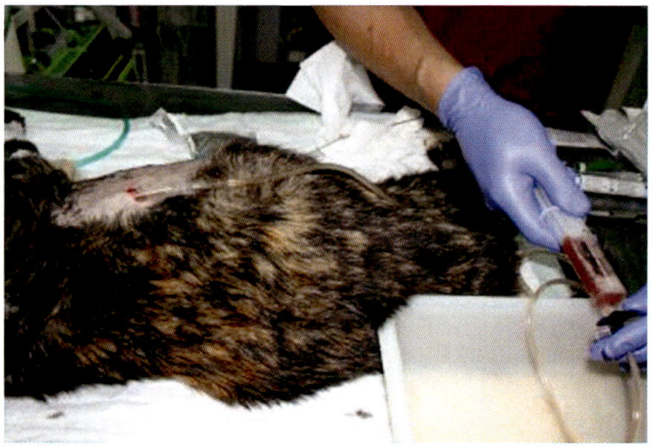

Figure 9. Drainage of chest cavity.

Open technique if trocar is not available

An open technique can be used for placement of a chest drain in the absence of a trocar. This involves the following stages:

» A curved Kelly forceps is inserted to create a subcutaneous tunnel from the 9th–10th **ICS** to the 7th–8th **ICS** by blunt dissection.

» Pressure is applied, keeping the tips of the forceps closed, in order to pass through the intercostal muscle between the ribs.

» The forceps is removed and closed onto the tip of the tube, which is then inserted into the subcutaneous tunnel created with the forceps, through the drainage hole created in the chest wall, and into the pleural cavity, after which the Kelly forceps is removed.

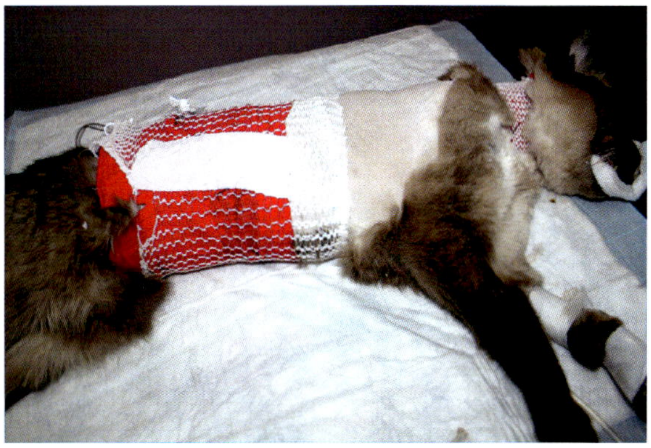

Figure 10. Protection of chest drain with comfortable bandage.

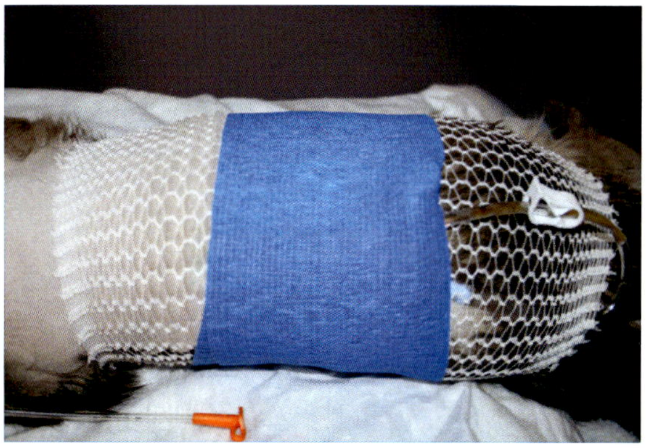

Figure 11. Daily examination and replacement of the bandage.

Postoperative care

The drain insertion point is dressed with antibiotic cream and covered with sterile gauze and a bandage that does not compress the thoracic region (Fig. 10). Radiographs are performed to verify correct placement of the drain for maximum efficacy. The dressing should be changed at least once per day and all connections should be checked (Fig. 11).

It is important to prevent re-expansion pulmonary oedema by carrying out re-expansion progressively, especially if large amounts of material need to be drained and the liquid has remained in the pleural cavity for more than 48–72 hours.

When should the drain be removed?

» When the pleural effusion is <2.2 ml/kg/day. This is the amount produced by placement of the drain itself.

» Absence of pneumothorax and confirmation of negative pressure in preceding 12 to 24 hours, as revealed by radiography.

» There is no need to suture the skin at the tube outlet, as this will close by secondary intention.

In cases of pyothorax, it is preferable to use a larger diameter tube and perform slow pleural washes 2 to 4 times daily using 10 ml/kg warm saline.

Applying these measures, the use of a protective Elizabethan collar is not necessary. Provided that the animal is comfortable and has received adequate analgesia, the likelihood of self-injury or removal of the tube or its various connections is minimal. Nonetheless, constant vigilance is required.

Abdominocentesis

Abdominocentesis or paracentesis is a procedure that involves the insertion of a needle or catheter into the peritoneal cavity to remove ascites fluid.

Indications

The main indications are:

- Sampling of peritoneal fluid for diagnostic purposes (performed using a simple blind technique), especially in cases involving large amounts of liquid.
- Removal of ascites fluid if an abundance of fluid is causing the animal discomfort or pain, respiratory difficulties, or compression of abdominal organs.

Complications

Potential complications associated with this technique include:

- Peritoneal infection.
- Bleeding and haemoperitoneum.
- Laceration of any abdominal organ.

The abdominocentesis area should be prepared aseptically (clipping, skin disinfection, and use of sterile gloves and drapes).

Local anaesthesia is applied, using either anaesthetic ointments applied in advance or by infiltrating the area with lidocaine or bupivacaine.

Needles or catheters of 18–22 G are required, as well as a closed drainage system, tubes in which to collect and study the liquid, extension tubes, and a three-way stopcock (Figs. 12–14).

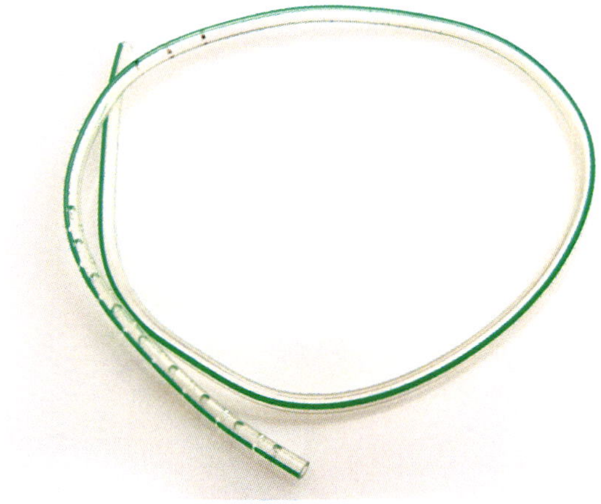

Figure 12. Simple tube without needle for abdominal drainage.

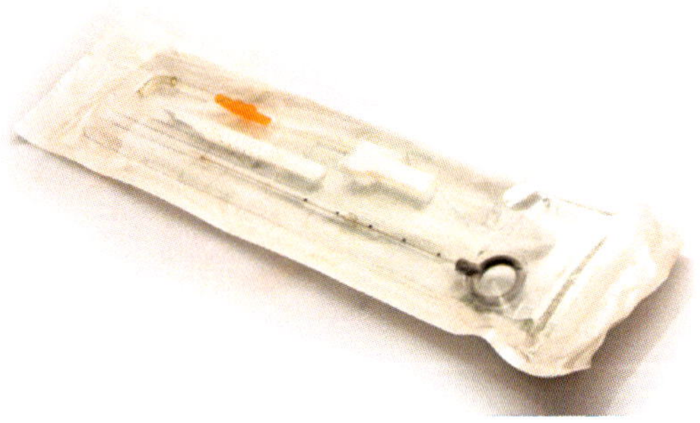

Figure 13. Peritoneal drainage tube with internal needle for abdominocentesis.

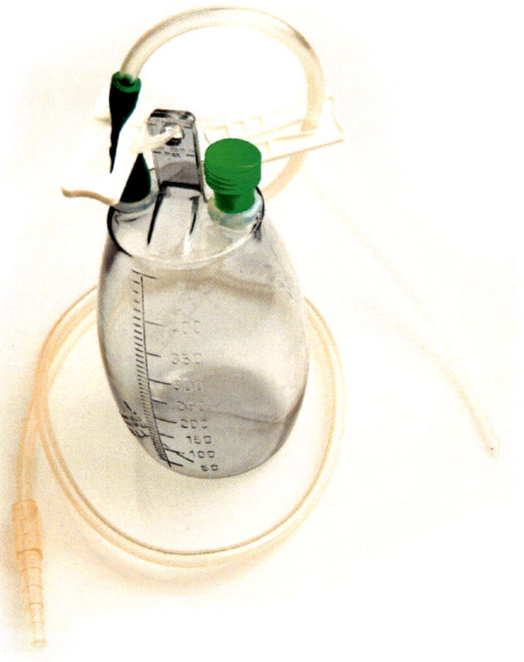

Figure 14. System for the collection of drained material.

Technique

If possible, the bladder should be emptied of urine in advance of the procedure, which should be performed with the animal in the supine recumbency position to avoid the risk of intestinal laceration (unless an ultrasound guided procedure is used).

The abdominocentesis site, after aseptic preparation of the area, should be about 0.5–1.5 cm caudal to the umbilicus and slightly lateral to the linea alba. The needle is inserted caudally (oriented toward the pelvis), at an angle of about 45 °, creating a subcutaneous tunnel before entering the peritoneal cavity (Fig. 5).

If an intravenous catheter is used, ideally a small cutaneous incision should be made with a needle or a scalpel blade to avoid damaging the teflon of the device.

Once inside the peritoneal cavity the needle is removed, the catheter advanced and connected to the drainage system with the extension tube, the three-way stopcock, and a collection bag or syringe.

When the procedure has been completed and the needle removed, pressure is applied to the area for a few minutes until the insertion point is sealed.

This entire procedure of inserting the needle or intravenous catheter can be performed either blind or using ultrasound.

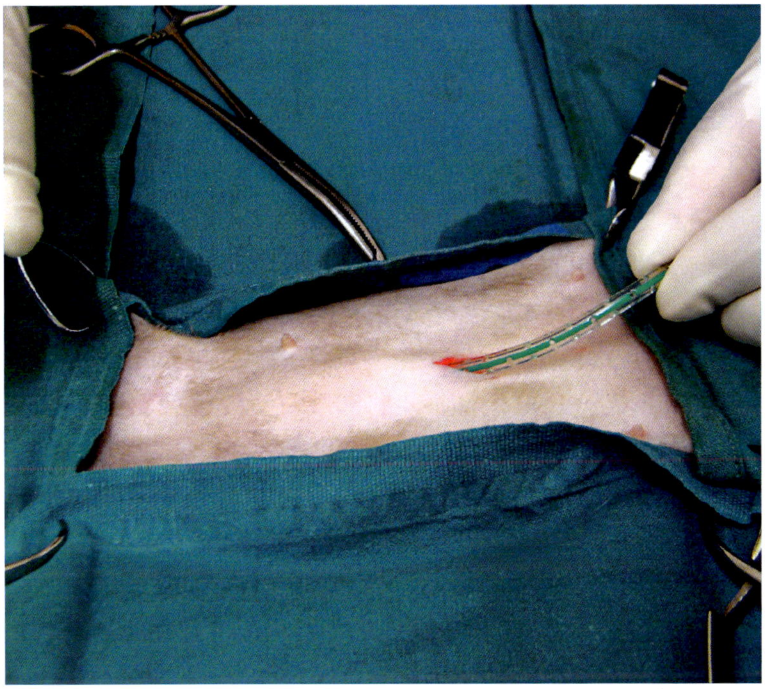

Figure 15. Placement of simple drainage tube without needle.

References

Crow, S.E., Walshaw, S.O., Boyle, J.E. *Manual of clinical procedures in dogs, cats, rabbits and rodents* (3rd ed.). Ed. Wiley Blackwell, 2009.

Tillson, M.D. Thoracostomy tubes. Part i. Indications and anesthesia. *Compend Educ Pract Vet*, 1997; 19(11):1258-1267.

Tillson, M.D. Thoracostomy tubes. Part ii. Placement and maintenance. *Compend Educ Pract Vet*, 1997; 12:1331-1338.

Walters, J.M. Abdominal paracentesis and diagnostic peritoneal lavage. *Clin Techn Small Anim Pract*, 2003; 18:32-38.

White, R. Emergency techniques. In: *Manual of canine and feline emergency and critical care*. Ed. Bsava, 1999; pp. 307-340.

Appendix 6

Feline oral disease

Oral diseases are common in feline medicine and have specific characteristics that can cause great pain and difficulty eating, resulting in anorexia, weight loss, and behavioural disturbances.

A study conducted in the United States in 1996 found that oral disease was the second most common diagnosis in cats aged 0 to 7 years, and the most common in older animals (Harvey, 1992; Holmstrom, 2005).

A detailed assessment, raising the lip of the animal, should be performed on every visit to a veterinary clinic.

There is a connection between oral and systemic disease. Severe kidney failure can cause oral ulcers as a result of ammonia produced by the decomposition of urea in saliva, exacerbating periodontal disease (Harvey, 1992; Holmstrom, 2005). Conversely, oral processes can cause systemic disease. Dental pathologies cause bacteraemia in cats, resulting in the dissemination of bacteria to distant organs, in which alterations occur (Quimby *et al.*, 2006).

Many types of diseases can affect the oral tissues: immune-mediated, degenerative, neoplastic, metabolic and traumatic diseases, as well as infections and chronic inflammation.

When the epithelial protection mechanisms (salivary and cellular) do not work properly and the epithelial surface has been damaged, exposed oral tissues are bathed in a medium rich in bacteria, to which they react. Therefore, inflammatory phenomena are practically universal in oral lesions. All cats with clinically evident oral disease should thus undergo a comprehensive examination to determine the nature of the problem.

Clinical signs

The following clinical signs may appear in cats with problems that affect the oral cavity (Harvey, 1992; Holmstrom, 2005):

- Halitosis.
- Hypersalivation.
- Bleeding from the mouth.
- Discomfort in the area (touching of the mouth).
- Dental hypersensitivity.
- Facial swelling.
- Sneezing.
- Nasal discharge.
- Altered eating habits.
- Dropping of food from the mouth.
- Behavioural changes.

Major oral diseases of cats

Periodontal disease

In general this develops as a result of the deposition of dental plaque. In their natural state, the abrasive effect of the cat's diet during chewing prevents the accumulation of plaque and the development of periodontal disease. Current feline diets are developed to be convenient for both the cat and for the owner, and thus may contribute to the development of periodontal disease, although this topic is a matter of some debate.

Initially, deposited dental plaque is soft and can be removed easily, and consists of bacteria within a biofilm. The mineral composition of saliva is responsible for the hardening of this plaque into tartar, which in turn favours further plaque deposition (Fig. 1).

This can be the result of less frequent cleaning (as occurs in cases of malocclusion), tooth loss, inadequate diet, and diminished defence against systemic diseases (uraemia, diabetes, liver disease) and viral diseases such as leukaemia, immune deficiency, and feline infectious peritonitis (Belows, 2010; Harvey, 1992; Holmstrom, 2005) (Fig. 2).

Predisposing factors

The following predisposing factors have been identified:

- **Bacterial flora:** bacteria occupy all structures of the mouth including the tongue, gums, teeth, and oral mucosa, although they are most abundant on the surface of the teeth, especially at the gingival margin. This is where the proteins from saliva and food are deposited and, together with polypeptides and lipids, form an abundant film over the gum margin. Specific bacteria have certain properties that facilitate adhesion to this film. These bacteria further promote the deposition of the biofilm and its transformation into calculus. These include bacteria of the genus *Bacteroides*, as well as *Pasteurella multocida*.
- **Gingivitis:** the gum is the part of the oral mucosa that covers and protects the crown of the tooth. Gingivitis or gum inflammation is reversible if the plaque is removed and the cat has a normal immune response.
- **Periodontitis:** the tooth is anchored to the mandible or maxilla by a connective tissue called the periodontal ligament. Inflammation of this ligament weakens the union of the tooth to the alveolar bone. This results in the loss of bone and gum, leading to gingival recession, or the formation of gingival pockets between the tooth and the gum, facilitating the accumulation of bacteria in the margin and therefore exacerbating the disease.

These two pathologies are in fact two different stages of the same process. Gingivitis is an inflammatory process induced by the accumulation of bacterial plaque, whereas periodontitis is a more established, chronic process indicative of a more advanced, and in many cases irreversible, pathology.

Treatment

Tartar removal and dental cleaning are essential for the initial management of the disease. This process should include careful examination of the teeth and the gingival margin, and measurement of the

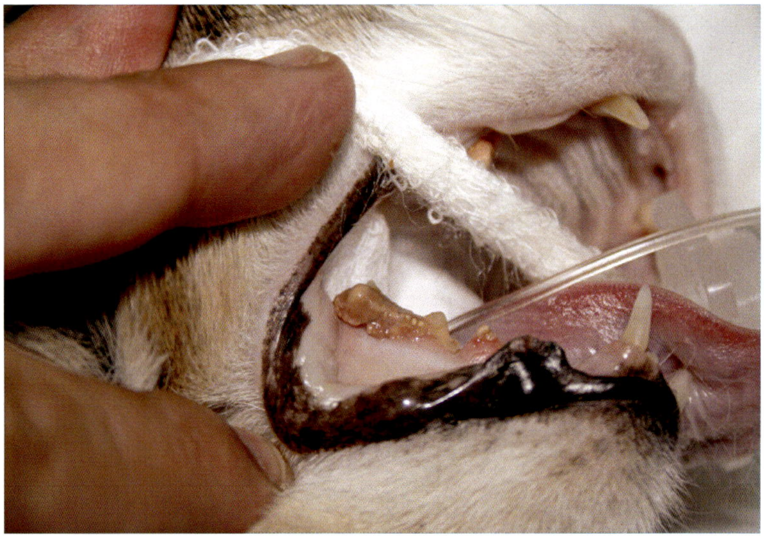

Figure 1. Oral examination of a cat with large amounts of dental plaque/tartar.

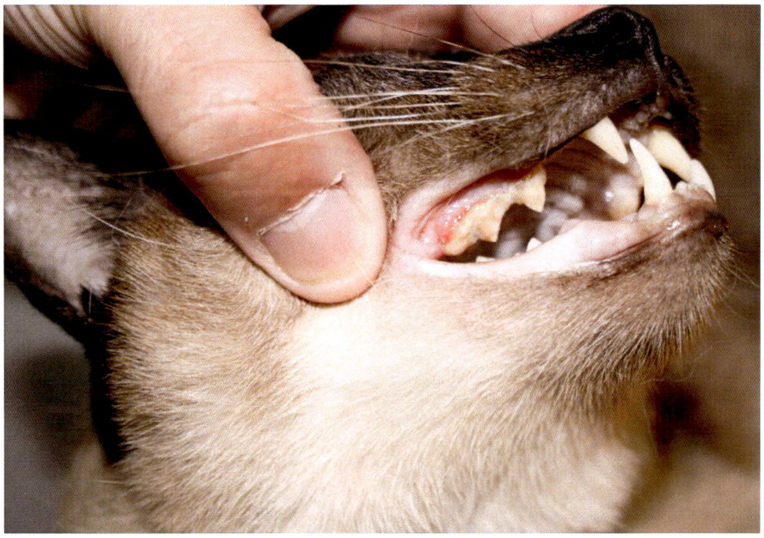

Figure 2. Periodontitis in maxillary molars with advanced gingival retraction and bone loss, and build-up of tartar.

depth of the pockets created (Fig. 3). If the pocket is deeper than 2 or 3 mm, cleaning (Fig. 4) and tartar removal will be insufficient. The same applies in cases involving bone loss and gingival recession exposing the furcation (the connection between the roots of a tooth).

In these cases, the best approach is dental extraction, before the teeth fall out of their own accord with the risk of root retention and consequent pain.

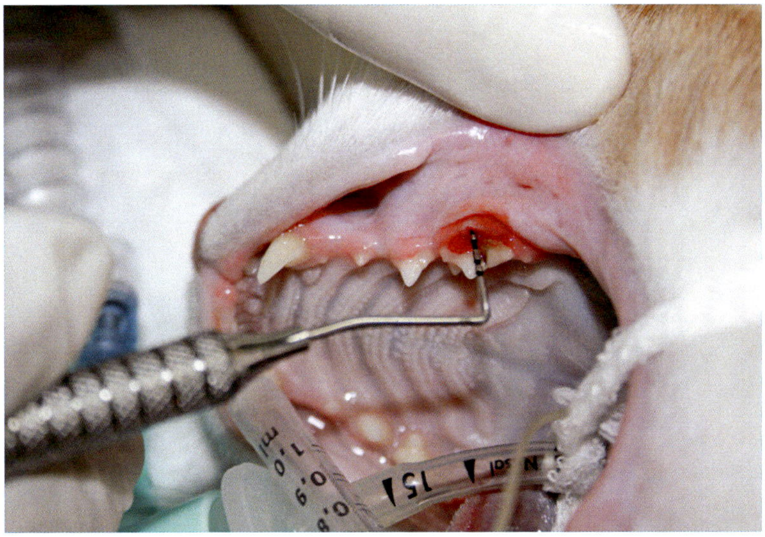

Figure 3. Use of a calibrated probe to measure gingival pockets formed as a consequence of gingival retraction.

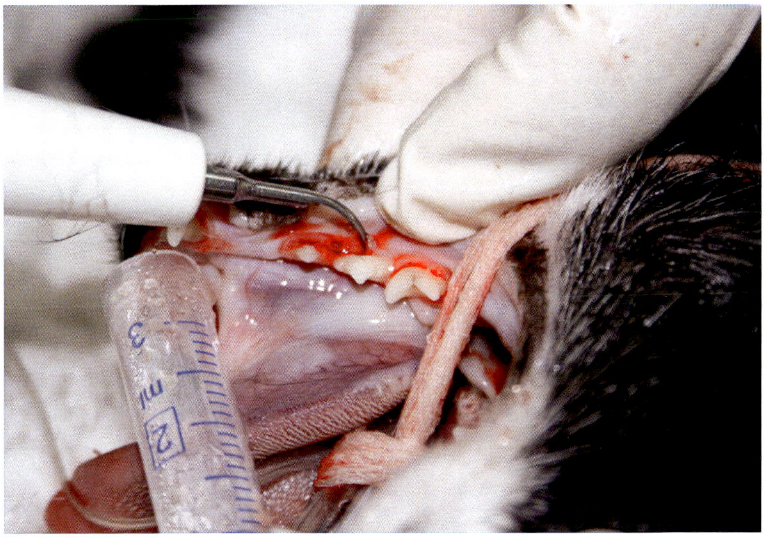

Figure 4. Ultrasonic scaling and subgingival scraping.

Some cats tolerate tooth brushing, which can be effective if performed assiduously. Certain commercial diets are designed to slow the build-up of tartar.

Chlorhexidine gel is the best antiseptic option for controlling bacterial colonisation. The use of antibiotics is controversial; while they are effective for the control of plaque-producing flora, continued use can cause bacterial resistance and exacerbate the condition.

Feline chronic gingivostomatitis

Feline chronic gingivostomatitis (FCGS) poses significant diagnostic and therapeutic challenges in daily feline medical practice (Belows, 2010). It is a multifactorial disease in which the host's immune system responds inappropriately to the stimulus caused by oral antigens of different origins, both oral and non-oral. Lymphoplasmacytic infiltration and hypergammaglobulinaemia are common findings (Hennet, 1997).

Associated dental problems such as periodontal disease and tooth resorption are chronic inflammatory processes that can play prominent roles in the pathogenesis of FCGS (Hennet, 1997).

The incidence of this disease is striking. While many consider this to be a common syndrome, it accounts for 3 % of all dental diseases in cats (Hennet, 1997), with a breed predisposition observed in Abyssinian, Somali, and Persian cats.

A 2007 study (Healey *et al.*, 2007) found that the prevalence of FCGS among animals attending general veterinary centres was only 0.3 %, with no clear sex, age, or breed-related predisposition.

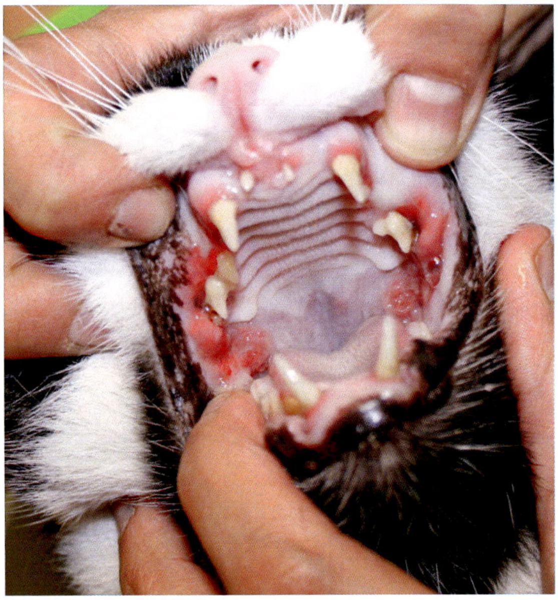

Figure 5. Oral examination revealing several pathologies: periodontitis in some canines and premolars and FCGS with ulceration and necrosis of the caudal oral mucosa.

Is it possible that many diagnoses of FCGS are incorrect? It is important to be able differentiate distinct dental pathologies in order to correctly address each problem (Fig. 5).

FCGS is characterised by severe and persistent (>6 months) inflammation or ulceration of the soft tissues, both gingival and non-gingival, the oral cavity, and in some cases the lateral mucosa of the palatoglossal arch, the pharynx, the tongue, and the caudal oral mucosa (Belows, 2010; Hennet 1997) (Figs. 6 and 7).

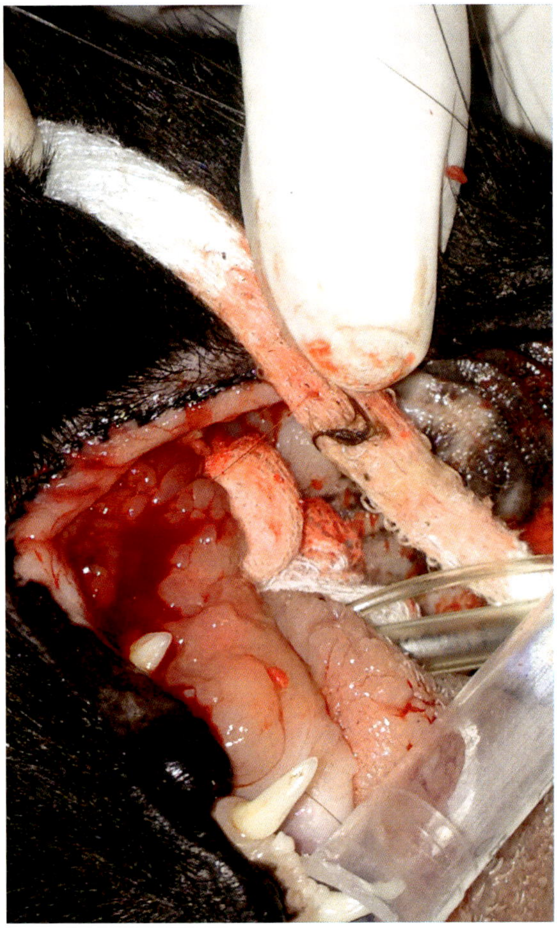

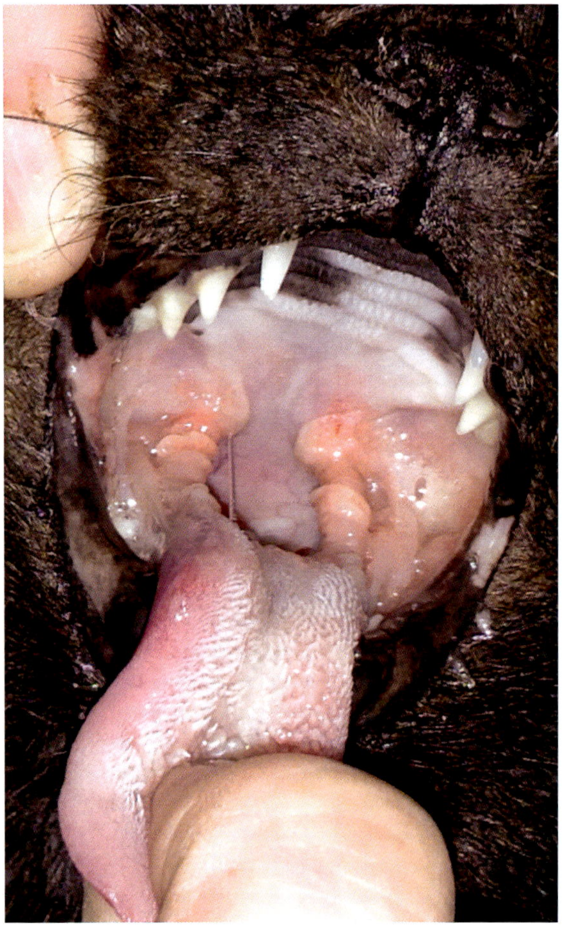

Figures 6 and 7. Marked necrosis of the caudal oral mucosa and palatoglossal arch.

Several terms are used to describe this process, including caudal stomatitis and buccal or alveolar mucositis. It is an extremely painful process.

Depending on the site of inflammation, this condition is classified as:

- Caudal stomatitis: inflammation of the caudal oral mucosa and palatoglossal arch.
- Alveolar stomatitis: inflammation affecting the alveolar zone of the teeth, extending to the gingival mucosa. Often inflammation is observed in the absence of tartar build-up on the teeth.
- Labial/buccal stomatitis: inflammation of the labial or cheek mucosa.

Factors involved

The main factors implicated in the onset of FCGS are:

- **Stress:** in colonies and homes with many cats, close contact between individuals facilitates the transmission of infectious agents and stress contributes to a decrease in immunity. In these environments the incidence of FCGS is increased (Addie *et al.*, 2003; Holmstrom, 2005).
- **Bacterial plaque:** oral bacteria present in plaque elicit a non-specific and abnormal inflammatory response. *Pasteurella multocida* is the bacteria most commonly isolated from oral cultures (Dolieslager *et al.*, 2010; Quimby, *et al.*, 2008). Furthermore, there is a close relationship between FCGS and the presence of *Bartonella* spp. (Dowers *et al.*, 2010; Sykes *et al.*, 2010) and *Chlamydophila* spp. (Dolieslager *et al.*, 2010; Quimby, *et al.*, 2008).
- **Feline calicivirus:** 70 % of cats with chronic inflammatory processes (>6 months) of the oral cavity test positive for the presence of FCV in the oropharynx (Knowles *et al.*, 2010; Quimby, *et al.*, 2008). FCV has been identified as a cause of ulcerative glossitis and inflammation of the palate, and can also cause acute diseases of the upper respiratory tract. The role of FCV in FCGS remains unclear, but it is thought that it may facilitate the penetration of other agents, causing damage to the cell membrane. However, given that 30 % of the cat population is estimated to carry FCV, other factors are necessary for the development of FCGS (Zicola *et al.*, 2009). Attempts have been made to induce caudal stomatitis in cats using oropharyngeal samples taken from affected animals, but this approach does not reproduce the inflammatory process in all animals. With the development of PCR it was demonstrated that only 30 % of cats with calicivirus have FCGS. It is thought that there may be a specific FCV biotype responsible for the development of caudal stomatitis in cats with FCGS. Moreover, it has been suggested that the development of chronic disease may depend on antigenic variation resulting from a series of mutations induced by pressure from the immune system. This antigenic variation could constitute a type of escape route for the virus.
- **Feline leukaemia and immunodeficiency viruses** (Belows, 2010; Hennet 1997; Hosie *et al.*, 2009; Quimby, *et al.*, 2008): studies of the relationship between FCGS and FeLV/FIV date back to 1989, when the incidence of retrovirus was greater, and indicated that 15 % of cats with FCGS were positive for FeLV or FIV. Today this percentage is lower, although cats with FIV-induced immunosuppression may develop secondary infections, a possibility that should be taken into account when deciding upon a disease management strategy. Feline leukaemia and immunodeficiency viruses contribute to the establishment of the disease, preventing an adequate immune system response to the formation of dental plaque. Although cats positive for FeLV develop gingivitis or stomatitis (presumably due to immunosuppression secondary to infection), FeLV infection is not associated with a higher prevalence of oral lesions. In addition to causing immunosuppression, this virus can promote a hyper-reactive immune response, leading to the development of immune-mediated diseases with the formation of antigen-antibody complexes, which in turn may play a role in FCGS. Evidence demonstrating a causative role of feline immunodeficiency virus is also lacking. Some cats with chronic stomatitis are positive for FIV. Oral inflammation is the most common clinical sign in FIV-positive cats. It seems likely that FIV-induced immunosuppression predisposes cats to the development of oral lesions, but there is no direct aetiologic relationship between FIV and chronic oral inflammatory disease in cats.

- **Dental diseases** (Belows, 2010; Harvey, 1992; Hennet 1997; Holmstrom, 2005): dental and other oral diseases are among of the main factors that influence the development of FCGS. The accumulation of plaque and tartar causes gingivitis or periodontitis, which trigger alterations in the oral mucosa. These processes are accompanied by an inflammation of varying extension that may elicit an immune reaction that perpetuates the oral process. In this situation, bacteria exacerbate the tissue damage (Belows, 2010; Dolieslager *et al.*, 2010; Hennet 1997; Quimby, *et al.*, 2010).
- **Immune system:** 50 % of cats with FCGS develop polyclonal hypergammaglobulinaemia compared with normal cats (Harley *et al.*, 2003). The immune response of animals without FCGS is a T *helper* lymphocyte type 1 (Th1) response. By contrast, those with FCGS exhibit a mixed Th1/Th2 immune response, indicating a poor cellular and humoural response. Immunohistochemistry of mucosal biopsies from animals with FCGS reveal a much higher proportion of CD8+ than CD4+ cells, which is indicative of a highly destructive cytotoxic immune response compatible with a viral aetiology (Harley *et al.*, 1999).
- **Systemic diseases:** the health of the oral mucosa depends on the balance between the oral bacterial flora and the immune system. Systemic diseases alter the immune response, and in turn the bacterial flora, contributing to the establishment, progression, or persistence of bacterial plaque and periodontal disease, with the development of oral inflammation (Belows, 2010).

Juvenile hyperplastic feline gingivitis

» Juvenile hyperplastic feline gingivitis (Fig. 8) appears in cats of less than 9 months of age, with a notable disposition in Siamese, Maine coon, and domestic shorthair breeds. These are "sickly" animals of small stature with chronic upper respiratory tract disease.

» Gingivitis of varying severity coincides with the eruption of permanent teeth. This is accompanied by marked deposition of plaque and calculus, bone resorption, gingival retraction, and even dental reabsorption (Belows, 2010; Hennet 1997). It can contribute to the development of FCGS in adulthood.

» Affected animals are often those that have had problems during growth, are smaller than the average size of their littermates, and have had respiratory infections.

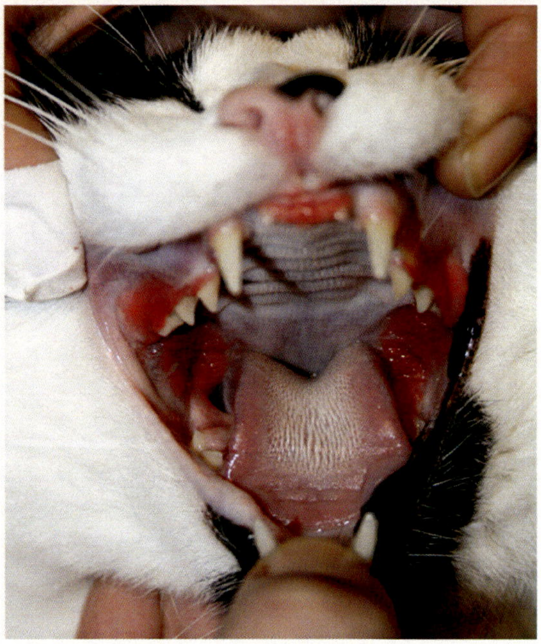

Figure 8. Advanced juvenile gingivitis.

Diagnostic tests

Various analytical and diagnostic imaging tests can be used to identify the factors underlying FCGS:

- **Analysis for virus detection:** the recent development and standardisation of the PCR technique has enabled easy detection of viruses such as FeLV, FCV, and FHV. The presence of FIV is detected using serological tests, since in Europe no vaccination plan has been implemented for this virus.
- **Bacterial cultures:** aerobic and anaerobic. Culture usually reveals a high proportion of *Pasteurella multocida* (Dolieslager *et al.*, 2010).
- **Haematology and biochemistry:** other systemic diseases should also be taken into account. About 10 % of cats with chronic kidney disease have FCGS (Hennet, 1997). It is important to plan treatment based on the underlying diseases, particularly when deciding upon anaesthetic protocols or long-term NSAID treatment.
- **Biopsy:** biopsy of the gingival mucosa is recommended when the extent, appearance, or severity of the lesions is unusual. It is important to select non-symmetrical lesions when performing biopsies to rule out the presence of squamous cell carcinoma, lymphoma, or other malignancies. In cases of FCGS, biopsy reveals lymphoplasmacytic infiltration, which is absolutely non-specific as it is indicative only of chronic inflammation of the mouth.
- **Dental examination:** examination and radiography of all teeth, present and absent.

Management of chronic feline gingivitis

The aim of most treatments for this disease is to reduce inflammation and pain, thus alleviating discomfort and favouring proper feeding (Belows, 2010; Hennet 1997).

> In all cases baseline treatment should be instituted to reduce the presence of oral antigen.

The following are the stages involved in initial management of FCGS.

Control of bacterial plaque

Descaling is beneficial, but the effects are short-term unless it is followed by regular and effective home care (Fig. 4).

Control of other dental diseases

Other dental diseases that should be treated when managing FCGS include periodontal disease and tooth resorption. This sometimes requires partial extractions of affected teeth in accordance with the specific clinical criteria for the management of these diseases (Girard and Hennet, 2005).

Analgesics and anti-inflammatories

Opioids and nonsteroidal anti-inflammatory drugs (NSAIDs) can be administered during the pre- and postoperative periods. Buprenorphine, butorphanol, and meloxicam can be administered pre-operatively in cases of dental extraction, which is the treatment of choice, or post-operatively in cases in which extraction results in incomplete resolution of clinical signs.

Control of inflammation

Corticosteroids have been widely used to effectively manage inflammation. However, they are not currently recommended as in the medium term they can increase viral replication of calcivirus and exacerbate the associated lesions (Southerden and Gorrel, 2007). NSAIDs are preferred for short and medium-to-long term control of inflammation (Belows, 2001).

Supportive therapy

Vitamins, fatty acids, and special recovery diets can be administered as required. In very weak cats, an oesophageal catheter can be used to aid recovery after dental extraction, followed by placement of an oesophagostomy tube.

Antibiotics

Antibiotic treatment is recommended to reduce the bacterial load in the mouth for a significant period of time. This in turn reduces inflammation and discomfort. Antibiotics are also used during the preoperative and postoperative stages for a minimum of 8 to 10 days (Belows, 2010; Dowers *et al.*, 2010; Hennet 1997).

Commonly used antibiotics include:

- Clindamycin: 11–22 mg/kg once daily.
- Amoxicillin-clavulanic acid: 12.5 mg/kg twice daily.

Metronidazole has also been used at doses of 10–15 mg/kg every 12 hours and fluoroquinolones such as marbofloxacin at doses of 2 mg/kg per day.

In some cases pulsed antibiotic treatment followed by a waiting period may be preferable.

Adjunctive treatment in specific cases

Repeated cleaning and polishing

In patients with juvenile gingivitis it is important to ensure minimal exposure to bacterial plaque during the first years of life and to resolve any anatomical defects as soon as possible. This may require professional cleaning every three months to minimise exposure to bacterial plaque and thus ensure minimal inflammation of the oral mucosa and reduced immune system activity.

Complete versus partial dental extraction

Complete dental extraction has been proposed as a treatment of choice, and tends to be the first choice of treatment, rather than a last resort (Fig. 9).

The following outcomes have been described for this treatment approach (Bellei et al., 2008; Girard and Hennet, 2005):

- Complete cure in 50–60 % of cats.
- Significant improvement in 27–33 % of cats, although additional anti-inflammatory treatment was required.

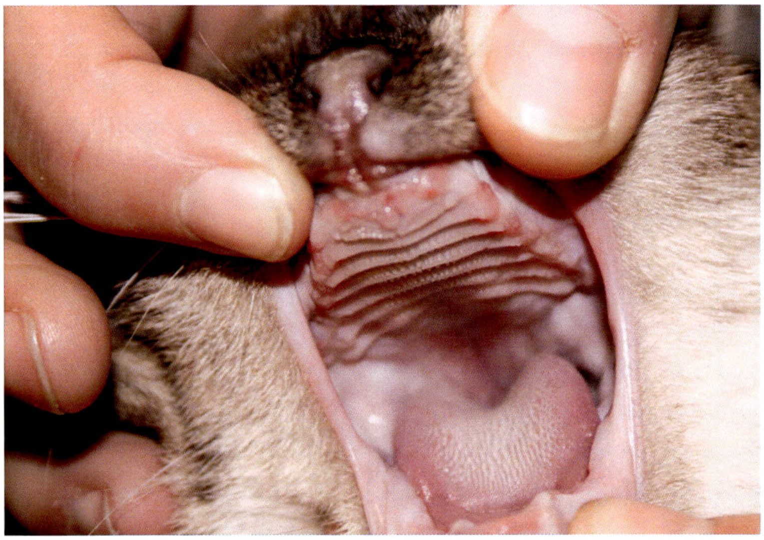

Figure 9. Mouth after a complete dental extraction.

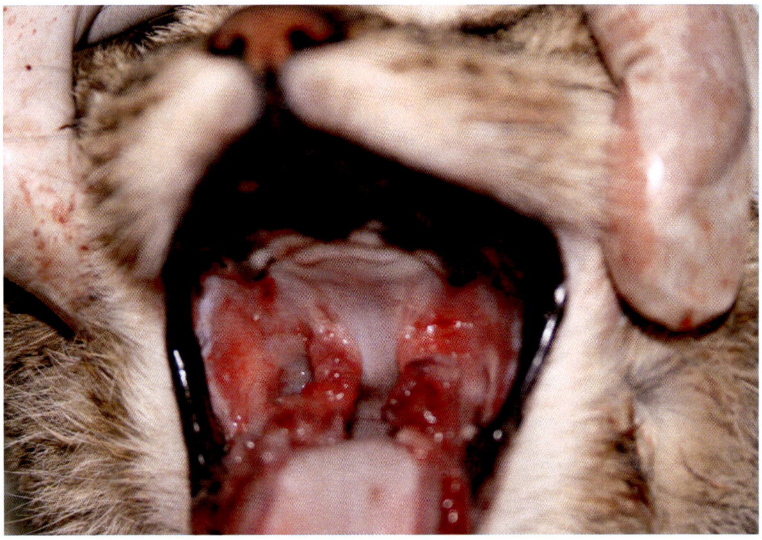

Figure 10. Cat showing inadequate response to dental extraction.

- Between 7 % and 13 % were refractory to dental extraction, with no improvement observed, or improvements observed in the gingival and oral mucosa surrounding the teeth but not in the caudal oral mucosa or palatoglossal arch (Figs. 10 and 11).

In these cases it is important to perform radiographic studies after dental extraction as any remaining root remnants can continue to stimulate an antigenic and inflammatory response by the immune system, preventing complete resolution (Fig. 12).

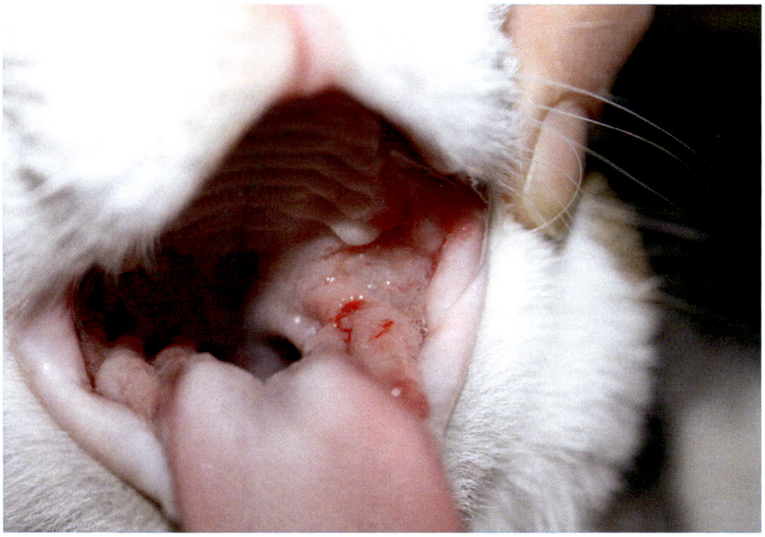

Figure 11. Cat showing inadequate response to dental extraction.

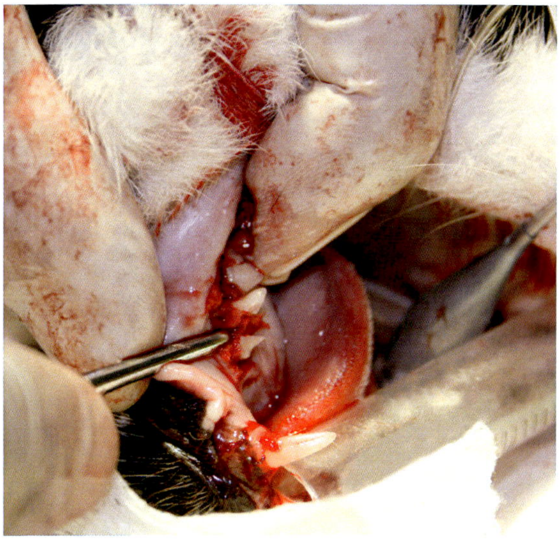

Figure 13. Closed extraction of double-root premolar with crown section to facilitate removal.

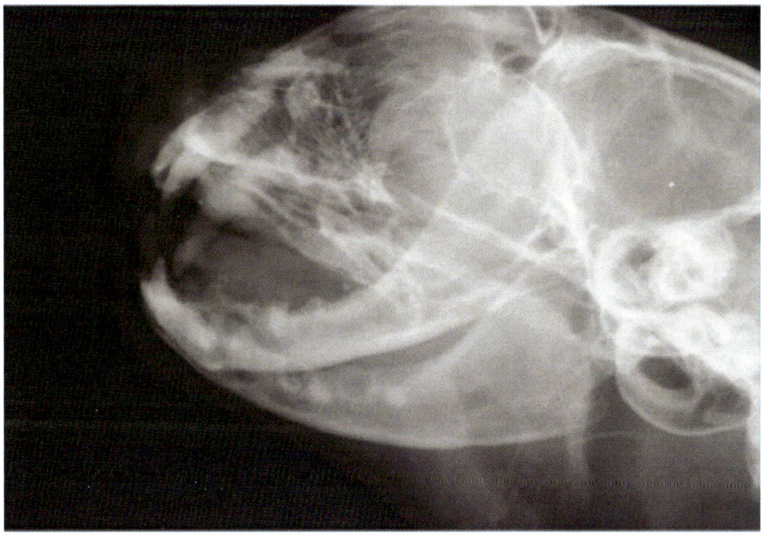

Figure 12. Radiograph of the head of a cat showing retention of root remnants following dental extraction.

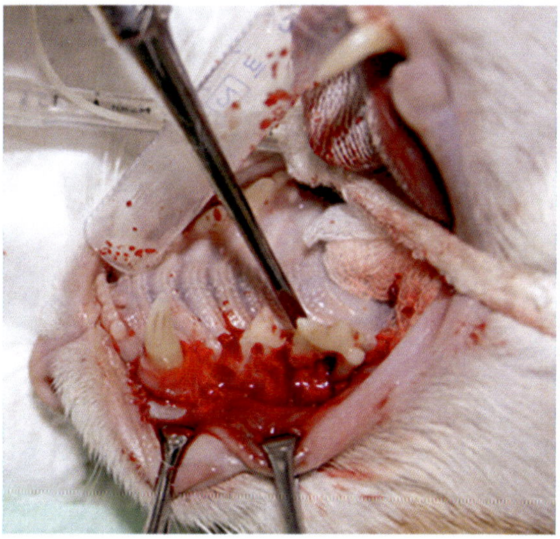

Figure 14. Extraction of multiple teeth in a case of FCGS using the flap technique.

Box 1. Radiographic criteria for selective extraction

- Poorly vascularised or sclerotic bone.
- Ossification of root in alveolar bone.
- Tooth with resorptive lesion.
- Retraction of alveolar bone with evident retraction of the gingival mucosa and visible furcation.

Partial dental extraction should be applied in cases involving specific radiographically detectable criteria (Box 1).

This involves the selective extraction of teeth which, as a result of dental resorption of any kind or advanced periodontitis, meet the clinical requirements for recommended removal (Figs. 13–15).

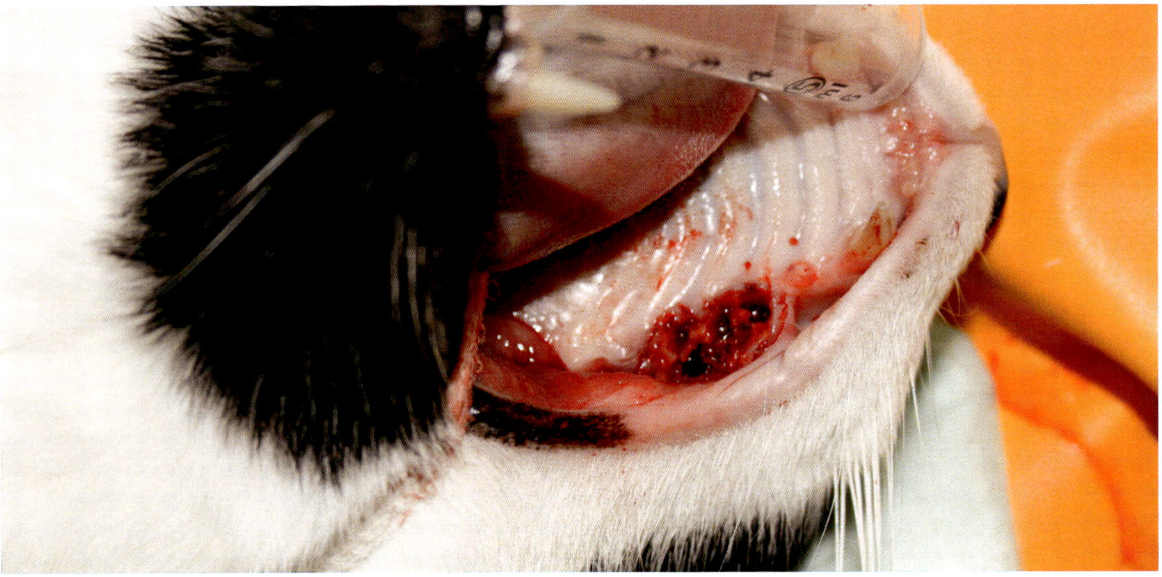

Figure 15. Mouth several weeks after dental extraction.

Dental extraction: postoperative management

Multiple extractions require analgesia, antibiotic therapy, and postoperative nutrition. Analgesics used include opioids, such as buprenorphine, and NSAIDs, such as meloxicam. Antibiotics selected should show good activity in bone and efficacy against anaerobic bacteria. Treatment should be instituted preoperatively. The antibiotics of choice are clindamycin and amoxicillin-clavulanic acid.

Feeding plans should provide short- and medium-term nutritional support. Although effective analgesic therapy and soft, palatable food is usually sufficient to encourage feeding, it is important to monitor the cat, and if no signs of appetite are observed in the first 24 hours assisted feeding should be considered.

Evaluation of other anti-inflammatory and immunomodulatory treatments

NSAIDs

The anti-inflammatory of choice is meloxicam, which is indicated for long-term use in the guide to long-term NSAID treatment in cats, published by the International Society of Feline Medicine (ISFM) and the American Association of Feline Practitioners (AAFP) (Sparkes *et al.*, 2010).

Recombinant feline interferon ω

In a randomised, double-blind study (Hennet *et al.*, 2010), conducted over 3 years with 39 FCV-positive cats that showed a poor response to partial dental extraction, interferon therapy provided a greater level of comfort than other treatments, including corticosteroids. In another study of a sterilised, eight-year-old, domestic shorthair cat with FCGS, initial treatment by extraction of premolars and molars was unsuccessful. However, lesions improved after six weeks of treatment with recombinant feline interferon ω (Southerden and Gorrel, 2007).

Oral administration

The treatment regimen is as follows:

- 10 MU (million units) are injected into 100 ml of physiological saline (0.9 %).
- The solution is aliquoted (10 ml each) and frozen. It can be stored frozen for 1 year and in the refrigerator at 4 °C for 21 days.
- It is administered orally at a doses of 1 ml/cat/day for 3 months.

Initial intralesional administration

According to the consensus established in October 2010 by the European Veterinary Dental Society, intralesional administration is not necessary to begin treatment, as recommended by the manufacturer of recombinant feline interferon ω.

In the aforementioned study of calicivirus-positive cats with FCGS and caudal stomatitis that were refractory to complete dental extraction (Hennet *et al.*, 2010), the effects of interferon treatment were compared with those of slow-release corticosteroids. Both treatments significantly reduced inflammation. However, cats treated with prednisolone showed a reduction in inflammation followed by a rebound effect, whereas those treated with interferon remained more stable and enjoyed a longer period without recurrence of clinical signs. Hennet recommended testing for calicivirus in cats with chronic gingivostomatitis that are refractory to complete extraction, and treating positive cats with feline interferon ω, antibiotics, and anti-inflammatories (Fig. 16).

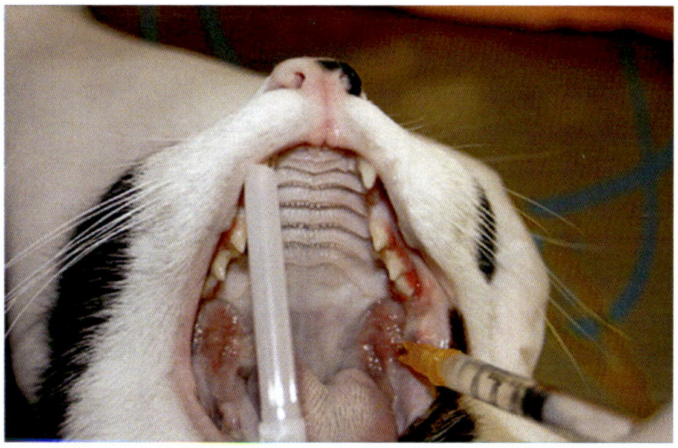

Figure 16. Intralesional injection of feline interferon ω.

Corticosteroids

Corticosteroids are widely used for the control of inflammation, especially in cases refractory to partial dental extraction. The outcome is no better than that observed with oral interferon, and corticosteroids are associated with many more side effects (Belows *et al.*, 2010).

Questionnaire for the evaluation of FCGS management

This questionnaire is used to objectively monitor the response to FCGS treatment.

The following are important considerations when administering a questionnaire on FCGS treatment response:

- The questionnaire should be administered periodically by the same person, if possible, accompanied by photos.
- Any changes in the treatment protocol should be noted, and the questionnaire re-administered one week after starting treatment.
- The first two questions should be answered by the owner.
- The questionnaire should be scored out of a maximum of 33, corresponding to the worst possible clinical situation.

PATIENT DATA

Weight	
Diet	
Date	

Evaluation score	
Appetite	• 3: eats only from the hand. • 2: eats only moist food. • 1: eats dry food but smaller than usual quantity. • 0: eats normally.
Activity level	• 3: uninterested in people or other pets and spends most of the time sleeping. • 2: low level of activity, but occasionally plays when stimulated. • 1: plays spontaneously. • 0: normal level of play and activity.
Grooming	• 3: does not groom. • 2: grooms occasionally, but not as before. • 1: grooms excessively. • 0: regular grooming.
Comfort	Evaluate comfort with 0 indicating maximum level of comfort and 3 indicating the minimum.
Inflammation of oral cavity	• 0: none. • 1: mild. • 2: moderate. • 3: severe.

FCGS ACTIVITY INDEX	0	1	2	3
Appetite				
Mobility				
Grooming				
Perceived comfort				
Inflammation of maxillary oral mucosa				
Inflammation of the mandibular oral mucosa				
Inflammation of the maxillary gingiva				
Inflammation of the mandibular gingiva				
Lateral inflammation of the palatoglossal arch				
Inflammation of the molar salivary gland				
Inflammation of the oropharynx				
TOTAL (maximum = 33)				

References

Addie, D.D., *et al.* Cessation of feline calicivirus shedding coincident with resolution of chronic gingivostomatitis in a cat. *J Small Anim Pract*, 2003; 44 172-176.

Belows, J. *Feline dentistry. Oral assessment, treatment and preventive care.* Ed. Wiley-Blackwell, 2010.

Bellei, E., *et al.* Surgical therapy in chronic feline gingivostomatitis (FCGS). *Vet Res Commun*, 2008; 32(1):S231-S234.

Dolieslager, S.M.J., Riggio, M.P., Lennon, A., Lappin, M., Johnston, N.W., Taylor, D., Bennet, D. Identification of the bacteria associated with feline chronic gingivostomatitis using culture-dependent and culture-independent methods. *Veterinary Microbiology*, 2011; 148(1):93-8.

Dowers, K.L., Hawley, J.R., Brewer, M.M., Morris, A.K., Radecki, S.V., Lappin, M.R. Association of Bartonella species, feline calicivirus, and feline herpesvirus 1 infection with gingivostomatitis in cats. *J Feline Med Surg*, 2010 Apr; 12(4):314-21.

Girard, N., Hennet, P. Retrospective study of dental extractions treatment of chronic caudal stomatitis in 60 positive cats. Proceedings of the 19th Veterinary Dental Forum, 2005; p. 447.

Harley, R., Gruffydd-Jones, T.J., Day, M.J. Salivary and serum immunoglobulin levels in cats with chronic gingivostomatitis. *Vet Rec*, 2003 Feb 1; 152(5):125-9.

Harley, R., Helps, C.R., Harbor, D.A., *et al.* Cytokine mRNA expression in lesions in cats with chronic gingivostomatitis. *Clin Diagn Lab Immunol*, 1999 Jul; 6(4):471-8.

Harvey, C.E. Manual of small animal dentistry. BSAVA, 1992.

Healey, K.A., *et al.* Prevalence of feline chronic gingivostomatitis in first opinion veterinary practice. *Journal of Feline Medicine and Surgery*, 2007 Oct; 9(5):373-8.

Hennet, P. Chronic gingivostomatitis in cats: Long-term follow-up of 30 cases treated by dental extractions. *J Vet Dent*, 1997; 14:15-21.

Hennet, P.R., Camy, G.A., Privat, V., McGahi, D. Comparative efficacy of a feline recombinant interferon omega in refractory cases of calicivirus-positive cats with caudal stomatitis: a randomised, multicentric controlled double blind study of 39 cats. Proceedings of the 19th European Congress of Veterinary Dentistry, Nice 2010; pp. 193-195.

Holmstrom, S.E. Veterinary Dentistry. *Veterinary Clinics of North America: Small Animal Practice*, July 2005; 35(4):763-1072.

Hosie, M.J., Addie, D., Belák, S., Boucraut-Baralon, C., Egberink, H., Frymus, T., Gruffydd-Jones, T., Hartmann, K., Lloret, A., Lutz, H., Marsilio, F., Pennisi, M.G., Radford, A., Thiry, E., Truyen, U., Horzinek, M.C. Feline immunodeficiency. ABCD guidelines on prevention and management. Review Article. *Journal of Feline Medicine & Surgery*, July 2009; 11(7):575-584.

Hosie, M.J., Addie, D., Belák, S., Boucraut-Baralon, C., Egberink, H., Frymus, T., Gruffydd-Jones, T., Hartmann, K., Lloret, A., Lutz, H., Marsilio, F., Pennisi, M.G., Radford, A., Thiry, E., Truyen, U., Horzinek, M.C. Feline calicivirus infection. ABCD guidelines on prevention and management. Review Article. *Journal of Feline Medicine & Surgery*, July 2009; 11(7):556-564.

Knowles, J.O., Gaskel, R.M., Gaskell, C.J., *et al.* Prevalence of feline calicivirus, feline leukaemia virus and antibodies to FIV in cats with chronic stomatitis. *Vet Rec*, 1989; 124(13):336-338.

Quimby, *et al.* Evaluation of the association of Bartonella species, feline herpesvirus 1, feline calicivirus, feline leukaemia virus and feline immunodeficiency virus with chronic gingivostomatitis. *J Feline Med Surg*, 2008; 10(1):66-72.

Southerden, P., Gorrel, C. Treatment of a case of refractory feline chronic gingivostomatitis with feline recombinant interferon omega. *Journal of Small Animal Practice*, 2007; 48(2):104-106.

Sparkes, A.H., Heiene, R. Lascelles, B.D.X., *et al.* Directrices de consenso de ISFM y AAFP. Uso a largo plazo de AINEs en gatos. *Journal of Feline Medicine and Surgery*, 2010; 12:521-538.

Sykes, J.E., Westropp, J.L., Kasten, R.W., Chomel, B.B. Association between Bartonella species infection and disease in pet cats as determined using serology and culture. *Journal of Feline Medicine & Surgery*, August 2010; 12(8):631-636.

Zicola, A., *et al.* Feline herpes virus 1 and feline calicivirus infections in a heterogeneous cat population of rescue shelter. *Journal of Feline Medicine & Surgery*, 2009; 11:1023-1027.

Appendix 7

When to stop treatment

It is important to know when a treatment has reached its limit of effectiveness. This point can be extremely subjective, depending not only on the cat, but also the other cats with which it lives.

The following are some criteria that should be taken into account when deciding when to end treatment:

- In cases with a poor short-term prognosis.
- In the absence of alternative therapies.
- When quality of life is markedly reduced (Fig. 1).
- In cats with visible pain or behavioural changes (Figs. 2 and 3).

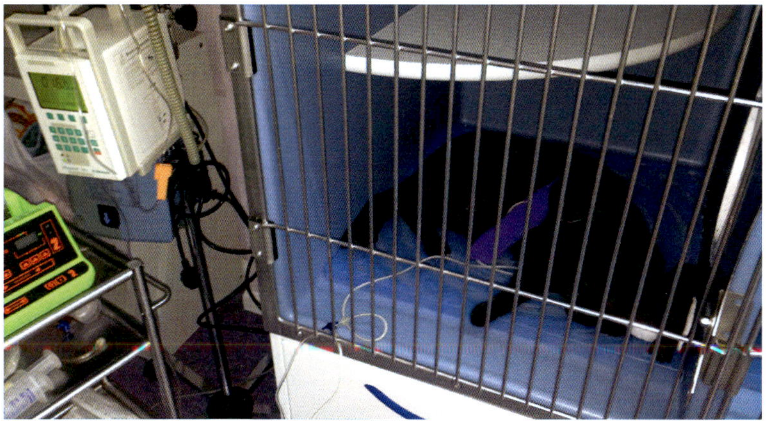

Figure 1. Animal in considerable pain, and in need of continuous infusion of large amounts of fluids and analgesia.

Many owners recognise that they are unable to pinpoint when their cat began to suffer. In these cases, quality of life surveys help objectify subjective concepts such as number of good versus bad days, movement, feeding, hygiene, etc.

End of life

Each veterinary surgeon has an ethical obligation and a moral commitment to ensure their patient's welfare. This is the first responsibility of the veterinary surgeon.

The veterinary surgeon should strive to help patients enjoy the five needs/freedoms outlined in the general guide on the welfare of feline patients of the American Association of Feline Practitioners (AAFP). It is crucial to prevent pain and suffering in animals.

It is unethical to deny veterinary care to a patient that needs it, or to seek to prolong an animal's life for other reasons.

The five freedoms, which were drafted in 1970 by the Farm Animal Welfare Council, still constitute the guide to the rules guaranteeing the quality of life of animals, and are used by many societies, associations, and international agencies to define the basic minimum standards of animal welfare.

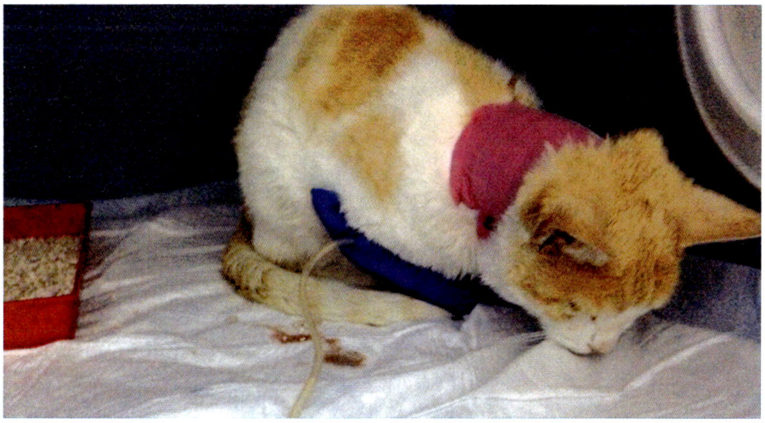

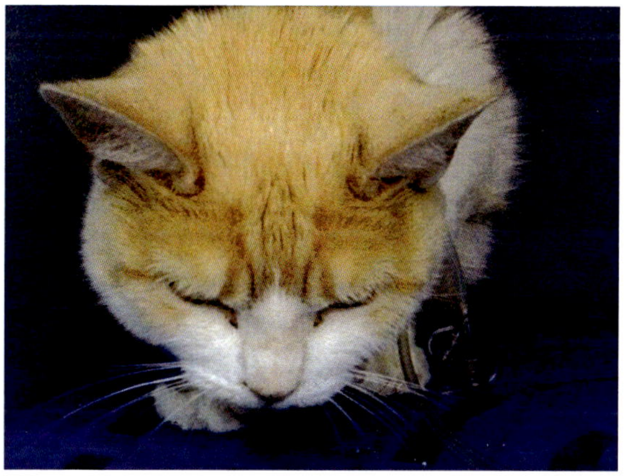

Figures 2 and 3. These cats are in considerable pain.

Responsibilities of the veterinary surgeon

Cats can provide important emotional support for the people they live with. Thanks to significant advances in modern medicine, in terms of both diagnostic methods and treatments, cats can be provided with an excellent quality of life (Figs. 4 and 5). Many customers seek these kinds of medical care, which we should be able to provide under any circumstances.

The close relationship between people and cats can be so intense that caregivers are unable to identify the moment at which their cat begins to suffer unnecessarily. It is the responsibility of the veterinary surgeon to advise caregivers in these circumstances to avoid prolonging unnecessary suffering and to provide cats with an excellent quality of life. However, the fact that advanced diagnostic techniques and treatments are available does not mean that they have to be used in all situations.

Quality of life

Preserving and promoting the quality of life of the patient is the primary objective of the veterinary surgeon (Fig. 6). Promoting quality of life entails providing cats with the essential resources necessary for the species: food, water, capacity and ability to walk, urinate or defecate, relief from all types of discomfort, freedom from disease, social interaction, and security and environmental stability.

It can be difficult to assess pain in cats, as this is influenced by both physical and behavioural factors. However, the fact that this may be difficult to assess does not mean it should be disregarded.

The old theory that pain in cats serves to limit their activity at a given time is incorrect and inappropriate and should be abandoned immediately. Failure to recognise and control pain in patients is unethical and implies a loss of quality of life for affected cats. Quality of life should always be part of the continuous dialogue between veterinary surgeons and cat owners.

The five freedoms of animals

- Freedom from thirst, hunger, and malnutrition, with access to fresh water and a diet that ensures full health and wellbeing.
- Freedom from discomfort in their environment, with a comfortable resting area and all necessary resources.
- Freedom from pain, injury, and disease through effective prevention, rapid diagnosis, and appropriate treatment.
- Freedom to express their natural behaviour, with sufficient space in an area suited to their needs.
- Freedom from fear and stress, with an environment free from emotional distress that does not promote the development of behavioural disorders.

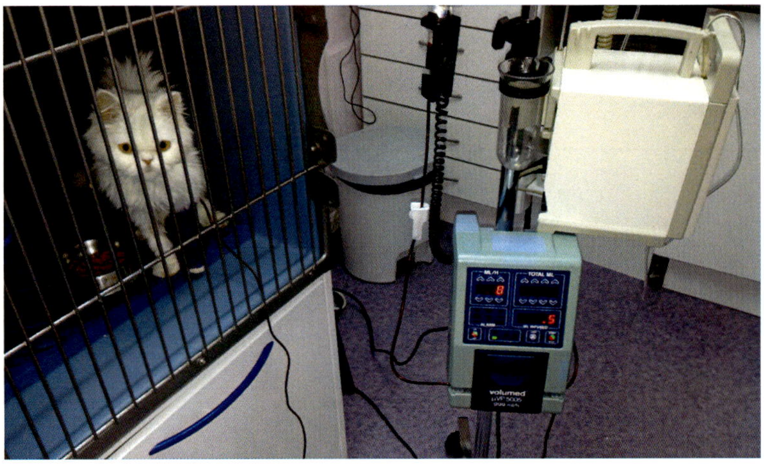

Figure 4. Patient in need of a blood transfusion due to terminal chronic kidney disease.

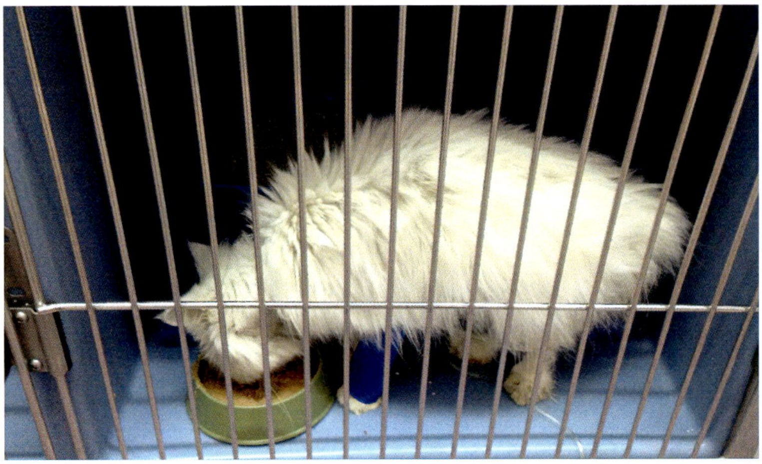

Figure 5. Cat from previous image after transfusion.

Euthanasia

Poor quality of life of patients is the most important factor influencing the decision to euthanise. In terminally ill patients euthanasia is a humanitarian act, as it puts an end to unnecessary suffering and pain.

In veterinary medicine, euthanasia should be selected for terminally ill animals that have no other options and those in which the loss of quality of life is so significant that euthanasia is necessary to avoid further suffering.

In some cases, owners of cats may seek euthanasia for their pet because they are unable or unwilling to provide proper care. Veterinary surgeons should not provide euthanasia for the sake of convenience; this is not in the best interests of the cat or the veterinary profession. The veterinary surgeon should remind owners that their cat is another member of their family, and should receive all the love, respect, and care they need.

If an owner persists in their decision to euthanise the animal after having been presented with all potential alternatives, it is the responsibility of the veterinary surgeon in charge to ensure the rights of the animal from an ethical and moral point of view, and to act accordingly.

Some owners may request euthanasia as a solution to behavioural problems in cats, such as aggression. In these cases it is up to the veterinary surgeon to propose alternatives other than euthanasia.

It may be the case that the owner is unable to afford even the most modest veterinary care for their cats. Alternatively, the caregiver may even be physically or emotionally unable to care for the cat. While it is not the role of the veterinary surgeon to make the decision for the owner, they should ensure that the patients' rights are upheld, and inform the owner about all available alternatives to try to improve the patient's situation and avoid euthanasia.

Rejection of euthanasia by owners

In some cases, despite all attempts to explain to the consequences of terminal illness for their cat, owners will persist in their intention to continue treatment or keep the animal alive, regardless of the suffering and loss of quality of life. If every effort has been made to improve the quality of life of a cat and the owner insists on continuing treatment, it is once again up to the veterinary surgeon to uphold the rights of the animal from an ethical and moral standpoint, and to act accordingly.

The main objective in veterinary medicine is quality, not quantity, of life. At this point, the use of a quality of life questionnaire can be useful.

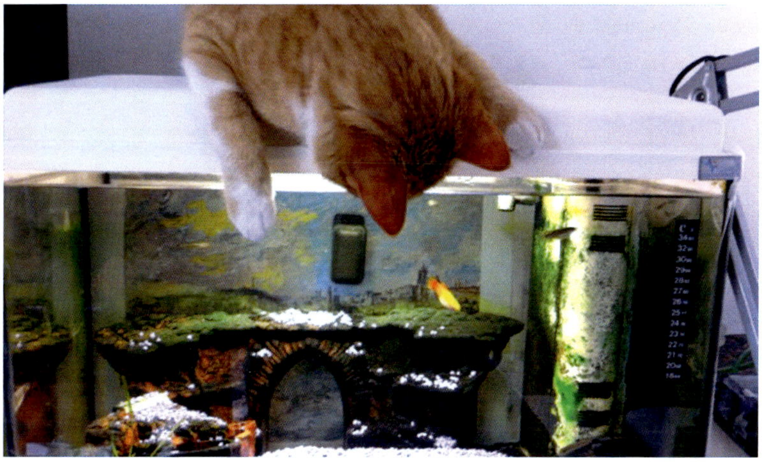

Figure 6. *Peteto* (see case studies on feline panleukopaenia). This is quality of life.

How can I know if my cat is suffering?

The greatest aspiration of veterinary surgeons and "companions" (rather than owners) of cats is to provide them with quality of life. However, this is an abstract concept and is difficult to define, and even more so when the cat's situation changes from one day to the next.

Those who live with and love the cat may have trouble perceiving these changes, or may not want to perceive them. Moreover, cats are skilled at hiding their symptoms.

Defining and establishing a scale to quantify quality of life is extremely complicated, as this involves subjective feelings, perceptions, and values. As such,

Table 1. Criteria for evaluating patient quality of life.

Criterion	Score	Observations in patient
PAIN	10	A score of 10 is assigned when the cat breathes normally, is relaxed when at rest, shows interest in the environment, has a "contented" facial expression, has non-slanted eyes, and shows no signs of body tension. Gentle palpation should reveal no signs of discomfort.
	5–10	A score between 10 and 5 is assigned if the cat has some difficulty breathing or shows abdominal movement while breathing.
	0–5	A score between 5 and 0 is assigned when the cat shows marked dyspnoea or requires oxygen and pain cannot be controlled.
APPETITE	10	Eats well.
	5	Only eats capriciously from the hand, with assistance.
	0	An oesophagostomy tube is required.
HYDRATION	10	Normal hydration status.
	5	Dull eyes, dry mouth, responds well to subcutaneous fluid therapy.
	0	Sunken eyes, skin tenting, requires intravenous fluid therapy.
HYGIENE	10	Clean haircoat.
	5	Cat fails to clean itself properly, or has an unkempt or poorly maintained haircoat.
	0	Traces of dirt are evident in the hair.
HAPPINESS	0–10	A cat is assigned a score of 10 if it plays, communicates with other cats in the environment both visually and using its body, purrs, and responds to the movement of objects.
MOBILITY	0–10	• Cats are considered to enjoy life when they have no pain, regardless of their degree of mobility. • It is important to evaluate whether they are alert and respond to stimuli including touch, sunlight, games, and smells (e.g. catnip). • It is important to move the cat bed to different areas of the house, always keeping it close to the feeding area, litter tray, and scratching post, and to ensure that the rest area is comfortable. • Mobility is scored on a scale of 0 to 10. However, unlike dogs, changes in mobility in cats may be unrelated to quality of life.
MORE "GOOD" DAYS THAN "BAD"	0–10	• "Bad" days are those on which clinical signs of the disease that cause discomfort are observed (vomiting, anorexia, seizures, falls, etc.) or days involving stressful activities (e.g. hospitalisation). • Recording "good" and "bad" days on a calendar is a good indicator of disease progression.

If the total score is **over 35** the patient is considered to have an acceptable quality of life.

while scales can be useful, they should be interpreted with caution (Table 1). Scales can help us identify signs of pain in the cat in order to determine when the animal is uncomfortable and how its quality of life can be improved. This cannot be done from the clinic, as a cat's behaviour changes when it leaves its own territory and is subjected to stress. Moreover, those who live with the cat are better able to observe these changes in behaviour, appetite, hydration, hygiene, mood, mobility, etc., and can inform the veterinary surgeon as to improvement or deterioration of the animal's status, or whether the animal has more bad days than good.

A scale of 0 to 10 is used, with 0 and 10 reflecting the minimum and maximum values for the criteria shown in Table 1.

While we have to think for the animal in question, it is they who suffer the effects of any given condition.

Weekday									
PAIN									
APPETITE									
HYDRATION									
HYGIENE									
HAPPINESS									
MOBILITY									
MORE "GOOD" DAYS THAN "BAD"									
TOTAL									

It is therefore our duty to provide them with a good quality of life.

Owners can be provided with a sheet similar to that shown below in order to collect information on the progression of their cat.

References

PITTARI, J., RODAN, I., BEEKMAN, G., GUNN-MOORE, D., POLZIN, D., TABOADA, J., TUZIO, H., ZORAN, D. American association of feline practitioners. Senior care guidelines. *J Feline Med Surg,* 2009; 11:763-78.

ROLLIN, B.E. Ethical issues in geriatric feline medicine. *J Feline Med Surg,* 2007; 9: 326-34.

SCHERK, M. Home care and end of life issues. *Veterinary Information Network. Http://vin.Com/members/cms/rounds/default.Aspx?Id=777.*

MCMILLAN, F.D. Rethinking euthanasia: death as an unintentional outcome. *J Ame Vet Assoc,* 2001; 219:1204-6.

MCMILLAN, F.D. Quality of life in animals. *J Ame Vet Assoc,* 216:1904-11.

TANNENBAUM, J. *Veterinary ethics: animal welfare, client relations, competition and collegiality.* 2Nd ed. Mosby, st louis, 1995.

ROBERTSON, S.A. Managing pain in feline patient. *Vet Clin North Am Small Anim Pract,* 2008; 38:1267-90.

AAFP FELINE WELFARE COMMITTEE. General principles welfare. *J Feline Med Surg,* 2007; 9: xiv. Http://catvets.Com/professionals/guidelines/position.

Appendix 8

Vaccination

Vaccination plays a critical role in preventing infectious diseases both in individuals and in the larger population. Routine vaccination plans have resulted in a marked decrease in the incidence of certain infections, including some highly infectious pathogens such as feline panleukopaenia.

However, the extent of the protection provided against these infections is dependent on many factors, and vaccination is not without risk, particularly the risk of developing the disease against which the vaccine is designed to protect. This depends on the patient's age and health status, the degree of exposure to the agent in question, and the pathogenicity thereof. There is also the possibility that the immune response elicited is insufficient, as occurs in certain diseases, situations that produce immunosuppression, or as a consequence of the interfering effect of acquired maternal immunity. Vaccination should not be viewed as a guarantee of protection. Even if animals are vaccinated, their exposure to infectious agents should be minimised.

Vaccination is a medical procedure and the decision to vaccinate or not, even in the case of vaccines included in the essential vaccine programme (core vaccines) should be based on assessment of the risk/benefit ratio.

Overall objectives of vaccination

1» Vaccinate only against infections to which the animals are exposed.

2» Vaccinate against infectious agents that cause serious disease.

3» Vaccinate only when the benefits outweigh the risks.

4» Vaccinate cats with the right frequency, and not more times than necessary.

5» Vaccinate as many at-risk cats as possible.

According to various international panels of experts, vaccines can be divided into two broad groups: those that are considered essential and those that are not. Moreover, some vaccines may not be recommended, or their use may depend on the prevalence of certain diseases in a given geographic area. Vaccines are classified as:

- **Essential (core) vaccines:** highly recommended for all cats, and include feline panleukopaenia (FPV), feline calicivirus (FCV), and feline herpesvirus type 1 (FHV-1).
- **Optional (non-core) vaccines:** these should be given to cats based on the risk/benefit ratio for both the individual and the population. This group includes vaccines for rabies, feline leukaemia virus (FeLV), *Chlamydophila felis*, and feline infectious peritonitis (FIP) virus.

The rabies vaccine is also subject to legal requirements, which vary between regions and countries.

Types of vaccines

In general, different vaccines contain distinct elements to immunise and protect against the same pathogens, using different technologies or routes of administration, and thus vary in terms of safety and effectiveness. Different types of vaccines against the same microorganism may be available in a given region. Alternatively, certain vaccines may not be available in all areas, as is the case with the FIV vaccine in Europe.

Inactivated vaccines

Vaccine agents are completely inactivated using various physical or chemical methods, eliminating the risk of replication of the microorganisms in question. These vaccines are more stable and safer than attenuated vaccines, but are less capable of inducing a potent immune response, and are thus always accompanied by adjuvants that may enhance or facilitate the immune response. These vaccines are only able to generate humoural (Th2) immune responses and very weak cellular (Th1) responses, unless specific adjuvants are used to enhance the latter (saponins, CpG DNA, Th1 cytokines, etc.). These adjuvants, in turn, can induce certain adverse reactions. Inactivated vaccines have been developed against panleukopaenia, herpesvirus type 1, calicivirus, FeLV, *C. felis*, and rabies.

Modified live (attenuated) vaccines

In these vaccines the pathogens are intact, but are modified so that they lose their virulence, but maintain the ability to replicate or multiply enough to elicit an effective immune response. These vaccines rapidly induce a strong immune response. However, in adverse conditions there is a possibility that they may revert to a virulent form, inducing the disease they are designed to prevent, although this phenomenon is extremely rare. These are mainly used to vaccinate in situations in which there is a high risk of pathogen transmission, in order to produce immunity much faster than other vaccine types. Modified live vaccines have been developed against panleukopaenia, calicivirus, herpesvirus type 1, *C. felis*, and *Bordetella bronchiseptica*.

Recombinant vaccines

These are created by isolating small genetic sequences from the microorganism that encode proteins, which in turn generate immunity. These vaccines can use viral vectors or can be subunit vaccines. These vaccines avoid all risks associated with vaccines, such as the possibility of the replication of microorganisms, making them very safe and allowing their use in extreme conditions, such as in animals with other pathologies that have potentially compromised immune systems. Recombinant vaccines against rabies and feline infectious leukaemia have been developed.

The protection afforded by these vaccines varies considerably from one vaccine to the next, and the associated risks should be evaluated by relevant panels of experts to establish appropriate recommendations. In general, recommended vaccination and revaccination regimens vary depending on the risk to a given population of cats.

Most current vaccines are licensed for annual revaccination. One exception is an inactivated FeLV vaccine recently marketed in Europe, which is licensed for revaccination every year or every three years.

Vaccination guidelines

House cats

In this group it is assumed that a low number of cats will coexist in a given territory, and thus the risk of infectious disease is low. However, the risk of infectious disease also varies depending on the lifestyle of the cats in question (whether they live exclusively indoors or also spend time outdoors).

In the case of vaccination against rabies, a single dose is administered, followed by annual revaccination according to the legal requirements of the region in question and depending on whether the cat will travel outside of the country.

In animals with leukaemia, immune deficiency, and other diseases in which the immune system is altered, it is recommended to use safer vaccines, such as inactivated or recombinant forms.

In pregnant females it is not recommended to vaccinate during the gestation period. Females should be vaccinated in advance so that they can transmit effective passive immunity to the litter.

Shelter cats

These cats live in an environment that generally has a high density of individuals. This can promote the transmission of infection, and thus the risk of disease is much higher than in other situations.

Vaccine recommendations should consider the prevalence of different diseases in a given shelter. In these circumstances the use of optional (non-core) vaccinations should be considered. Vaccines against *Bordetella bronchiseptica* and *C. felis* should only be administered if these diseases are concurrent and pose a serious problem (Fig. 1).

Essential (core) vaccine recommendations are the same as for house cats.

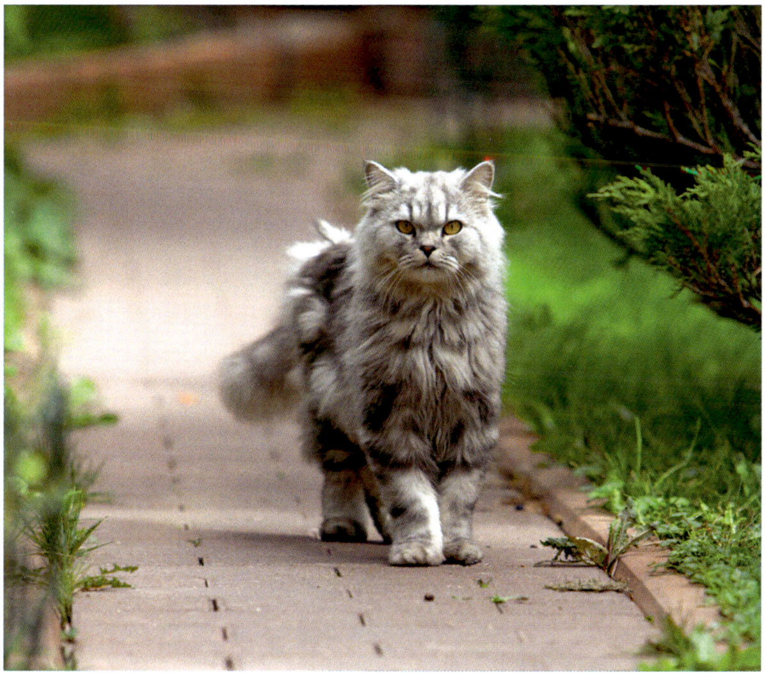

Figure 1. All cats should receive the essential (core) vaccines, as well as the optional (non-core) vaccines that the veterinary surgeon considers necessary depending on the factors relating to the patient in question (Anna Utekhina, Shutterstock.com).

If the prevalence of upper respiratory tract disease or feline panleukopaenia is high, it is advisable to rapidly implement a vaccination programme to protect new arrivals. In animals with mild illness and those of less than 8–9 weeks of age, the same vaccination scheme applies, using safer vaccines (recombinant or inactivated forms).

Trap-neuter-return (TNR) programme cats

Since these animals are only seen once by a veterinary surgeon, the general recommendation is to administer the essential vaccines. The considerations are the same as described for shelters: it is recommended to vaccinate very young animals (from 2–3 weeks of age) and those with mild clinical signs, even without prior deworming, using inactivated or recombinant vaccines. It has been shown that this vaccine regimen produces a suitable degree of immunisation, even with single dose vaccination.

An exception can be made to the rule that sick animals, with possible parasitosis or unknown levels of maternal antibodies, should never be vaccinated, given that this may be the only vaccination the animal will receive. Although revaccination is not possible, the use of inactivated vaccines may provide better results than no vaccination at all.

Cats in catteries

Vaccine recommendations for catteries are similar to those for house cats. Although the size of the colony may be large, segregation into smaller groups makes the two situations comparable.

In general, vaccination against feline leukaemia is recommended based on the specific risk of exposure of a given cat population. The FeLV status of all cats should be determined, as vaccination can never replace the analysis and isolation of positive

Table 1. General recommendations for vaccination of cats.

Vaccine	Initial vaccination: Kittens <16 weeks	Initial vaccination: Adults >16 weeks	Revaccination	Comments
Panleukopaenia + herpesvirus type 1 + calicivirus (FPV, FHV-1, FCV) Modified live and inactivated vaccines for parenteral administration.	• First dose administered from 8–9 weeks of age. • Revaccination every 3–4 weeks up until 16 weeks of age.	Two doses at 3–4 week interval.	One year after initial vaccination.	Cats that are subjected to stress, exposed to pathogens, or that will be housed in shelters should be revaccinated 7–10 days earlier.
Feline leukaemia (FeLV) Inactivated and recombinant.	Two doses at 3–4 week interval beginning at 8–9 weeks of age.	Two doses at 3–4 week interval.	• One year after initial vaccination. • Subsequently every 2 (3–4) years in low-risk situations.	• First it is recommended to verify that the cat is negative for FeLV. • Always vaccinate kittens up to one year of age and at-risk adults.
Rabies Inactivated and recombinant. Compulsory in endemic regions.	One dose after 12 weeks of age.	One dose.	• One year after initial vaccination. • Subsequently one per year (depending on the type of vaccine).	It is important to be aware of local regulations.

animals. This vaccine may be unnecessary if an effective testing and isolation programme has been implemented.

Vaccination against feline infectious peritonitis has not been shown to elicit strong immunity.

Table 1 lists the recommendations for general vaccination of cats.

Update on feline injection-site sarcoma

» Injection-site sarcoma has been recognised since the early 1990s. It was initially associated with the administration of inactivated vaccines for rabies and feline leukaemia containing aluminium adjuvants. Subsequently it was demonstrated that this reaction is unrelated to the type of vaccine. Rather, chronic inflammation can occur in response to repeated injections of multiple products in a single location, particularly in predisposed animals (Fig. 2).

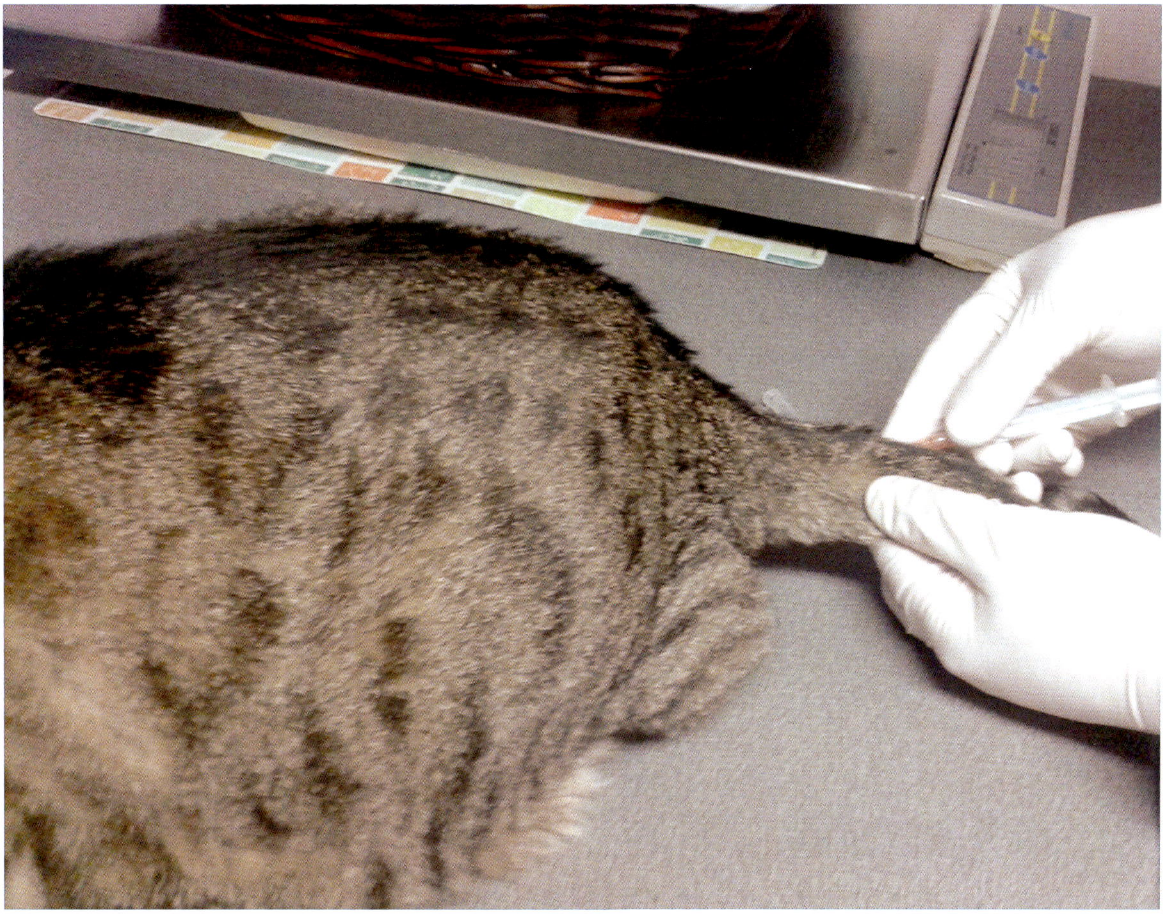

Figure 2. Administration of a vaccine into the tail of a cat. If an injection-site sarcoma develops following vaccination, the tail can be easily amputated with wide margins, preserving the animal's life.

References

Hendricks, C., Levy, J., Tucker, S., Olmstead, S., Crawford, P., Duvoy, E., Hanlon, C. Tail vaccination in cats: a pilot study. *J Fel Med and Surg*, 2014; 16:275-280.

Horzinek, M., Addie, D., Belak, S. *et al.* ABCC: Update of the 2009 guideline on prevention and management of feline infectious diseases. *J Fel Med Surg*, 2013; 15:530-539.

Hosie, M., Addie, D., Belak, S., *et al.* Matrix vaccination guidelines. ABCD recommendations for indoor/outdoor cats, rescue shelter cats and breeding catteries. *J Fel Med Surg*, 2013; 15:540-544.

Möstl, K., Egberink, H., Addie, D., *et al.* Prevention of infectious diseases in cat shelters: ABCD guidelines. *J Fel Med Surg*, 2013; 15:546-554.

Scherk, M., Ford, R., Gaskell, R., Hartman, K., Hurley, K., Lappin, M., Levy, J., Little, S., Nordone, S., Sparkes, A. 2013 AAFP Feline Vaccination Advisory Panel Report. *J Fel Med Surg*, 2013; 15:785-808.

Published by Servet Editorial - Grupo Asís Biomedia S.L.